Animals and Alternatives in Toxicity Testing

The proceedings of a Meeting held at the Royal Society of London on 1-3 November 1982 to discuss the Report of the FRAME Toxicity Committee

Animals and Alternatives in Toxicity Testing

Editors

Michael Balls
Rosemary J. Riddell
Alastair N. Worden

1983

ACADEMIC PRESS
A Subsidiary of Harcourt Brace Jovanovich, Publishers
London New York
Paris San Diego San Francisco
São Paulo Sydney Tokyo Toronto

ACADEMIC PRESS INC. (LONDON) LTD.
24/28 Oval Road
London NW1

United States Edition published by
ACADEMIC PRESS INC,
111 Fifth Avenue
New York, New York 10003

British Library Cataloguing in Publication Data
Animals and alternatives in toxicity testing
1. Drugs—Great Britain—Toxicology—Congresses
2. Veterinary toxicology—Great Britain—Congresses
3. Laboratory animals—Great Britain—Congresses
I. Balls, M. II. Riddell, R.J.
III. Worden, A.N.
615.9'07 RH1238

ISBN 0-12-077480-1

LCCCN 83-70946

Printed in Great Britain by
Whitstable Litho Ltd., Whitstable, Kent

CONTENTS

GENOTOXICITY

HUMAN STUDIES

REGULATIONS

DEVELOPMENT OF ALTERNATIVES

DISCUSSIONS

APPENDIX

CONTRIBUTORS

Van ABBÉ, N.J. Beecham Products Research Department, Leatherhead, Surrey, England
BALLS, Michael. Department of Human Morphology, University of Nottingham Medical School, Nottingham, England
BAWDEN, David, Pfizer Central Research, Sandwich, Kent, England
BENNETT, P.N. Department of Pharmacy and Pharmacology, University of Bath, Bath, Avon, England
BERRY, C.L. Department of Morbid Anatomy, London Hospital Medical College, London, England
BRIDGES, J.W. Robens Institute of Industrial and Environmental Health and Safety, University of Surrey, Guildford, Surrey, England
BROOKS, G.T. ARC Institute of Invertebrate Chemistry and Physiology, University of Sussex, Brighton, Sussex, England
BROWN, N.A. MRC Laboratories, Woodmansterne Road, Carshalton, Surrey, England
BROWN, R.C. MRC Pneumoconiosis Unit, Llandough Hospital, Penarth, South Glamorgan, Wales
BROWN, V.K.H. Shell Toxicology Laboratory, Sittingbourne Research Centre, Sittingbourne, Kent, England
CARSON, E.R. Department of Systems Science, The City University Northampton Square, London, England
CHANTER, D.O. Huntingdon Research Centre, Huntingdon, Cambridgeshire, England
CHASSEAUD, L.F. Huntingdon Research Centre, Huntingdon, Cambridgeshire, England
CLARK, D.G. Shell Toxicology Laboratory, Sittingbourne Research Centre, Sittingbourne, Kent, England
CLAYTON, Ruth. Institute of Animal Genetics, University of Edinburgh, Edinburgh, Scotland
COCKBURN, Andrew. Beechams Research Centre, Harlow, Essex, England
COHEN, G.M. Department of Pharmacology, School of Pharmacy, University of London, London, England
CONNING, D.M. British Industrial Biological Research Association, Woodmansterne Road, Carshalton, Surrey, England
DEAN, B.J. Shell Toxicology Laboratory, Sittingbourne Research Centre, Sittingbourne, Kent, England
DEARDEN, J.C. School of Pharmacy, Liverpool Polytechnic, Liverpool, England
DEWAR, A.J. Strategic Planning Division, The Shell Centre, London, England
FACCINI, J.M. Institut Français de Toxicologie, L'Arbresle, France
FOWLER, J.S.L. ICI Pharmaceuticals Division, Mereside, Alderley Park, Macclesfield, Cheshire, England

GOLBERG, Leon. Duke University Medical Center, Durham, North Carolina, USA
GOLDBERG, A.M. The Johns Hopkins Center for Alternatives to Animal Testing, Baltimore, Maryland, USA
GOULDING, Roy. 36 Ashley Court, Morpeth Terrace, London, England
GRIFFIN, J.P. DHSS Medicines Division, Market Towers, Nine Elms Lane, London, England
GUILLOT, J.P. Institut Francais de Toxicologie, L'Arbresle, France
HEALEY, G.F. Searle Research & Development, High Wycombe, Buckinghamshire, England
HESS, Robert. Ciba-Geigy, Basel, Switzerland
HEYWOOD, Ralph. Huntingdon Research Centre, Huntingdon, Cambridgeshire, England
HODGES, Peter. Pfizer Central Research, Sandwich, Kent, England
INMAN, W.H.W. Drug Surveillance Research Unit, University of Southampton, Southampton, England
KIRKLAND, D.J. Toxicol Laboratories, Ledbury, Herefordshire, England
KNOX, Peter. Department of Biochemistry, St. George's Hospital Medical School, London, England
KRINKE, G. Ciba-Geigy, Basel, Switzerland
LEE, P.N. 25 Cedar Road, Sutton, Surrey, England
LEGG, Nigel. Royal Postgraduate Medical School, Du Cane Road, London, England
LONGSTAFF, Eric. ICI Central Toxicology Laboratory, Alderley Park, Macclesfield, Cheshire, England
MACHIN, David. Department of Community Medicine, Southampton General Hospital, Southampton, England
MARKS, Ronald. Department of Medicine, Welsh National School of Medicine, Heath Park, Cardiff, South Wales
MILLER, Klara. British Industrial Biological Research Association, Woodmansterne, Road, Carshalton, Surrey, England
ÖBRINK, K.J. Institute for Physiology and Medical Physics, University of Uppsala, Uppsala, Sweden
PALMER, A.K. Huntingdon Research Centre, Huntingdon, Cambridgeshire, England
PARKE, Dennis V.W. Department of Biochemistry, University of Surrey, Guildford, Surrey, England
PARRY, J.M. Department of Genetics, University College of Swansea, Swansea, South Wales
POOLE, Alan. MRC Pneumoconiosis Unit, Llandough Hospital, South Glamorgan, Wales
PURCHASE, I.F.H. ICI Central Toxicology Laboratory, Alderley Park, Macclesfield, Cheshire, England
READING, H.W, MRC Brain Metabolism Unit, University of Edinburgh, Edinburgh, Scotland

ROE, F.J.C. 19 Marryat Road, Wimbledon, London, England
SCAIFE, M.C. Johnson & Johnson Limited, Cosham, Portsmouth, Hampshire, England
SCHAEPPI, J. Ciba-Geigy, Basel, Switzerland
SHEPHARD, N.W. Medical Science Research, 19 London End, Beaconsfield, Buckinghamshire, England
SNELL, Keith. Department of Biochemistry, University of Surrey, Guildford, Surrey, England
SWANSTON, D.W. Medical Division, Chemical Defence Establishment, Porton Down, Salisbury, Wiltshire, England
TATTERSALL, M.L. Fisons Limited, Loughborough, Leicestershire, England
TURNER, Paul. Department of Clinical Pharmacology, St. Bartholemew's Medical College, London, England
TUTE, M.S. Pfizer Central Research, Sandwich, Kent, England
VINE, R.S. Shola, Fielden Road, Crowborough, East Sussex, England
WALKER, C.H. Department of Physiology & Biochemistry, University of Reading, Reading, Berkshire, England
WALKER, S.R. Centre for Medicines Research, Woodmansterne Road, Carshalton, Surrey, England
WEISBURGER, J.W. Naylor Dana Institute for Disease Prevention, Valhalla, New York, USA
WILLIAMS, S.J. Haskell Laboratory for Toxicology and Industrial Medicine, Newark, Delaware, USA
WORDEN, A.N. Cantab Group, Cross Keys Orchard, Hemingford Abbots, Cambridgeshire, England
YORK, Michael. Unilever Research, Colworth House, Sharnbrook, Bedfordshire, England
YOUNG, A.R. Institute of Dermatology, Homerton Grove, London, England

PREFACE

The aims, philosophy and policies of FRAME are indicated in the Introduction to the Report of the FRAME Toxicity Committee, which, together with the list of members of that Committee, their general conclusions and main recommendations, and summaries of working party reports, forms an Appendix to these Proceedings.

The Meeting at the Royal Society of London on 1-3 November, 1982 was held in order to present and discuss the Report. The main sections of these Proceedings consist of a contribution by a member of the Committee, the comments of a number of independent discussants, and a summary of the main points made in discussion. Professor Karl Öbrink has provided a summary of the concluding general discussion, and this is followed by a personal summing-up by Professor Leon Golberg.

It was realised by the Committee that the Meeting could best serve to highlight the inadequacies and excesses of conventional toxicity testing procedures and to point a way forward: we may in all modesty suggest that these aims were largely achieved, even if the road ahead is a long one. While much of what was said had been put forward before, and there were clear conflicts of ideas and interpretation in some of the discussions, there was nevertheless a concerted attempt to recommend elimination of the unnecessary and to elevate the scientific status of such work as must, for the time being at least, continue to be carried out with experimental animal models. Examples include the modification of acute toxicity studies, with the virtual elimination of the LD50 test in its present form; the refinement of long-term and carcinogenicity studies; the much greater use of man in dermal toxicity testing; the modification of ocular irritancy testing procedures; the widespread introduction of metabolic and kinetic studies; a more constructive approach to neurotoxicity testing, and the placing of reproductive toxicity in its proper perspective. The need for a better understanding with informed regulatory bodies and for the international harmonisation of regulatory guidelines and requirements was repeatedly stressed.

The role of the so-called "alternative" (mainly in vitro) procedures was also seriously and rationally addressed. It was appreciated that much disservice to sensible progress could result from uncritical, blanket attempts to press for the introduction of alternative procedures as wholesale replacements for living animal models before their specific value had been objectively established and independently confirmed. Nevertheless, there was enthusiasm for the continuation and inauguration of research programmes and controlled studies that would serve to promote the development, validation and acceptance of non-animal methods, not only as alternatives, but also to supplement or complement necessary conventional procedures and human studies.

While FRAME is not an animal welfare organisation, it is clear that the recommendations emerging from the Report and these Proceedings should lead to a reduction in the numbers of animals used in toxicity testing, and should ensure that those that have to be employed are used in a more humane, scientific and less wasteful manner.

The FRAME Toxicity Committee will continue to meet to seek the greater rationalisation of current methods in toxicology and safety evaluation, and to promote the introduction of valid alternatives. FRAME's periodical journal, ATLA (Alternatives to Laboratory Animals), will be devoted to discussion of the concept of alternatives and to the widest possible dissemination of original research and critical reviews and comment. FRAME will also continue to work with industry and with academic research scientists in co-ordinated research aimed at the development and assessment of alternative methods.

FRAME and the Editors of these Proceedings wish to thank the Royal Society and the Reform Club for their hospitality; the Cancer Research Campaign, Ciba-Geigy PLC, the Dulverton Trust and the Maurice Laing Foundation for their generous financial support; the chairmen, speakers, discussants and members of the Toxicity Committee; the staff of Academic Press Inc. (London) Limited; and all those who have contributed in any other way.

Michael Balls
Rosemary Riddell
Alastair Worden

June 1983

FRAME (Fund for the Replacement of Animals in Medical Experiments), 5b The Poultry, Bank Place, Nottingham NG1 2JR, England.

Acute Toxicity Testing

V. K. H. BROWN

INTRODUCTION

Acute toxicity testing in laboratory animals is potentially one of the most severe procedures forming part of the conventional assessment of products. It is the purpose of this report to define the problems associated with acute toxicity testing and to review the possibilities for relieving the situation.

Some Definitions

Toxicity is the inherent property of a product to cause an adverse biological effect.

Acute implies short-term. The term acute can be applied to the nature of the exposure or to the form of the response (1), but for the purpose of this report the former definition is more relevant.

Acute toxicity tests are frequently carried out to aid hazard assessment and risk prediction. Hazard is the potential for the occurrence of an adverse effect under specific conditions. (N.B. There are, of course, hazards other than toxicity associated with chemical products, e.g. explosiveness, flammability.) Risk represents the probability of the hazard being experienced (2).

Symptomatology is the overall manifestation of toxic effects. Signs of intoxication are overt and can be observed (e.g. convulsions, elevated body temperature). Symptoms are apparent only to the subject of the intoxication and cannot be observed by others (e.g. headache, blurred vision). The term symptomatology is generally considered to describe both signs and symptoms.

The LD50 test is the procedure by which one determines the

LD50 value. The LD50 has been defined as being a numerical index which gives some information about the acute toxicity of a chemical substance in experimental animals (3). The definitive LD50 is a best estimate with statistically-established confidence limits.

A limit test is one in which a maximum dose-level is fixed and, if the test animals have not succumbed from that exposure, then further, larger, doses are not investigated (3,4). The accepted maximum for the test will be dependent on the nature of the product being tested.

There is a common misconception that the LD50 test is synonymous with acute toxicity testing. We regret that the difference was not emphasised more strongly by the Home Office Advisory Committee on the Administration of the Cruelty to Animals Act, 1876 (3). The difference has been recognised by the Royal Society for the Prevention of Cruelty to Animals (4), but the essential fact remains that the LD50 value is widely used as a numeric index of acute toxicity, albeit with constraints on its intrinsic value. Acute toxicity testing is concerned with the wider implications of the response to short-term exposure to products than just a numeric index (5,6); some perspective on this is to be found in the scientific literature (1,7), and has not been wholly overlooked in the popular press (8).

Not all acute toxicity testing requires the use of large numbers of animals, and for some purposes it is the accepted practice to obtain an approximate range for the index of acute toxicity (i.e. the LD50 value is estimated to lie between x mg kg^{-1} and y $mgkg^{-1}$) or to employ a limit test. Clinical observations form an integral part of the design of acute toxicity studies, and the investigation should include scrutiny of the organs and tissues from at least a selection of the exposed animals, unless the investigator has good reason for omitting this procedure. To this end, a small subacute study may be more helpful than the ritualistic acquisition of numeric data based on larger experimental populations. The idea that the LD50 estimation automatically debars the possibility of obtaining information on symptomatology and organ-directed or tissue-directed effects is fallacious.

A further misconception is that all acute toxicity testing is carried out in laboratory animals with the sole objective of creating data that can be extrapolated to man. The majority of acute toxicity tests do have this objective, but a proportion of them are carried out so that domestic animals, animals of economic significance and wildlife can be protected (7). Some forms of sublethal acute toxicity testing are carried out in humans, but the ethical and legal constraints are obvious (9).

In this report, we shall present an objective review of the current situation with regard to acute toxicity testing, together with our perception of the possibility for devising alternatives to the use of living animals or at least reducing the numbers of animals that need to be used. The bibliography provided with this report is clearly not exhaustive, but the references that are quoted have been chosen to illustrate facets of the review and to provide a guide to further reading. It must be realised that acute toxicity testing is not to be considered as an exclusive area of toxicology and that there are matters of relevance that will be dealt with in other chapters in this book.

OBJECTIVES OF ACUTE TOXICITY TESTING

Acute toxicity tests involving the use of vertebrates are carried out for the following purposes:

a. to assess toxic potential;
b. to aid the prediction of hazard;
c. to generate data for use in risk-benefit assessments;
d. to provide information on the mechanism of acute toxic action.

Although it is sometimes cited as an objective, in reality, toxicologists rarely determine acute toxicity data solely for the purpose of fixing dose-rates for longer-term exposure studies, as the data are generally required for one or more of a. to d., above. There is no a priori reason for assuming any direct relationship between acute and long-term exposure effects in toxicology, and this difference is fundamental to the problem of seeking alternatives to the conventional laboratory animal testing methods. Acute exposures may swamp the normal physiological processes of the exposed subject, to produce an effect that is often pharmacological, whereas long-term exposure may allow for metabolism (i.e. toxification and/or detoxification) and excretion. The consequences of these two different mechanisms can be critical to the nature of the response. Fig. 1 shows, in simplified form, an example of the difference between the acute and the long-term exposure toxicology for the carbamate, aldicarb. Other differences between the effects observed in acute and long-term toxicity are common.

Within the context of a. and b., LD50 values are commonly used for the purpose of classification of products (e.g. labelling requirements).

SOME PRACTICAL CONSIDERATIONS

The processes of acute toxicity testing can be expressed as a flow diagram (Fig. 2). If the sequence in this diagram is followed, some of the major practicalities of acute toxicity testing can be considered in a logical order.

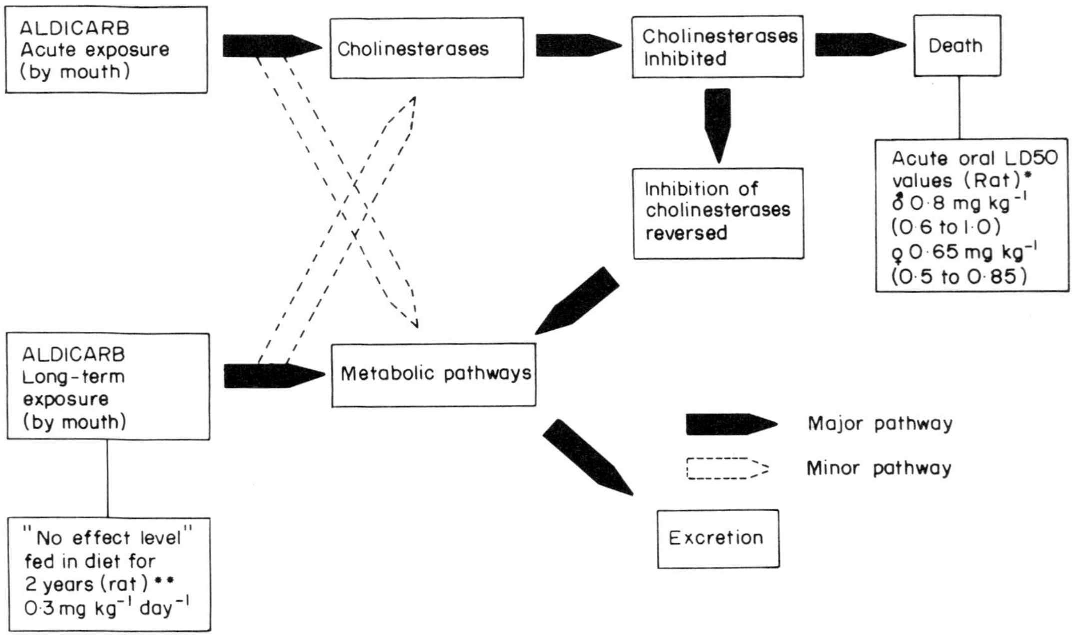

Figure 1

An Example of Difference Between Responses to Acute and Long-term Exposure to a Chemical (a Simplified Flow Diagram)

*Gaines, T.B. (1969). Toxicology & Applied Pharmacology 14, 515-534.
**"The Pesticide Manual". British Crop Protection Council.

Choice of Target Model

The ideal choice of experimental model must be the species for which acute toxicity data are required. If the information is required for the purpose of assessment of hazard to man, then the problems associated with assessing acute toxicity in man are founded in both ethical considerations and in the law (9). Other ethical and legal constraints are applicable if the tests are to be carried out to assess hazard to wildlife by using some feral animals.

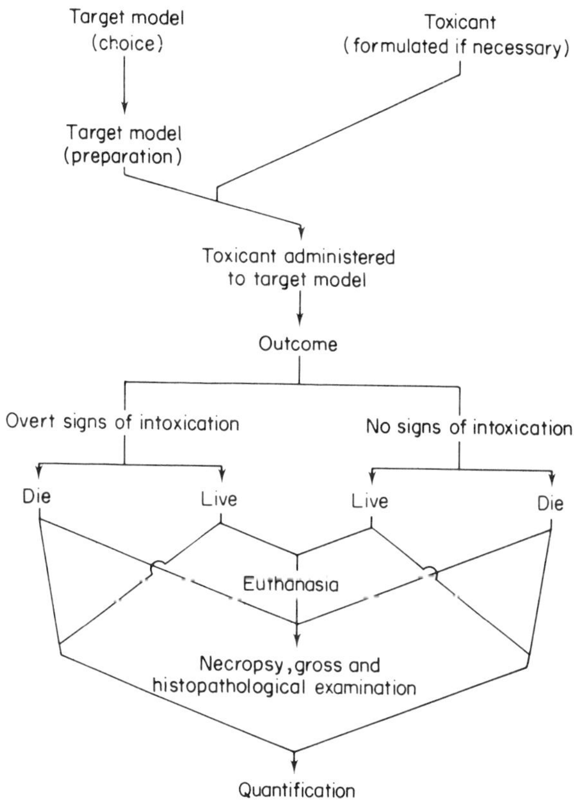

Figure 2 Acute Toxicity Testing - a Flow Diagram

No species completely mirrors the total physiological complexity of another species (this is a fundamental phylogenic principle), but an experimental model has to be capable of generating information that can be extrapolated to other species. However, by the application of reasoned selection, the use of a living animal model is bound to provide a closer approximation to another living animal than any other model system (10). All too frequently, acute toxicity data are the subject of facile extrapolations between species without adequate thought for the biological principles involved (11).

Many animal models have been used in the determination of acute toxicity (7), but, primarily for reasons of expediency, the laboratory rat (*Rattus norvegicus*) has become the most commonly used model for predictive acute toxicity testing (10,12). This use of a relatively inexpensive model in a test procedure that is not particularly labour-intensive does mean that there is little incentive to seek alternative test methods, but the ethical considerations make the search for an alternative imperative.

Preparation of the Target Model

The minimum preparation for an acute toxicity test involves the selection and weighing of each animal. For peroral exposure, food is generally withheld from the animals for a time before the product is administered, so that the gut contents do not influence absorption of the toxicant. Percutaneous toxicity necessitates the removal of hair from the area to be treated with the product under test and the use of either restraint or an occlusive dressing to prevent grooming (14). Exposure by other routes (e.g. inhalation, parenteral administration, etc.) generally involves some physical restraint, although this is minimised to avoid stress.

The Toxicant

The physical presentation of a toxicant to an animal can be critically important to the outcome. Bioavailability can be influenced by the physical characteristics of the product and can be substantially affected by formulation (1,7). Although every chemical has an intrinsic acute toxicity, it must be emphasised that bioavailability is often capable of being manipulated, and modification of the bioavailability will change the acute toxicity associated with the chemical.

The Outcome

It must be emphasised that toxicologists are concerned with predicting adverse effects and not only death (7,11). Animals, other than humans, are unable to describe symptoms, so all animal tests are dependent on overt signs of intoxication and morphological changes recorded at necropsy, and these experiments do not provide information on the symptoms associated with poisoning. Some aspects of linking predictive acute toxicity testing with pharmacological (i.e. therapeutic effects) experiments have been discussed elsewhere (1,11,13).

The sequel to exposure is critically important. Good observation for overt signs of intoxication, together with timing of the onset of observed events and, where appropriate, their regression, are essential. More-detailed studies of clinical events (e.g. ECGs) can be made, if required. The cumulative mortality can be used for quantification purposes. Detailed necropsies of those animals that die and also of some or all of those that survive the intoxication can be used to detect organ-directed toxicity.

Since there may be important differences in the qualitative as well as the quantitative responses elicited by a product in different species (7), this possibility must be considered by the toxicologist in the design and interpretation of the investigation (11).

At its simplest, acute toxicology has been considered by some people to equate to the application of the quantal nature (i.e. two possible outcomes: "all or none") of the living or dead situation in order to produce an index of acute toxicity. It is this narrow view of acute toxicology that has been manifested as an obsession with the LD50 test. Many toxicologists have strong reservations about the importance of the LD50 value for a product when it is considered in isolation (1,5,6,7,14), and there is some evidence that this concern is being noticed by those in legislative toxicology (15). There is now increasing acceptance of the idea of using smaller numbers of animals in each acute toxicity test by the application of modified experimental design (16-19) and also by the more realistic use of limit tests. For some classes of products, particularly new pharmaceuticals and food additives, the need for statistically-defined LD50 values has been superseded, at least in part, by an acceptance of data from limit tests supported by pharmacokinetics and other relevant information. Sometimes a study in which a few animals are dosed repeatedly with a product can reveal more than a conventional acute toxicity test and may be more economical in terms of the number of animals used.

DISCUSSION

Quantification

On the subject of life and death, any debate is infinite. The philosopher, theologian and scientist, Benedictus de Spinoza (1632-1677), stated, "There is nothing which a free man ponders less than death; his wisdom is to meditate not on death but on life". The inclination of those concerned with acute toxicity has tended to be directed at preserving the life of humans and other selected animals at the expense of "expendable" laboratory animals. Arguably this is without adequate meditation on the need for so many deaths (8). As to whether the experimental toxicologist is a "free man" is debatable, for we are frequently reminded that the LD50 test is demanded by some form of legislative requirement, even when the toxicologist considers that some less-demanding test might be more appropriate.

There have been many published comments on the limited value of the LD50 as a meaningful quantification of acute toxicity (17,19). However, the eminent physicist, Lord Kelvin (1824-1907), expressed the opinion that, "When you measure what you are speaking about and express it in numbers you know something about it, but when you cannot measure it, when you cannot express it in numbers, your knowledge is of a meagre and unsatisfactory kind". This desire to quantify findings has been adopted by those concerned with acute toxicology and this has been apparent in the demand for the LD50 test (15).

It is unrealistic to consider that humans could be used for routine acute toxicity testing (19), but the value of data generated from human exposure can be very helpful and sometimes serves to put the data generated from experimental models into perspective (20). It is an often quoted fact (8), with substantial support in the scientific literature (7), that species differences in susceptibility to the acute toxic properties of products may take the form of qualitative differences and that these may not be apparent in the form of an index of toxicity (i.e. the LD50 value). To the toxicologist, this last observation is of paramount importance and one logical sequel to this would be an extension of the number of species used for testing purposes. The use of animals of more species for acute toxicity tests, albeit in small numbers, is more logical than the desire for quantification of results.

If we could do away with the artificial respectability of the LD50 value (9), then it would be possible to diminish the number of animals required to assess acute toxicity by the use of more-appropriate experimental design (17-19). At this time, the use of mathematical modelling (20-23) as a tool for assessing acute toxicity as numeric values is very limited (24,25), and in qualitative terms is impractical.

Some General Considerations

It has already been stated that studies involving animals other than man cannot be expected to detect symptoms, and that symptoms may be an important part of the toxic effect. Studies that are carried out _in vitro_ cannot provide information on symptoms or the overt signs of intoxication. The _in vitro_ approach is therefore at a disadvantage when compared with _in vivo_ studies, for the latter does provide some information on the signs of intoxication.

Some chemicals are toxic because of a well-defined physiological interaction when they get into an animal. Sometimes this interaction may be demonstrable using *in vitro* methodology, but correlation with *in vivo* effects may be poor. This is well illustrated by the very poor correlation that has been found between the inhibition of the cholinesterases *in vitro* and the acute toxic effects of cholinesterase inhibitors *in vivo* (25).

Interactive toxic effects of exposure to more than one product *in vivo* cannot be predicted by *in vitro* experiments. However, the use of available historical data can sometimes allow useful predictions about interactive effects to be made from data obtained *in vitro* (e.g. the adverse reponse to some foods by patients undergoing treatment with drugs that are monoamine oxidase [MAO] inhibitors would alert any toxicologist to be cautious if the product under investigation was shown by *in vitro* tests to be an inhibitor of MAO).

Interactive effects of chemicals on bioavailability can influence the acute toxicity of a product by very large amounts. Occasionally, the toxicologist can anticipate a change in the toxicokinetics from precedents (e.g. some vehicles will tend to facilitate absorption by particular routes). The magnitude of the effect on bioavailability is only realistically measurable by *in vivo* experimentation, but there are some useful *in vitro* techniques that can give helpful data for different routes of exposure (e.g. skin (26), lungs (27)).

Neither the *in vivo* nor the *in vitro* techniques currently available are helpful in predicting idiosyncratic or low level atypical responses to acute intoxication (11,20).

Current Areas of Endeavour

The search for alternatives to the use of vertebrates in acute toxicology is being undertaken in several different ways:

In vitro culture techniques. The value of *in vitro* tissue and organ culture techniques is well established for some types of toxicological investigations (28-34). Acute toxicity is often associated with the swamping of the normal physiological mechanisms rather than by organ-directed cellular interaction, and there is no logical reason for expecting that organ or tissue culture techniques will be capable of predicting these toxic effects.

Even with products that are acutely toxic because of organ-directed effects (e.g. 2,4,7,8-tetrachlorodibenzo-*p*-dioxin), it has been shown that tissue culture techniques are not good predictors of acute toxicity (34).

There is no conceivable way by which the toxicokinetics of the whole animal *in vivo* can be mimicked in tissues *in vitro*. The value of the contribution of information obtained using tissue or organ culture to the knowledge of the acute toxicity of a product will vary in each case and will often prove to be very limited.

Embryotoxicity techniques. The use of the developing chick embryo as a model for use in acute toxicity testing is not new (36,39). Recently published data from the Czechoslovakian Academy of Sciences (40) suggest that their chick embryotoxicity screening test (CHEST I) has a high predictive value when compared with data from conventional rodent acute toxicity tests with some classes of compounds (e.g. mycotoxins). The outcome of future research involving bird embryos may prove to be of considerable interest.

Isolated organ techniques. The use of isolated organ techniques has long been established practice in pharmacology for the elucidation of some mechanisms of action, and this approach can be of value in predicting the mechanism of toxic action of some products. Toxicokinetic data can be partially elucidated by the use of isolated organs (e.g. isolated skin for predicting skin absorption characteristics (26), isolated perfused lungs for respiratory uptake (27)), but the limitations of the methodology are readily apparent.

Isolated enzymes. Some chemicals are highly specific in their toxic action, e.g. by the inhibition of an enzyme system. Inhibition of the various cholinesterases by some organo-phosphorus and carbamate compounds is an example of this activity, but, although cholinesterases are readily isolated, the inhibition of the various cholinesterases *in vitro* has proved to be a poor correlate of acute toxicity (25). The use of isolated enzymes in this context presumes that the toxicant has unhindered access to the enzyme system *in vivo* and that there is no metabolism of the toxicant or breakdown *in vivo* of the inhibited enzymes. These are not meaningful assumptions.

Invertebrate animals. Some, but not all, objectors to animal experimentation distinguish between vertebrates and invertebrates as being acceptable for the use of living whole animals for experimental purposes. The philosophy of this has been vexatious and there is a school of thought that even some invertebrates, and certainly the Cephalochordate molluscs, should be included within the laws enacted to protect animals (41).

Many of the physiological characteristics of invertebrates differ widely from those of vertebrates. Although parallels may be found between the acute toxicity of a few products to some invertebrates and the acute toxicity of the same products to vertebrates, the response is never uniform to all species (42). Indeed, the variation between the sensitivity of different insects to insecticides illustrates this point, and where there has been an attempt to correlate acute toxicity data obtained for invertebrates with those obtained for vertebrates, the results have not been valuable (43).

The use of Daphnia and other invertebrate species in ecotoxicology has become important, but these invertebrate species are not providing data that reflect the acute toxicities of products to fish (44).

Plants. Obviously, plants do respond to some toxic chemicals, but the magnitude of the differences between the physiology of plants and that of vertebrates restricts the idea of a plant model for acute toxicology to only a few scientists (45). It will be a long time before there are adequate data available to convince the sceptics that there should be a major expenditure of effort on that line of research. However, there are areas of related endeavour in which plant-derived systems are showing promise as models for animal systems (e.g. The use of Moong beans for the screening of drugs with anti-convulsant properties (46)), but the application of this approach to acute toxicity testing is remote.

Mathematical modelling. The mathematical modelling of chemical/biological interactions is of such importance in toxicology (22) that it is the subject of a separate chapter in this book. There is already a commercial computerised method available for predicting LD50 values on the basis of a number of physical and chemical characteristics (21). The validity of this system has been criticised (23,24), and there is a need for increased research in mathematical modelling in relation to acute toxicology. Some toxicokinetic processes have been modelled using computerised techniques (47-54) and, because of the added incentive that has been provided by pharmacokinetic modelling successes, these are likely to contribute to the quest for alternatives to living animal experimentation, though there are still many problems to be overcome.

Data-banking. Although data-banking does not provide an alternative to animal experimentation, it can significantly reduce the replication of tests. There are several data-banks accessible either direct from computers or published as reference books (55,56). The monitoring of the quality of the input to data-banks is a major problem. Currently, the majority of the information residing in data-banks has been obtained from publications in the open literature; this means that the data source can be checked, whereas a system that depends on data being banked without review is clearly unacceptable.

CONCLUSIONS

The foregoing has led us to the following conclusions:

1. There is a need for those concerned with advising on matters of toxicology to be knowledgeable about the meaning of acute toxicity testing.

2. There is a need for a detailed justification of the purpose that is achieved in acute toxicology by quantifying what is essentially qualitative information. The objective of diminishing the numbers of animals used for this purpose is attainable by improved experimental design. Thorough clinical examination of a few animals, coupled with the information on the toxicity at necropsy, can provide a lot of valuable information on the toxicity of a chemical, and this is not necessarily improved by the use of large numbers of animals to obtain apparent statistical respectability.

3. Any biological testing that involves extrapolation of findings from one species to another is fundamentally weak. Most acute toxicity testing falls into this category. This could imply a need for more, rather than less, animal testing (i.e. the use of more species in each test), and the validity of this argument needs constructive rebuttal.

4. There has not been a sufficiently rigorous approach to investigating the consequences of not acquiring or possessing knowledge of the acute toxicity of products in laboratory animals, albeit this information is too often represented by no more than an LD50 value with all its shortcomings. For some classes of products (e.g. pharmaceuticals and food additives), the need for definitive LD50 values has been superseded, at least in part, by the acceptance of data from limit tests supported by pharmacokinetics and other relevant information. Sometimes, a repeated-dose study can be more informative than a conventional acute toxicity test.

5. A total alternative to the use of living animals in predictive acute toxicity testing has yet to be achieved. The most acceptable conclusion at this time is that the so-called "alternatives" should be considered as adjuncts to conventional acute toxicity testing. This could have the effect of improving the data-base and so reducing the numbers of animals required in acute toxicity tests.

6. The search for "alternatives" needs impetus coupled with restraint. It is naïve to believe that this objective is attainable without the impetus of substantially more research. Restraint must come with the realisation that there are no easy solutions to the problem.

in pharmacokinetics. Federation Proceedings 39, 54-59.
11. Dayan, A.D., (1981). The relative worth of animal testing. In "Risk-benefit Analysis in Drug Research" (ed. J.F. Cavalla), pp. 97-112. Lancaster: MTP Press.
12. Noakes, D.N. & Sanderson, D.M. (1969). A method for determining the dermal toxicity of pesticides. British Journal of Industrial Medicine 26, 59-64.
13. Fowler, J.S.L., Brown, J.S. & Bell, H.A., (1979). The rat toxicity screen. Pharmacology & Therapeutics 5, 461-466.
14. Zbinden, G. & Flury-Roversi, M. (1981). Significance of the LD50 test for the toxicological evaluation of chemical substances. Archives of Toxicology 47, 77-99.
15. Griffin, J.P. (1981). Referring to the paper by Zbinden & Fluri-Roversi. Archives of Toxicology 49, 99-103.
16. Tattersall, M.L. (1982). Statistics and the LD50 test. Archives of Toxicology, suppl. 5, 267-270.
17. Brown, V.K. (1981). The "up-and-down" approach to dose fixing in acute toxicity tests. ATLA 9, 49.
18. Chanter, D.O. & Heywood, R. (1982). The LD50 test: some considerations of precision. Toxicology Letters 10, 303-307.
19. Weatherall, M. (1982). An end to the search for new drugs? Nature, London 296, 387-390.
20. Enslein, K. & Craig, D.N. (1978). A toxicity estimation model. Journal of Environmental Pathology and Toxicology 2, 115-121.
21. Dunn, W.J. & Wold, S. (1980). Relationships between chemical structure and biological activity modelled by SIMCA pattern recognition. Bioorganic Chemistry 9, 505-523.
22. Eschenroeder, A., Irving, E., Lloyd, A., Tashima, C. & Tran, J. (1980). Computer simulation models for assessment of toxic substances. In "Dynamics, Exposure and Hazard Assessment of Toxic Chemicals" (ed. R. Hague), pp. 323-368. Michigan: Ann Arbor Science Publishers.
23. Rekker, R.F. (1980). LD50 values: are they about to become predictable? TIPS (October issue), 383-384.
24. Tute, M. (1981). Computer prediction of LD50 values. ATLA 9, 50-52.
25. Mager, P.P. & Seese, A. (1980). Quantitative struktur - toxizitats - beziehungen bei phosphorsaureestern. Pharmazie 35, 806-808.
26. Grasso, P. & Lansdown, A.B.G. (1972). Methods of measuring the factors affecting percutaneous absorption. Journal of the Society of Cosmetic Chemists 23, 481-521.
27. Mehendale, H.M., Angevine, L.S. & Ohmiya, Y. (1981). The isolated perfused lung: a critical evaluation. Toxicology 21, 1-36.
28. Rowan, A.N. & Stratmann, C.J. (eds.) (1980). "The Use of Alternatives in Drug Research". 190 pp. London: Macmillan.
29. Ekwall, B. (1980). Screening of toxic compounds in tissue culture. Toxicology 17, 127-142.

30. Ord, M.J. (1981). A cell system for use in toxicology studies. ATLA 9, 7-13.
31. Rees, K.R. (1980). Cells in culture in toxicity testing: a review. Journal of the Royal Society of Medicine 73, 261-264.
32. Krasovskii, G.N. & Ilnitskii, A.P. (1967). The question of the use of tissue culture methods in sanitary and toxicological studies (in Russian). Gigiena I Sanitariya 32, 66-70.
33. Elizarova, O.N. & Nuzhdina, D.P. (1971). Application of tissue cultures for determining the toxicity of pesticides. Gigiena I Sanitariya 36, 83-87.
34. Knutson, J.C. & Poland, A. (1980). 2,3,7,8-tetrachlorodibenzo-p-dioxin: failure to demonstrate toxicity in twenty-three cultured cell types. Toxicology & Applied Pharmacology 54, 377-383.
35. Ekwall, B. (1980). Preliminary studies on the validity of in vitro measurement of drug toxicity using HeLa cells. II. Drug toxicity in the MIT-24 system compared with mouse and human lethal dosage of 52 drugs. Toxicology Letters 5, 309-317.
36. Marliac, J-P. (1962). Injection of chemicals into chicken eggs as a toxicity test. Federation Proceedings 21, 450.
37. Marliac, J-P. (1963). Use of the chick embryo technique for detecting potentiating effects of chemicals. Federation Proceedings 22, 188.
38. McLaughlin, J. & Mutchler, M.K. (1962). Toxicity of some chemicals measured by injection into chicken eggs. Federation Proceedings 21, 450.
39. McLaughlin, J., Marliac, J-P., Verrett, M.J. Mutchler, M.K. & Fitzhugh, V.H. (1963). The injection of chemicals into the yolk sac of fertile eggs prior to incubation as a toxicity test. Toxicology & Applied Pharmacology 5, 760-771.
40. Vesely, D., Vesela, D., & Jelinek, R. (1982). Nineteen mycotoxins tested on chicken embryos. Toxicology Letters 13, 239-245.
41. Report to the Secretary of State on the Framework of Legislation to Replace the Cruelty to Animals Act, 1876, by the Advisory Committee on Animal Experiments. (1981). 40 pp. London: Home Office.
42. Kaiser, H.E. (1980). "Species-specific Potential of Invertebrates for Toxicological Research". 224 pp. Baltimore: University Park Press.
43. Krueger, H.R. & Casida, J.E. (1957). Toxicity of fifteen organophosphorus insecticides to several insect species and rats. Journal of Economic Entomology 50, 356-358.
44. Johnson, W.C. & Finley, M.T. (1980). Handbook of Acute Toxicity of Chemicals to Fish and Aquatic Invertebrates. Resource Publication No. 137 of Fish and Wildlife Service. 120 pp. Washington: US Department of the Interior.

45. Kordan, H. (1981). Responses of whole plant systems to pharmacological agents. ATLA 9, 24-37.
46. Anon. (1982). Moong beans may replace animals for drug screening. New Scientist 94, 702.
47. Dagani, R. (1981). Toxicologists seek structure - activity links. Chemical Engineering News (9 March issue), 26-29.
48. Ashford, J.R. (1981). Biological and mathematical models. Chemistry & Industry (1 August issue), 521-525.
49. Pla-Delfina, J.M. & Moreno, J. (1981). Intestinal absorption-partition relationships: A tentative fundamental non-linear model. Journal of Pharmacokinetics and Biopharmacology 9, 191-215.
50. Metzler, C.M. & Tong, D.D.M. (1981). Computational problems of compartment model with Michaelis-Menten-type elimination. Journal of Pharmacological Science 70, 733-737.
51. Luecke, R.H., Thomason, L.E. & Wosilait, W.D. (1980). Physiological flow model for drug elimination interactions in the rat. Computer Programs in Biomedicine 11, 88-98.
52. Colburn, W.A. (1981). Simultaneous pharmacokinetic and pharmacodynamic modelling. Journal of Pharmacokinetics and Biopharmacology 9, 367-388.
53. Carson, E.R. (1983). The role of mathematical models in biomedical research. In "The Role of Animals in Scientific Research" (ed. P. Turner). London: Macmillan (in press).
54. Wold, S. (1981). Computer methods for the assessment of acute toxicity. In "The LD50 and Possible Alternatives" (ed. M. Thelestam). Stockholm: CFN (in press).
55. Toxic Substances List (published periodically). Rockville, Md: US Department of Health, Education and Welfare (NIOSH).
56. Fairchild, E.J. (1978). "Agricultural Chemicals and Pesticides: a Handbook of the Toxic Effects". 229 pp. Tunbridge Wells: Castle House Publications.

Short-term Testing in Drug Development

J. S. L. FOWLER

INTRODUCTION

In this century, the use of drugs as medicines has considerably improved the length and the quality of life. With this increased use of drugs has grown the recognition that the undoubted benefits may, on occasion, be accompanied by disadvantages, including hazards to health. Such hazards have been extensively publicised and are subjects for public concern and interest. Each year many entirely novel chemical entities possessing intrinsic pharmacological activity are evaluated as potential medicines. Of the many new chemicals that are made, the vast majority are discarded on the basis of structure-activity studies. Those that remain are tested in vitro and, if necessary, in animals, to help predict their usefulness in preventing or treating diseases of man and animals. One in every hundred chemicals progresses to short-term testing and about 1 in 1000 to rigorous testing by methods such as the median lethal dose assay (LD50 test).

In our work, which is concerned with the safety evaluation of new medicines, we believe that it is essential to study carefully the acute toxic effects of new drugs and, before giving them to people, to establish the safe margins that exist between effective and toxic doses (1). The patient is not the only person who may suffer ill-effects from the distribution of a new chemical; each year the United Kingdom and Republic of Ireland National Poisons Information Services receive 40,000 telephone enquiries on acute poisoning, and half of these concern misuse or accidents with drugs (2). Pharmaceutical companies are required to supply doctors in the United Kingdom with data on likely effects of overdose (3), and we note that the National Poisons Information Service believe that these data are frequently inadequate (4).

OBJECTIVES OF SHORT-TERM TOXICITY STUDIES

Short-term toxicity studies must be designed so that they produce a maximum amount of useful information.

Several important drugs have small margins of safety but have an important role in the treatment of disease. For this reason, it is necessary to determine the nature of the adverse effects and to quantify them so that appropriate advice may be given to the clinician. In addition to protection of the patient, all new substances which are considered for possible use must be manufactured, transported and distributed safely: their useful life may extend to several decades. During this time many people will be intentionally or accidentally exposed to these chemicals, their side-effects and beneficial actions, whether as formulated medicines, bulk chemical or intermediate chemical needed during synthesis of the new medicine.

Short-term tests are intended to provide:

a. quantitative data of reasonable accuracy, including lethality information (5);

b. qualitative data regarding the cause of death, time of death, incidence, severity and reversibility of important abnormalities (6);
c. a basis for design of subsequent studies (6).

LIMIT TEST OR SLOPE OF THE DOSE-RESPONSE CURVE

If there is no knowledge available concerning a new substance, then small "ranging studies" must be done first. When these are complete, it is found that compounds of "high pharmacological activity" and "low toxicity" are better studied using a limit test. In this approach a small number of animals are given a range of doses that are multiples of the dose proposed for use: even if no severe toxicity or lethality occurs at a high limiting dose, then this limit will not be exceeded. In the case where the limit is reached, the main objective of the study becomes the thorough investigation of acute effects, other than death, that ensue. We recognise that reliance upon such limit test data assumes that the slope of the lethality dose-response curve is predictable and confers a sufficient safety margin. There will be occasions when confidence in this slope may only be established by execution of an LD50 test using conventional numbers of animals. For example, occasionally the slope of a dose-response curve is very steep or almost flat. A steep slope indicates rapid extensive absorption, poor detoxification and severe toxicity; a flat slope indicates poor or very slow absorption, effective detoxification and/or insidious toxicity ((6), Fig.1).

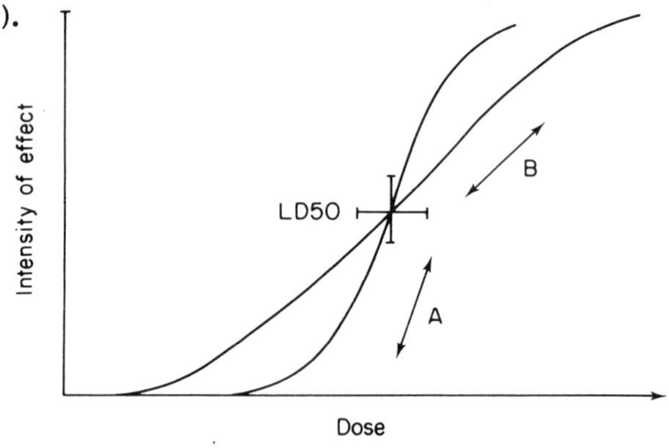

Figure 1 Illustration of Importance of Slope in Lethality Studies

Key: Slope A illustrates rapid distribution, slow elimination.
Slope B illustrates variable distribution, variable elimination.

In many cases, reliable definition of the lethal dose-response curve is necessary in order to establish the highest doses that may be given safely in order to achieve the desired effect. The ratio of the median effective dose (ED50) to the median lethal dose (LD50) is the so-called therapeutic index (LD50/ED50). It would be better if this safety margin was calculated by using the minimal toxic dose and the maximal effective dose. Although these doses cannot be discovered directly, a good guide can be obtained by comparison of the slopes of the effective and toxic dose-response curves (Fig. 2).

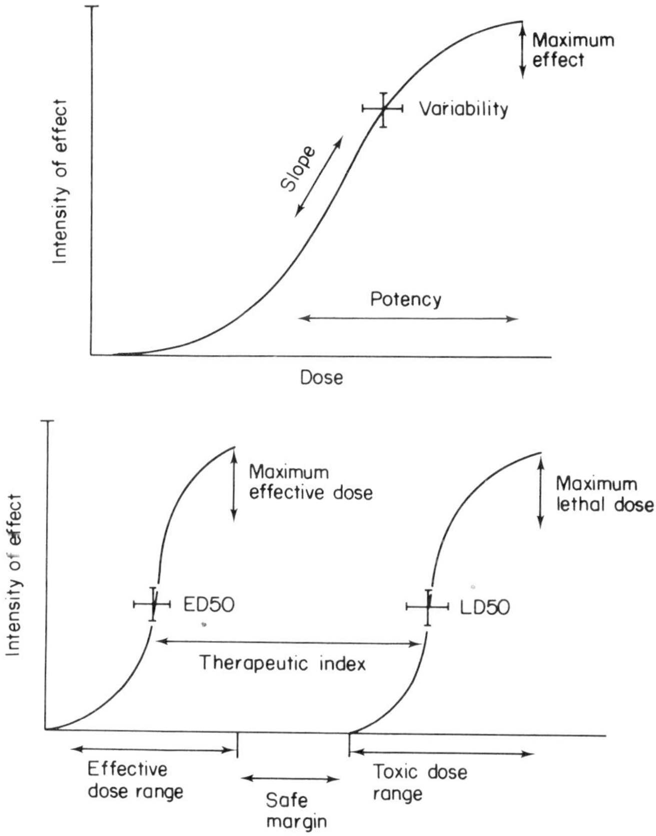

Figure 2 Representative Dose-effect Curves (taken from Goodman & Gilman (7)).

It is clear that the smaller the ratio between the likely effective dose of the drug and the lethal dose in animals, the greater the need for a high degree of accuracy and precision in determining this margin. This is an argument for attainment of sufficient precision in establishing the slope of the dose-response curve and its confidence limits. To make a choice between a limit test or a formal test designed to provide an estimate of the slope of response which corresponds to dose (the LD50 test is an example), several factors must be considered. What is the medicine for and to whom will it be given? How dangerous is it to make and to dispense? What should be done if excessive quantities are accidentally or intentionally ingested?

There has undoubtedly been an overemphasis on the numerical results obtained from acute toxicity testing: these values, which are of use in classification of new chemicals, must be accompanied by a description of the nature and time of appearance of changes in animals which have been given large doses. This information must be reported to doctors so that they can guard against the appearance of such side-effects in man. The formal LD50 study is necessary on occasions when a comparison of effective and toxic doses is required, particularly when the safety margin of a new drug is likely to be small: the formal LD50 study is reserved for that stage in a drug's development when we consider it is most likely to proceed to the clinic.

DESIGN AND CONDUCT OF STUDIES

Utilisation of animals in the testing of new drugs is a regulatory requirement and reflects the underlying "presumption in favour of humans over animals" (8).

Short-term tests must be designed and conducted so that:

a. the information or knowledge to be obtained is required for a serious and necessary purpose;
b. the number of animals used is restricted as far as is practicable;
c. in achieving the purpose of the study, any pain is kept to a minimum.

Studies are usually with rodents, such as rats and mice, and, rarely, with species such as the guinea-pig or rabbit. Scientific or legislative requirements for LD50 studies in such species can normally be completed to the satisfaction of all parties by other assessments of acute toxicity, for example, the stepwise increase in dosage from an acute no-effect level to a maximum tolerated dose or first incidence of mortality.

A strict policy must be defined which states the maximum volumes and doses which may be employed. Some examples which are based on results of practical work have been presented previously (9).

Limit doses are recommended independent of volume and should not exceed 5g/kg. For potent pharmaceutical agents suitable doses may safely be set at much lower limits.

Species	Route	Volume	Limiting Factor
Mouse (20g)	oral	1.0ml	stomach distension
	i.v.	0.5ml	hyperpnoea
Rat	oral	3ml/100g	stomach distension
	i.v.	2ml/100g	lung changes

In order to avoid unnecessary suffering, all animals which are moribund or considered to be in pain must be humanely killed without delay. In the numerical handling of data these will be recorded as "deaths", all details being faithfully recorded in the original data. Although this will have the effect of slightly overestimating the toxicity of new drugs, it is generally deemed a responsible and humanitarian attitude.

In short-term toxicity studies, a minimal number of tissues (if any) will be required for histopathological evaluation. The aim of taking such tissues must be to reach an understanding of the perilethal effects and to identify target organs for possible further study.

REPORTING OF SHORT-TERM STUDY DATA

In general, there has been an overemphasis of the numerical value for LD50. Reports of such investigations must always include:

a. the nature of the toxic response: the important signs of toxicity and likely target organs or systems;
b. the time at which the toxic responses appeared and disappeared: allowing separation of reversible from irreversible effects;
c. the median lethal dose including an estimate of the range of doses in terms of slope, enabling safety predictions to be made.

A variety of approaches have been reported for describing temporal as well as dose-relationships of toxicity (10).

CONCLUSIONS

We strongly advocate the thoughtful application of acute testing methodologies, including, on occasion, the LD50 test. Also, we note that it is current practice to discard a large number of potential new drugs on the basis of structure-activity studies, in vitro tests or very small-scale animal studies. We hold that it is necessary to develop further alternative methods for study of the acute toxic effects of new drugs in animals, although the LD50 test has an important role in defining the dose-range over which adverse effects will be encountered. However, this extensive testing should be used in circumstances when it can be scientifically justified and when other simpler approaches are insufficient.

On those occasions when the formal LD50 test is required, the use of higher animals should be prohibited: strict limits should be applied to the volumes and doses of test article that may be administered, and in all cases the scale of the study must be sufficient to provide the precision of data that is required.

We should not, however, throw the baby out with the bath water. In order to minimise the consequences of misuse or abuse of drugs, it is vital that new drugs are classified, not only according to the numerical indices of their toxicity, but also according to the type and temporal aspects of adverse effects.

The dangerous dose-range, the nature of the danger, and the time-course of effects should be communicated for each new drug, and the method by which this is achieved should be the subject of international agreement.

REFERENCES

1. Pharmaceutical Manufacturers Association (PMA) (1982). "The Role of the LD50 Determination in Drug Safety Evaluation". 8 pp. Washington: PMA.
2. Volans, G.N., Mitchell, G.M., Proudfoot, A.T., Shanks, R.G. & Woodcock, J.A. (1981). National Poisons Information Services: report and comment 1980. British Medical Journal 282, 1613-1615.
3. Illingworth, R.N. & Prescott, L.F. (1980). Inadequate information about drug overdosage in manufacturers' data sheets. British Medical Journal 280, 1418.
4. Jefferys, D. & Volans, G.N. (1981). Ketotifen overdose: surveillance of the toxicity of a new drug. British Medical Journal 282, 1755-1756.
5. Griffin, J.P. (1981). Referring to the paper by Zbinden & Flury-Roversi. Archives of Toxicology 49, 99-103.
6. Organisation for Economic Cooperation and Development (OECD). (1982). Final Report of Working Party on Health Effects. 52 pp. Washington, DC: Environment Committee, Chemicals

Group, OECD Hazard Assessment Project.
7. Fingl, E. & Woodbury, D.M. (1975). General principles. In "The Pharmacological Basis of Therapeutics" (ed. L.S. Goodman & A. Gilman), 5th edn., pp. 1-46. New York: Macmillan.
8. Report on the LD50 test presented to the Secretary of State by the Advisory Committee on the Administration of the Cruelty to Animals Act, 1876. (1979). 31 pp. London: Home Office.
9. Fowler, J.S.L. & Rutty, D.A. (1981). Methodological aspects of acute toxicity testing, particularly LD50 determinations: present use in development of new drugs. In "LD50 and Possible Alternatives" (ed. M. Thelstam), Stockholm: CFN (in press).
10. Fowler, J.S.L., Brown, J.S. & Bell, H.A. (1979). The rat toxicity screen. Pharmacology & Therapeutics 5, 461-466.

Alternatives in Acute Toxicity Testing

M. C. TATTERSALL

An acute or short-term toxicity study is an all-embracing term that must often give the impression of being a specific test that is done in the same way and for the same purpose, whether it is carried out on an industrial chemical or on a new cosmetic. In this presentation I would like to draw attention to this misconception and then to talk about the implications of the introduction of alternatives.

It is fairly easy to make general classifications of chemicals based on their use. For example, they could be divided into industrial chemicals, agricultural chemicals, household products, cosmetics, and pharmaceutical products. Anyone could probably make a slightly different list. The point to be made is that acute studies should be designed, evaluated, considered and replaced in relation to the contact that human beings will have with the chemical, or in relation to subsequent toxicity studies which rely on the acute data. For example, human contact with an industrial chemical is going to be accidental or incidental. The main requirement is a knowledge of the order of toxicity, i.e. non-toxic, very toxic, etc. Some indication of suitable treatment for accidental poisoning may also be required. Some sort of numerical data probably need to be generated to provide this classification and an approximate LD50, a minimal lethal dose or a maximum non-lethal dose using a minimum of animals can provide this information. There is certainly no need for confidence limits and statistics. The requirements for drugs differ dramatically from industrial chemicals. The main difference arises because drugs are intended for human contact. Industrial chemicals and household products basically require only a measure of their toxicity; it does not really matter what the toxic level is as long as it is known. Although this may be considered a gross simplification, it does contrast with pharmaceuticals, where a particular specified quantity of the chemical must be safe. This point illustrates quite clearly that the requirement of acute toxicity testing of pharmaceuticals (i.e. a safe dose) is quite different from that of industrial chemicals (i.e. a knowledge of the toxic dose).

Some implications of the word "alternative" are worth considering. It is unlikely that we can completely replace all animal studies with alternatives in the near future. It is, however, a target well worth striving for. There appears to be a notion in the lay-press and hence in the minds of the general public that scientists oppose the use of alternatives. This is simply not true. If an alternative can be found that can be scientifically justified, that can provide the relevant answers to the questions being asked <u>and</u> is acceptable to regulatory authorities, most toxicologists would welcome it. Two distinct advantages are likely to result from the use of alternatives, in terms of cost and variability. Alternatives are likely to be less expensive than animal tests. To take an extreme example, if a bacterial test was suitable as an alternative to carcinogenicity studies (which it is not and I will return to this point later), then we could be comparing a cost of £1000 for a bacterial test with half a million pounds for two carcinogenicity studies. In reality, alternatives are unlikely to have such a financial advantage, but the evidence to date is that they will tend to reduce rather than increase costs. The second advantage likely to result from the use of alternatives is a reduction in variation. One of the most problematical areas of toxicology is evaluating variable results. The whole concept of the LD50 and the arguments concerning its merits are concerned entirely with variability between animals. By using non-animal models, variability is almost certain to be reduced, thus increasing the reliability of results. However, it must be borne in mind that there is a counter-argument that variability is important, and that losing it would be detrimental to safety assessment.

To completely replace acute animal studies is not practical at present, and I believe that what we will see is alternative studies being used as either complementary studies or, more importantly, as screening tests. I want to say more about non-animal screening tests because I think it is very important for those people who are actively engaged in seeking alternatives and those promoting, encouraging and financing such work that they do not, first of all, waste time looking for alternatives that cannot yet be found or, secondly, become disillusioned with either their own efforts or the apparent opposition of toxicologists to accept alternatives. The ultimate aim should remain the replacement of animal experiments.

I also believe that as far as alternatives are concerned most success will result initially, not in a reduction of the number of animals used, but in a reduction of any potential for suffering that might occur in current studies. This alone must be a worthy achievement. There are no real alternatives at present to acute toxicity studies, and at the rate things are progressing it will be a long time before there are. I suggest that the problem is approached differently. As there are no examples in the acute toxicity field, I shall illustrate this method from other areas of toxicology where it is occurring because of the nature of the successes being achieved, rather than by design.

I have already referred to bacterial tests attempting to replace carcinogenicity studies. These in vitro tests do not replace carcinogenicity studies, but any chemical that is shown to be very positive in a number of bacterial tests is not worth progressing to carcinogenicity testing. This is now a fairly well accepted conclusion for new products. So, what happens? A product is still required, another chemical is tested in vitro, found to be negative and hence is progressed to carcinogenicity studies. So, a thousand animals are going to be subjected to carcinogenicity testing whether the bacterial tests had been used as a screen or not. However, let us look at the potential for suffering that may occur in the two situations. Without the initial screening, a chemical that had a very high chance of being a carcinogen would have been incorporated in the animals' diet and may have induced tumours in some of the animals. Tumour development in old rats is normal, but inducing them earlier, or of different types, or in greater numbers, may in some circumstances cause suffering. In the latter case, where the mutagenic chemical has been discarded and replaced by a non-mutagenic chemical, there is a higher chance that the chemical will not induce tumours and thus a reduction in potential suffering will have been achieved. A second example is even simpler. The rabbit eye test for cosmetics has been widely criticised. Most rabbit eye tests, in fact, do not cause irritation and the rabbit suffers no more than the discomfort of application. For example, any chemical with a low or high pH is going to be irritant to the eye and it is pointless testing it. A single piece of litmus paper can therefore be considered in this case to be a useful, and acceptable, screening test to precede an eye test. There are also other physical characteristics of a chemical that would similarly preclude its use where it might come into contact with human eyes.

Can this type of approach be applied to acute toxicity testing? I see it as the only approach. There is so much information that can be obtained from acute studies, and the whole animal is such a mass of interactive effects, that anyone seeking an out-and-out replacement is unlikely to achieve it in one step. By looking for non-animal screening methods that will detect chemicals that are too toxic for their intended use, a reduction in potential suffering should be achieved. I want to emphasise intended use. It would, as I mentioned at the beginning, result in opposition from scientists, if a screening method was developed which would detect chemicals that would be unsuitable for, say, cosmetic purposes, and we find that regulatory authorities apply it to every other sort of chemical. It should be realised that screening methods like those advocated here are an additional expense to the manufacturer, and if they are not appropriate for particular types of chemicals they are bound to be resisted by both scientists and manufacturers.

In summary, I would like everyone who has an interest in acute toxicity studies, be they toxicologists, regulators or members of organisations such as FRAME, to bear in mind that there are many different requirements for these studies, and not to consider them all as one identical test with one result, just because they are all called acute toxicity tests. For those actively engaged in the search for alternatives, I believe more success will be achieved in the short-term by actively looking for screening methods that may initially reduce the potential to cause pain, but in the more successful cases may, with further development and experience, eventually fulfil the ultimate requirement of a real replacement of animal use.

General Discussion

ROY GOULDING

Rapporteur

Dr A. CALVIN opened by saying that most medicinal compounds are administered on a repeat-dose basis to man and that he would submit that the important safety margin is the one that is obtained from repeat toxicity studies, not from acute studies.

Nevertheless, it should be recognised that many regulatory authorities throughout the world do like to see a number presented as the LD50. Experience over the past few years had shown that using quite small groups of animals, 3 male and 3 female rats, and perhaps no more than 2 or 3 groups of animals, enabled an estimate of an LD50 to be calculated by using the method of moving average rather than probit analysis, which would not work with small numbers of animals. The regulatory authorities accepted these figures, and there had been no comeback from them, asking for repeat LD50s with larger numbers of animals.

Dr S. WILLIAMS said that Dr Brown's talk had given a definition of toxicity as being an inherent property of a chemical to cause an adverse biological effect, but that he personally considered that toxicity had very little to do with the inherent properties of materials: it would be more properly defined as being a measure of an adverse response of a biological system to a chemical insult. It should be realised that when numbers obtained from a biological test, especially from a toxicity test, were applied, they could not be used in the same way as an engineering measurement is made as a material property. Toxicity numbers are not material properties, but are dependent, as Dr Brown went on to discuss later, upon the system in which they are tested, the species, the rate of administration, etc.

The following points were made by Dr L. TURNER. First, that the development of alternatives was going to be a fairly slow business, therefore, maybe one should not be looking quite so closely at what the legislatory requirements are today, because they are going to be very different in 10 years time as experience accumulated. Secondly, from the few speakers that had been heard so far, there seemed, in his view, to be another limitation creeping in, in that there was a tendency to look for packages of tests that corresponded to the packages of tests we had today, i.e. one package to replace acute tests, another to replace long-term tests, etc. This was not a good way of thinking, since toxicologists thought of all tests together when they were looking at the toxicity of a compound.

Ms Sheila SILCOCK said that Dr Brown had suggested that data-banking might be one of the most helpful ways we had of reducing toxicity tests, but would problems of commercial confidentiality occur when such data, even perhaps negative data on no-effect levels, were put into the banks, at least while the substance was being developed?

Professor R. HESS added that he considered the issue of animal numbers to be important; the use of the limit test as outlined in the OECD guidelines made it possible, in his laboratory, to cut the number of animals used for acute toxicity testing for identical chemicals by about half.

Dr M. BALLS continued by saying that, in his opinion, one of the purposes of these discussions should be to consider any differences in views or approach as they emerged. One of the recommendations in the Report of the FRAME Toxicity Committee was that, in the case of most pharmaceuticals and other chemicals, formal LD50 tests should no longer be required. An end to the requirement for formal tests could lead to a significant reduction in the number of animals used without a reduction in the quality of the information obtained. The PMA in the States produced a report which reads very much like this part of the FRAME Toxicity Committee report. They say that the precise determination of an LD50 value should be limited to those rare cases where it was scientifically necessary to compare the different batches of the same chemical or chemicals with very different structures or activities. Since there were so many people from the British pharmaceutical industry present, he wanted to ascertain whether they could join FRAME and the PMA in calling for an end to the formal LD50 test for pharmaceuticals.

The Chairman then put the question to the Meeting, whether, at least for pharmaceutical compounds, there was any real advantage in insisting upon a formal LD50 in every instance on a show of hands, this was overwhelmingly rejected.

Dr FLETCHER said that he was intrigued that every time a meeting such as this took place, the LD50 came in for a lot of heavy comment, despite the fact that most toxicologists agreed that it was practically useless. Despite this, in a recent six year OECD exercise, the LD50 was yet again enshrined by a committee of toxicologists. There was therefore, in his view, either a certain amount of hypocrasy involved here or else the people who are devising the regulations were not at this Meeting.

Dr FOWLER said that he had been working in this area of short-term testing for 10 years, and his first objective was to use a very small number of rats, in fact far smaller than the company would even believe meant anything - 4, at 4 different dose-levels - in order to reduce the numbers of other animals that were used, including, in particular, dogs. He went on to say that initially he had made quite a fool of himself since the rat did not, in fact, reveal very much that was relevant. However, as he and his colleagues became used to handling data from these short-term studies, they eventually realised that certain manifestations in the rat could also apply to the dog. The extension of that was that certain data would extend through to man. Some examples confirmed that both the rat and the dog in major respects would model for man, although not in absolute detail and certainly not in respect of the precise dose emphasis. The importance of the steepness of slope of the dose-response curve should be emphasised and also the gap, if any, between the dose which would do the maximum good to the largest number of people and the dose which would start to harm people.

Dr BROWN suggested that the answer to Dr Fletcher's point on the LD50 test was that it was not so much two-facedness, but cold feet, in coming to grips with this problem. One had hoped at the very least that the regulations were internationally beginning to show signs of a little commonsense and rationalisation. The point that Professor Hess made about the OECD guidelines was, of course, absolutely right, and was an outward visible sign of Dr Turner's point. Dr BROWN went on to say that both Ms Silcock and himself looked upon data-banking as being a very important and positive step forward: however, it was nothing like as simple and straightforward as it sounded, and anybody who had any experience of handling data, even within one organisation, would know the problems encountered. These were multiplied when one was attempting to deal with data from innumerable sources. However, it was an area in which much was going on in the world and in which we would see big steps forward in the future.

Dr GOULDING finished by saying that the final summing-up must be left to the experts at the end of the Meeting, but that he thought it fair to say that there was no clear way ahead to abandon acute toxicity testing in animals. It might be refined, it might be abbreviated, it might be designed to be more informative, but we were left with it for the moment, with the reservation that probably the classical LD50 as it had been demanded was probably unnecessary from now on. There was a particular meaning in the comment that we were trying to concentrate too much on producing some tests which would substitute for acute toxicity, short-term toxicity, long-term toxicity, carcinogenicity, inhalation toxicity, etc., instead of going right back to the beginning and saying that chemicals should be assessed for their possible harm to man or other species. If we had no animals, how would we go about it?

Application of Pharmacokinetics

J. W. BRIDGES, L. F. CHASSEAUD, G. M. COHEN and C.H. WALKER

INTRODUCTION

The toxicity caused by a substance may arise at the site of exposure and/or systemically. It is important both in the assessment of hazard and in the understanding of how toxicity arises to consider three aspects of the overall process (Fig. 1): the chemical (stability) phase; the pharmacokinetic (distributive or toxicokinetic) phase, and the pharmacodynamic (toxicodynamic or interactive) phase (see Glossary of Terms).

The chemical phase describes the actual chemical and physical form(s) of the xenobiotic(s) under study to which the biological organism(s) is exposed. It includes consideration of chemical stability, water solubility, particle size, etc. For acute oral administration of a drug to a patient under medical supervision, the chemical phase is often very simple, whereas for chronic exposure to a xenobiotic in the environment the situation may be extremely complex, and an accurate description of the chemical phase may not be possible. For particulates it is often very difficult to ascertain the actual extent of exposure of tissue sites sensitive to toxicity and/or involved in uptake and accumulation.

The pharmacokinetic phase describes the relationship between the total dose of the xenobiotic to which the organism is exposed and the resulting concentrations of the xenobiotic and/or its metabolites (including both biotransformation products and chemical breakdown products) which are achieved in body tissue and tissue fluids. Thus, the study of the pharmacokinetic phase involves an assessment of the absorption, biotransformation, binding to tissues and tissue fluid components, and excretion of xenobiotics and their metabolites.

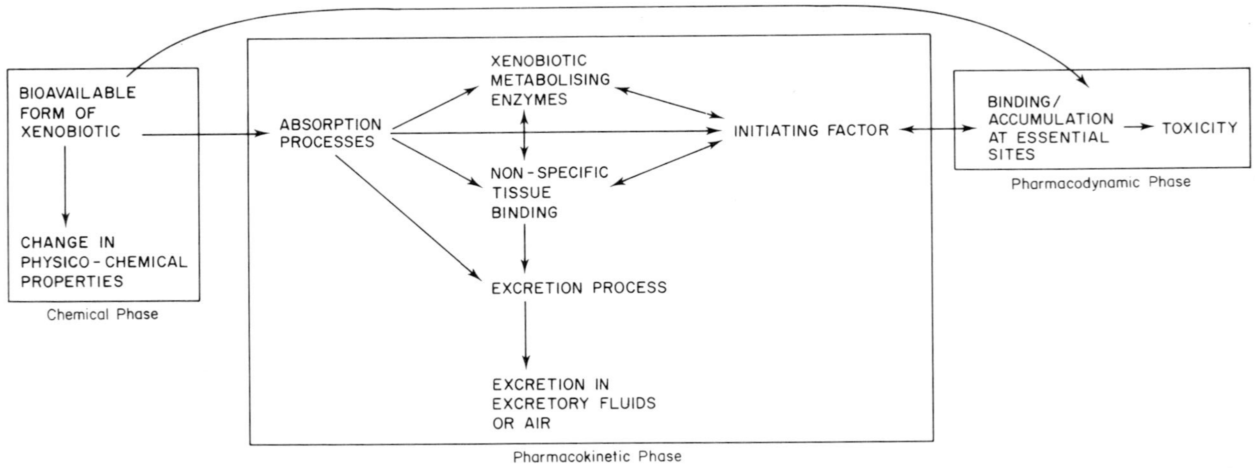

Figure 1 Phases in the Toxic Process

The pharmacodynamic phase describes the interaction of the xenobiotic and/or its metabolites with those cellular or extra-cellular components (receptors, sites of action) whose modified functions are involved in the immediate or later expression of toxicity.

The extent of the initial toxic interaction and its tissue location is typically directly related to the concentration of the xenobiotic and/or its metabolites at the actual sites of toxicity. (N.B. Hypersensitivity reactions are atypical in this respect.) Under apparently identical conditions of administered dose, organisms may vary considerably in the toxic response between species and between individuals of the same species. The principal cause of this variation can, in many instances, be ascribed to differences in the pharmacokinetic phase. Proper characterisation of the pharmacokinetic phase is therefore essential to the extrapolation of toxicological data from one organism to another. Unfortunately, in conventional toxicity testing consideration of the pharmacokinetic and chemical phases is frequently ignored and only the dose administered and the toxic effects encountered are determined.

Pharmacokinetic investigations can provide answers to the following important questions:

1. Is the xenobiotic absorbed or is it first metabolised or degraded and the products absorbed, and what proportion of the absorbed material reaches the systemic circulation?

2. Does the xenobiotic and/or its metabolite(s) accumulate or diminish in body tissues on repeated dosing, what is the cause of any accumulation (e.g. irreversible binding, binding to specific tissue components), are the organs having the highest concentrations of xenobiotic-related material the principal target organs for toxicity?

3. Are metabolites of known toxicity formed?

4. Does saturation of any rate-limiting process occur which might be expected to significantly affect the dose-response relationship? (N.B. If biotransformation is crucial to the detoxication of the xenobiotic, saturation of the metabolising enzymes may lead to a rapid increase in toxicity.)

5. How does the dose regimen influence the levels of the xenobiotic and related material in the tissue? (Such data is very relevant in deciding whether to administer a xenobiotic in the diet, by gavage, etc.)

6. What is the relationship between the dose administered and

the levels and persistence of xenobiotic and metabolite(s) achieved in tissue fluids and/or tissues in the various animal models used for toxicological investigations, and in man?

Ideally, some pharmacokinetic information should be obtained in the appropriate animal model(s) before any medium-term to long-term toxicological investigations on a particular xenobiotic are undertaken. In practice, this is often frustrated by the difficulty either of developing quickly an analytical method of suitable sensitivity and specificity or of synthesising a suitable radioisotopically-labelled material. Even if a suitable analytical method is available, there are a number of technical and ethical problems which can compromise the design and conduct of pharmacokinetic studies of a potentially toxic entity, namely:

a. It is rarely possible to identify the critical molecular targets for toxicity.
b. For ethical and practical reasons, it is frequently not possible to sample the target tissue(s) during the *in vivo* development of a toxic lesion, so monitoring of tissue fluids must be used instead.
c. In many instances, the metabolite(s) which are responsible for toxicity have a very short lifetime because they are chemically unstable or readily metabolised further. This may frustrate the direct identification of their structure and their role in initiating toxicity.

THE *IN VIVO* MONITORING OF BODY FLUIDS AND EXHALED AIR

Sampling Considerations

If tissues which are sites of toxic action cannot be sampled, it is usually possible to sample tissue fluids or, for volatile xenobiotics, exhaled air. In all cases it is important to establish sample storage characteristics and the reliability of the assay procedures before embarking on a pharmacokinetic study. The fluid most often sampled for pharmacokinetic purposes is blood, and levels of xenobiotics are commonly determined in plasma. Careful consideration must be given to the most relevant site for blood sampling, if valid predictions are to be made about the levels of xenobiotics in particular tissues. Ideally, samples should be taken of the arterial blood entering and the venous blood leaving any particular tissue, but this is not usually practicable. It is also important to establish the clearance of the xenobiotic and its metabolites from the body. For this purpose, both urine and bile should be sampled, as well as blood. Urine collection is usually straightforward, though care must be taken that the samples are not contaminated with faeces, which may also contain the xenobiotic and/or its metabolite(s). If the xenobiotic is administered in the food, food contamination of urine must also be avoided. Bile collection is best done from an animal fitted with a re-entrant bile duct cannula, in the absence of anaesthetic. Terminal cannulation of anaethetised animals is less satisfactory in pharmacokinetic work.

Most tissue fluids are separated from blood by permeability barriers, e.g. cerebrospinal fluid, testicular fluid, fetal tissue fluids and breast milk. The first three are more difficult to sample than blood. A number of xenobiotics are either volatile or are converted to volatile metabolites, including CO_2. In establishing the pharmacokinetic behaviour of a xenobiotic it is important to consider exhaled air as a potential excretory route.

The Relationship Between Tissue Levels of Xenobiotics and Levels in Body Fluids

Blood. The distribution of xenobiotics between blood and tissue is dependent upon the lipophilicity of the compound, its binding to plasma proteins, the permeability of the membrane barriers that separate blood and tissue, and the binding characteristics of the tissue itself. The octanol:water partition coefficient is often used as an index of lipophilicity. In general, xenobiotics with relatively high partition coefficients can readily cross membrane barriers by passive diffusion, as long as their molecular size is not too large. Xenobiotics vary considerably in their tendency to bind to plasma proteins. Some, such as the trypanocidal agent suramin, are very strongly bound, and this restricts their movement into tissues. There is evidence of substantial species differences in the ability to bind drugs to plasma proteins (3,4). There are also differences in the permeability of the membrane barriers between blood and different tissues. For example, the liver is freely permeable to most liposoluble xenobiotics, and it is also readily permeable to lipoprotein fragments of chylomicrons which may carry xenobiotics. The blood-cerebrospinal fluid and blood-brain barriers are also readily permeated by liposoluble xenobiotics, but not by large or ionised molecules. Finally, the uptake of xenobiotics may be influenced by binding within the tissue. Apart from covalent binding, which is discussed elsewhere, certain compounds may bind reversibly to cellular macromolecules, e.g. quinacrine is strongly bound in the liver, gentamicin is slowly but strongly bound in the kidney (see 1).

The relationship between blood and tissue levels has been investigated in some detail with liposoluble xenobiotics, such as dieldrin (5) and polychlorinated biphenyl (PCB) isomers (6). Because of their chemical and biological stability, it is relatively easy to obtain accurate assessment of the tissue levels of such xenobiotics *in vivo*. In the case of dieldrin given to the male rat, elimination occurred in two phases. These phases, which corresponded to long and short half-lives, were found to be similar in blood, adipose tissue and liver. In other studies, dieldrin half-lives were similar in four different tissues (depot fat, liver, brain and muscle) in both the rat and the feral pigeon (7,8).

Lutz *et al.* (6) have attempted to develop a pharmacokinetic model, in order to predict levels of PCB isomers in various tissues of the rat following administration of a single intravenous injection. The model was designed to account for each parent compound and its major metabolite. Partition coefficients between blood and different tissues were first determined experimentally, then employed in the model. Used in this way, the model provided a good simulation of the pharmacokinetic situation over a period of at least 4 days for two highly chlorinated PCB isomers in blood and four other tissues. The simulation was distinctly less effective for monoisomers and dichloroisomers, which are metabolised much more rapidly than dieldrin and the highly chlorinated biphenyls. These and other studies indicate that, in certain instances, it is possible to provide a reasonable forecast of the tissue levels of xenobiotics and metabolites which will be attained with time, based on the levels found in blood, but that such models cannot be applied generally (see subsequent sections). Some useful information may also be derived, in many cases, from a study of the pharmacokinetics of a xenobiotic using *in vitro* organ perfusion, but there is no guarantee that findings from such studies will accurately reflect the *in vivo* situation.

Bile and urine. The monitoring of levels of a xenobiotic and its metabolites, including conjugates in bile and urine, may give an indication of the concentrations achieved in the liver and kidney, but it is generally not useful for establishing the xenobiotic and metabolite levels attained in other organs. The liver has a dominant role in the biotransformation of most xenobiotics to produce water-soluble and excretable conjugates, and monitoring of bile therefore provides a means of studying these metabolic processes (9).

In one investigation, rats were dosed with the dieldrin analogue, HCE (10). Using data from studies with microsomal fractions, and knowing the concentration of substrate in the hepatic endoplasmic reticulum under *in vivo* conditions, an estimate was made of the rate of liver metabolism *in vivo*. This figure corresponded fairly closely with the rate of excretion of conjugates in bile, suggesting that for certain xenobiotics, at least, it is possible to obtain reasonable estimates of rates of hepatic metabolism by monitoring concentrations of metabolites in bile.

Relationship Between Xenobiotic Levels in Target Tissues and Toxic or Pharmacological Response

For xenobiotics and their metabolites which form readily reversible interactions with target sites for toxicity (e.g. receptors), the peak level of unbound compound present in the immediate vicinity of the target site should be directly related to the biological response over a considerable concentration range. For very reactive xenobiotics and their metabolites, the amount of compound present over a period is often more important than the peak level. For a number of compounds, a direct correlation between total covalent binding to cellular proteins and the extent of hepatocellular necrosis has been established. Similarly, for several carcinogens, DNA alkylation has been shown to be directly related to their carcinogenicity potency, although in some cases such a correlation is not observed with total binding but rather with specific adducts (e.g. dimethyl nitrosamine). There are a number of reasons why the concentration of a xenobiotic and its metabolites that are achieved in a tissue may not correlate with the biological response observed. Common causes are:

a. The xenobiotic and/or its metabolites may be strongly bound to cellular macromolecules which are not involved in the expression of biological activity. For example, cadmium is very strongly bound in both liver and kidney to the protein metallothionein; therefore, the measurement of total cadmium levels does not correlate well with the extent of adverse change.
b. The toxic effect on the tissue may be mediated indirectly, e.g. at a site which is distant from the observed site of biological activity. For example, the primary target may be the nervous or endocrine system.
c. The biological action may be of an "all or none" kind, e.g. initiation of antibody production.
d. The sampling technique for determining xenobiotic and metabolite levels may be inappropriate. This is common when the biological action is in a minority cell-type in a particular tissue.
e. More than one form of the xenobiotic is responsible for the biological activity.

For practical and ethical reasons, it may not be possible to obtain direct information on the levels of active molecules in target tissues in vivo. However, quantitation of a toxic or pharmacological response may allow an assessment of the concentration of a labile compound in the tissue or organ in which it acts, provided that there is only one active form of the xenobiotic and that the biological action is largely or entirely at one site.

Quantitation of a toxic response is most readily attained if the magnitude of the lesion can be assessed by monitoring *in vivo* biochemical changes. Organophosphate insecticides, for instance, which act by inhibiting acetyl cholinesterase in the brain, can provide an index of the concentration of the active form of an organophosphate present *in vivo*, even though the active metabolite is so unstable as to escape detection by ordinary chemical analysis.

GENERAL ASPECTS OF THE USE OF *IN VITRO* STUDIES

There are serious limitations to the extent to which the study of pharmacokinetic processes can be performed upon live animals. Apart from ethical issues, practical questions, such as cost and the difficulty of keeping many species, greatly restrict what can be done. There are also serious scientific limitations to the usefulness of purely *in vivo* experiments. For example, it is not possible to properly identify and characterise the enzyme systems involved in xenobiotic biotransformation by *in vivo* techniques alone. A particular problem of methodology arises with compounds (e.g. certain carcinogens) which are converted to unstable active metabolites, which either bind rapidly to cellular macromolecules and other cellular constituents or are destroyed very effectively by detoxication enzymes and therefore do not appear in blood or excreta. Here, critical species differences in metabolism are unlikely to be found by *in vivo* techniques alone.

In vitro studies permit the investigation of metabolic processes under controlled conditions, allowing the identification and characterisation of both the enzymes involved and the formation of stable and unstable metabolites. If toxicity in man is due to the parent compound, a number of *in vitro* model systems should be able to detect such toxicity, provided that the half-life of the compound is similar in man and in the model system(s) employed and there is no qualitative biochemical abnormality in man which predisposes him to such toxicity. If, as is often the case, toxicity is due to a reactive metabolite, then the nature of the drug metabolising system involved in its formation and degradation needs to be similar in the *in vivo* and *in vitro* situation.

Various *in vitro* drug metabolising systems are available, which differ mainly in their levels of cellular and tissue integrity. These systems include tissue homogenates, subcellular fractions, isolated perfused organs and cells, cell lines, and organ cultures. Two particular aspects of the metabolism in these systems must be considered: the qualitative nature of the metabolites produced, and the time-course of metabolite formation.

The majority of *in vitro* systems will, with varying degrees of success, mimic, at least qualitatively, the in vivo formation of metabolites. The disruption of the cellular integrity of any test system, e.g. the use of microsomes, often enables the optimum generation of reactive metabolites to be expressed. However, in vivo and in intact cells there are several defences to protect against the formation of such reactive metabolites or to inactivate these metabolites, if formed. Thus, model systems, such as organ cultures or isolated perfused organs or cells, which retain cellular and/or tissue integrity, will generally reflect the in vivo situation more closely than in vitro systems, such as homogenates or subcellular fractions, where cellular integrity has been disrupted (Fig. 2).

It must be emphasised that cell lines are generally deficient in a number of drug metabolising enzyme activities, particularly those dependent on cytochrome P-450 (phenobarbitone type), and this may restrict their value as in vitro models for toxicity testing (12). To some extent the problem may be overcome by the addition of an in vitro drug metabolising system (e.g. 9,000 x g liver supernatant, microsomes or intact hepatocytes) to the cell line (13). However, this approach is not always valid, since the two systems may be incompatible, metabolites produced in this way may not be able to reach the target sites for toxicity in sufficient concentrations, etc. A particularly difficult problem with any in vitro system is to realistically reflect in vivo situations with regard to tissue-tissue interactions. For example, the lack of both an excretory system and the dynamic equilibria of the in vivo system often leads to exaggerated in vitro effects which are not seen in vivo.

A number of extra-hepatic organs may also bring about the biotransformation of xenobiotics (14). Although these organs are generally less effective in the overall metabolism of xenobiotics, this is by no means always the case. Studies on the in vitro biotransformation of xenobiotics by extra-hepatic organs have been much less extensive than liver studies. Methods for preparing subcellular fractions and isolating those cells with particularly high concentrations of xenobiotic metabolising enzymes are far from ideal for most organs. Much of the published quantitative data on xenobiotic biotransformation activity in extra-hepatic organs is probably suspect, because inappropriate methodology was employed during tissue preparation.

CONDITIONS UNDER WHICH PHARMACOKINETIC PROCESSES MAY BE SATURATED

The metabolism and excretion (and hence the elimination) of most xenobiotics from the body follows first-order kinetics. The pharmacokinetic parameters (such as half-life [$t\frac{1}{2}$] and clearance) of such xenobiotics are independent of dose and thus

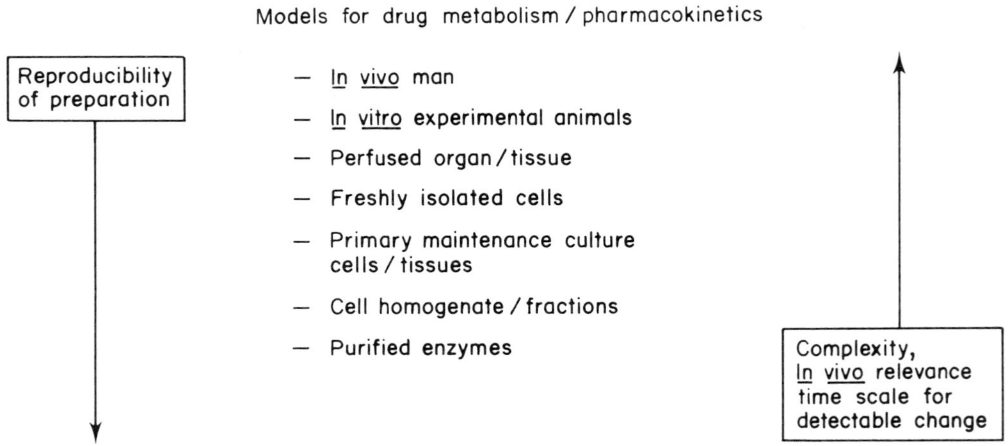

Figure 2 Models for Drug Metabolism/Pharmacokinetics

availability to the tissues of such substances (as measured by the area under the curve [AUC]) increases linearly with increasing dose. However, a number of xenobiotics have been demonstrated to show dose-dependent pharmacokinetics, i.e. the pharmacokinetic parameters vary with the exposure dose of xenobiotic. This is indicative of the saturation of one or more pharmacokinetic processes within the dose-ranges studied. As a consequence of saturation, a disproportionate change with dosage in the availability of xenobiotic and/or metabolites to the target sites for toxicity may occur, with a consequent sharp change in the observed quantitative and/or qualitative toxic effects (15).

A variety of metabolic processes may become saturated with increasing dose or multiple dosing, including those involved in transport, binding, biotransformation and excretion. In order to confidently predict the potential toxicity of a xenobiotic for another species, it is important to establish whether saturation of rate-limiting pharmacokinetic processes is likely to occur in either species over the dose-range of interest.

Theoretical Basis for the Saturation of Pharmacokinetic Processes

The effects of substrate concentration on the rate of enzymic formation of metabolites can be described by the Michaelis-Menten Equation:

$$v = \frac{V_{max} \quad S}{K_m \ + S}$$

where v = velocity of the reaction, V_{max} is the maximal velocity, S is the substrate concentration, and K_m is the Michaelis constant.

At low substrate concentrations:

$S << K_m$, and therefore $K_m + S$ approaches the value of K_m, thus:

$$v = \frac{V_{max} \quad S}{K_m}$$

i.e. the rate of excretion is first-order.

At high substrate concentrations:

$S >> K_m$, and therefore $K_m + S$ approaches the value of S, thus:

$$v = V_{max}$$

i.e. the rate of reaction is independent of the substrate concentration and is, therefore, a zero-order process.

It is evident from the above that as the substrate concentration is increased from a low value to a high value and the metabolic process becomes saturated, the reaction velocity will correspondingly change from first-order to zero-order kinetics. All enzymic processes will show this phenomenon if exposed to a sufficiently high concentration of substrate. (N.B. The K_m's of the drug metabolising enzymes are frequently in the range of 0.1 to 10mM.)

In addition to biotransformation enzymes, other processes which obey Michaelis-Menten type kinetics include active and facilitated transport (e.g. biliary excretion and kidney tubular secretion) and protein binding (e.g. albumin).

Effect of Route of Administration on Other Saturable Processes

Both the degree and the nature of toxicity may be affected by the route of administration. Thus, one route or form of administration may lead to sufficiently high concentrations of a substrate reaching the enzyme or other saturable pharmacokinetically important site to cause its saturation, whereas such saturation may not occur by an alternative route or form of administration (16). Saturation of pharmacokinetic processes is, for example, much more likely to occur when a xenobiotic is administered by injection or by gavage than if a comparable dose is administered in the diet.

The Practical Relevance of Saturation of Pharmacokinetic Processes

With highly toxic compounds, saturation of pharmacokinetic processes may be of little concern, because lethality occurs before saturation is reached. However, it can be of great relevance with xenobiotics of relatively low intrinsic toxicity. For example, studies with vinyl chloride monomer have demonstrated the importance of saturation for the expression of at least one aspect of its chronic toxicity, namely, angiosarcoma of the liver. Similarly, the importance of saturable processes in mediating the acute toxicity of 1,1-dichloroethylene and several other compounds has recently been recognised. The saturation of particular xenobiotic metabolising enzymes may result in a change in metabolite profiles. Consequently, metabolite profiles obtained at low dose-levels in man may often be difficult to relate to data obtained at high dose-levels in experimental animals.

Identification of Situations Where Saturation of Pharmacokinetic Processes Occur

Several criteria can be used to indicate that saturation of crucial pharmacokinetic processes for the elimination of a xenobiotic from the body is occurring (17-19):

a. The decline of the blood or plasma levels of the xenobiotic following cessation of dosing is not exponential.
b. The rate constant of elimination decreases with increasing dose.
c. The availability of the xenobiotic (as measured by the AUC) increases disproportionately with increasing dose.
d. A change in the relative amounts of the excretory products occurs with increasing dose.
e. The pharmacological or toxicological effects of the xenobiotic increase disproportionately with increasing dose.
f. Reaction of the xenobiotic or its reactive metabolites with critical "receptor" macromolecules, such as DNA, RNA or protein, increases disproportionately with dose.
g. Other xenobiotics at relatively low concentrations, which are either metabolised or transported by the same saturable processes, competitively inhibit the elimination and/or metabolism of the xenobiotic under study.

In Vitro Studies

Individual processes which may be saturated can usually only be characterised fully in vitro. The apparent K_m values of individual enzymes or tissue binding proteins are most readily determined using cell fractions or purified constituents, whereas to ascertain the saturated kinetics for active or facilitated transport processes, intact cell preparations are usually required.

It should be noted that physiological factors, such as blood flow, may sometimes limit the rate at which a xenobiotic reaches particular tissue sites, and that this may cause the observed pharmacological or toxicological response to plateau. Investigation of phenomena of this type is difficult to mimic in vitro.

SPECIES DIFFERENCES IN PHARMACOKINETICS

In the case of vertebrates, species differences in pharmacokinetic processes are usually quantitative rather than qualitative. Large quantitative differences in the biotransformation of a xenobiotic and/or in other pharmaceutical processes occur commonly between the different species normally employed in toxicity testing. (N.B. Species variations in biotransformation have received most attention and therefore will be given the major focus here. However, the paucity of studies of species differences in other pharmacokinetic processes should not be taken as evidence that they are insignificant for particular xenobiotics.) Because a compound may be converted to both active and inactive metabolites, species differences in biotransformation can be important factors in determining variations in susceptibility to drugs, pesticides and other chemicals. Such metabolic differences should be taken into account when selecting species to be used as models for man in toxicity testing and when choosing indicator species to assess the hazards of pesticides and pollutants to beneficial organisms such as domestic and farm animals, parasites and predators of pest species, and wildlife. Apart from the question of the response of living animals to xenobiotics, species differences in xenobiotic transformation also need to be taken into account in certain types of in vitro testing, e.g. the choice of microsomal systems in in vitro toxicity tests, such as the Ames test for bacterial mutagens.

Species differences in metabolism and pharmacokinetics are important for several reasons in addition to their basic scientific interest. They need to be taken into account when:

a. attempting to use animals as models for man in safety evaluation;
b. designing and testing drugs and pesticides for veterinary use;
c. designing selective pesticides which will not have undesirable side-effects (including the build up of residues) upon beneficial organisms.

Thus, the selection of species for toxicity testing is dependent in the first place upon the use to which a xenobiotic is to be put. In the cases of b. and c., a major concern is to find suitable models for species other than man (beneficial organisms).

Xenobiotics are usually eliminated more rapidly by animals than by man. Therefore, the general practice of once-a-day dosing in long-term toxicity studies in animals often means that each daily dose is eliminated before the next day's dose is administered. This often contrasts with the conditions of human exposure, e.g. to a pollutant where exposure may be continuous or to a therapeutic agent where the regimen used is often designed to maintain steady state levels of drug in the body.

Species Differences In Vivo

The sites of biotransformation and the rate at which biotransformation occurs are influenced by the factors which determine uptake and distribution. Thus, the course of metabolism may be dependent upon the route by which a compound is administered. An important source of species variation in metabolism is the tendency for a compound to be bound, e.g. to plasma proteins, or to be stored in fat deposits. The availability of a strongly liposoluble xenobiotic tends to be greatly increased during such processes as hibernation, migration and egg laying, all of which involve the mobilisation of fat reserves.

The route of excretion may also vary between species. Many xenobiotics are excreted as anionic conjugates, and there are marked species differences with regard to the preferred excretory route (9). For all vertebrates so far studied, urinary excretion of anions predominates at low molecular weight (<300), but biliary excretion predominates at high molecular weight (>500). Between these limits, different species show contrasting molecular weight thresholds for biliary excretion of anions; these are relatively low in the rat (c. 325), dog and hen, and rather high in the guinea-pig (c. 400), rabbit (c. 475), Rhesus monkey and man. (N.B. These values indicate the molecular weights above which most compounds undergo significant (>10%) biliary excretion in a particular species.) The gastrointestinal toxicity of indomethacin and related compounds in rats and dogs has been ascribed to the high local concentrations of the drug reached in the gut as a consequence of the extensive biliary excretion of this type of drug (20). These species differences in biliary excretion, taken in conjunction with the fact that toxic reactive metabolites will generally not be excreted *per se*, emphasise that comparisons of species differences in drug metabolism based solely on urinary metabolite profiles may give a very poor indication of species differences in tissue metabolism. These thresholds for biliary excretion are also important in determining the course of *in vivo* metabolism. Conjugates in the bile are frequently broken down when they reach the gut, and the metabolic fragments so released can undergo reabsorption and be returned to the liver (enterohepatic circulation). This raises the possibility of further metabolism either in the gut or within the animal after reabsorption (9,21). Chloramphenicol, for instance, is extensively excreted as a glucuronide in the rat (30-60% of dose), but not in man (<3%). In the rat, significant levels of toxic metabolites are generated by bacterial metabolism in the gut (21), with consequent systemic toxicity (e.g. to the thyroid gland). Sometimes, species differences in the flora of the gut result in differences in metabolism, as in the case of quinic acid. In man and Old World monkeys, this compound is extensively converted into benzoic acid following oral administration, whereas in New World monkeys and other species, this conversion is small or unmeasurable (22). In animals which practice coprophagy, the stomach and small intestine may be occupied by microorganisms. As a consequence, some xenobiotics may be metabolised prior to absorption in these species; e.g. carbenoxolone is hydrolysed by the microflora to enoxolone which is the predominant form which is absorbed in rats, whereas in man carbenoxolone is absorbed largely intact (23).

Species differences have been found in the oxidative metabolism of amphetamine and coumarin, although no clear phylogenetic trends have yet emerged (22). These differences are probably due to species variations in the distribution of forms of microsomal monooxygenase. Marked differences have also been found in conjugation reactions. For example, there is great species variation in the conjugates produced from phenol and its metabolite, quinol. At the extremes, the pig produces only phenol glucuronide and no sulphates, whereas the cat produces two sulphates, but no glucuronide (22). Carnivores are also deficient in hepatic glycine conjugation of benzoic acid and in the acetylation of aromatic amines, compared with other species (24).

Correlation Between Comparative Metabolism *In Vivo* and Toxicity

Some of the differences mentioned in the foregoing section are correlated with differences in toxicity. Thus, aniline is more toxic to the cat, dog and other carnivores than it is to herbivores, and this toxicity is related to the more extensive production of the toxic o-aminophenol by the carnivores and the failure in the case of dog to acetylate it (25). Also, many phenols and benzoic acid are more toxic to the cat than to non-carnivores.

Species Differences in Enzymic Activity *In Vitro*

Hepatic Microsomal Enzymes

Much work has been done on the oxidative metabolism of xenobiotics by the hepatic microsomes of vertebrates. In a survey of the literature, data were collected for hepatic microsomal monooxygenase activity measured using 10 different substrates in 65 different vertebrate species (26). To enable comparison between assay procedures employing different substrates, all activities were expressed relative to those of the male rat. In mammals, activities were negatively correlated with body weights, the highest values being found in the mouse and hamster, and one of the lowest in man. Comparing species of the same body weight, mammals showed higher activities than fish in all cases, the average difference being 10-13 fold. The activities in birds were widely scattered between those of mammals and fish, the fish-eating bird species having the lowest activities which were similar in most cases to those of fish.

The two microsomal enzymes, epoxide hydrolase and glucuronyl transferase, were also more active in mammals than in fish (27). Birds showed lower epoxide hydrolase activities than mammals (26).

Plasma Enzymic Activity

Mammals have an esterase in plasma which degrades the active forms of certain organophosphate pesticides. Activity of this kind was very low or non-detectable in the plasma of 14 species of birds representing 6 different orders (28).

Extra-hepatic Metabolising Enzymes

In contrast to the situation with hepatic enzymes, only a very limited number of reliable investigations have been made on species differences in extrahepatic tissues. Benzo[a]pyrene hydroxylation has been the subject of most of these studies (14).

The Use of *In Vitro* Systems to Predict Species Differences *In Vivo*

One approach has been to compare the biological half-lives of drugs in different species with rates at which they are degraded *in vitro*. For instance, half-lives of hexobarbitone, antipyrine, phenylbutazone, and dieldrin have been compared in different species. There is an inverse relationship between their half-lives and the oxidative capacity of liver microsomes towards these compounds and other relevant substrates (26). The longest half-lives and lowest oxidative capacities were typically found in man, whereas the shortest half-lives and the highest oxidative capacities were usually found in the mouse or rat. However, although this would appear to be a general trend, it is by no means inevitably the case that human microsomes are much less active in oxidation than those of rodents (29). Comparative toxicity may correspond to the metabolic rates *in vivo*. For example, organophosphates, such as diazinon, primiphos-methyl, and coumaphos, are considerably more toxic to birds than to mammals (28,30). This appears to be mainly due to a comparative deficiency of 'A' esterase in birds (31). It is also noteworthy that birds, which tend to have lower monooxygenase activity than mammals, are also more sensitive to carbamate insecticides than are mammals, presumably because most carbamates are detoxified by this enzyme system (32).

A direct comparison between *in vitro* and *in vivo* metabolism has been carried out with the dieldrin analogue HCE in the rat, rabbit, Japanese quail and pigeon (10,33). All the major metabolites formed by hepatic microsomes of a particular species were also found in the urine, bile and faeces of that species. This study indicates that in a number of other situations it might be possible to predict species differences *in vivo* from *in vitro* data.

Correlation Between Comparative Metabolism *In Vitro* and Toxicity

As the understanding of mechanisms of toxicity improves, so greater use can be made of such information for the elucidation of the processes of activation and deactivation for particular types of xenobiotic.

Different species exhibit marked differences in their susceptibility to the hepatotoxicity of paracetamol. For example, the mouse is markedly susceptible, whilst the rat is relatively resistant. These differences in susceptibility correlate with the relative abilities of microsomes from these species to metabolically activate paracetamol to covalently-bound species (34). The rate of activation of paracetamol by human liver is similar to that of the mouse, in agreement with the known susceptibility of humans to the hepatotoxicity of paracetamol.

2-Acetylaminofluorene is known to be a potent hepatocarcinogen in most species, except the guinea-pig, steppe-lemming and rainbow trout (36). Species which are susceptible to the hepatocarcinogenicity are able to N-hydroxylate 2-acetylaminofluorene, whereas resistant species do not excrete significant amounts of the material as N-hydroxy derivatives. The carcinogenicity of this compound in man is unknown, but man is able to form the N-hydroxy metabolite, leading to the expectation that 2-acetylaminofluorene would be a carcinogen in man.

Use of Pharmacokinetic Models

Although the use of mathematical modelling is discussed in detail elsewhere in this volume, it is appropriate to mention here some particular applications of mathematical modelling to pharmacokinetics (see also (37)). A potentially very useful approach is to utilise *in vitro* results on the nature of the metabolites formed and their kinetic characteristics, together with pharmacokinetic models, to predict pharmacokinetic behaviour of chemicals in man and other species which have well-documented anatomy and physiology. This approach has been used with some success for a number of compounds, including cytosine arabinoside, ethoxybenzamide, diphenylhydantoin and polychlorinated biphenyls (38). The relationship between inter-species variation in pharmacokinetics and body size (allometry) has also been investigated (39) and this approach may be of value in future studies on the extrapolation of animal data to man.

PHARMACOKINETICS IN MAN

The capacity of an individual to metabolise a particular xenobiotic expresses the interplay between genetic, environmental, physiological and pathological factors which influence the activity of drug metabolising enzymes and therefore the disposition of the xenobiotic. As these factors vary between individuals, so also will the response of those individuals vary to xenobiotics. The extent of human variability in pharmacokinetics should be an important factor in the selection of systems to be used in the toxicity evaluation of a particular xenobiotic.

On the basis of xenobiotic elimination studies in twins, Vesell et al. (40) suggested that the genetic factor was a more important determinant of xenobiotic metabolism than the environmental factor. Thus, xenobiotic metabolism was similar in monozygotic twins, but could vary greatly between dizygotic twins. In a series of patients receiving 75mg per day of the antidepressant, nortriptyline, a 50-fold variation occurred in steady state plasma levels (41). Peak plasma concentrations of the anti-anginal drug isosorbide dinitrate can vary over 5-fold in a group of human subjects (Huntingdon Research Centre, unpublished data), and similar variation for certain other drugs means that some subjects do not even achieve therapeutic levels whilst others may have toxic levels. Less variation occurs with many other drugs, but 3-fold intersubject variations in plasma drug levels are common. For xenobiotics that are not well absorbed from the gastrointestinal tract or are subject to considerable hepatic first-pass metabolism (42), intersubject variability is likely to be particularly great. Other pharmacokinetic parameters of xenobiotics are also subject to considerable variation (Table I). Such variability is of special importance when drugs with a low therapeutic index, such as digoxin, are administered. The possibility of intersubject variability for a xenobiotic is difficult to predict from studies in animals generally used for toxicity testing, since they are bred to be very uniform. Only rarely are very young, very old or diseased animals or a range of genetic types used in pharmacokinetic studies.

Genetic Variation

A proportion of the population differ considerably from the remainder in their ability to metabolise particular xenobiotics. One well-studied example, involving oxidation at the carbon atom, is the hypotensive drug, debrisoquine. The effective dose of this drug in different individuals may vary between 20-400mg per day. Individuals sensitive to the drug are deficient in their ability to hydroxylate the drug in the 4-position. The ratio of unchanged drug excreted in urine to 4-hydroxylated drug excreted in urine provides a means of dividing the population into 2 groups which differ in their ability to 4-hydroxylate the drug. Typical ratios are 0.7 for extensive metabolisers and 23 for poor metabolisers (43). Another example is that of slow and fast acetylators of drugs such as isoniazid and hydrallazine. The British population comprises almost equal numbers of both types, whereas almost all Canadian Eskimos are fast acetylators and Egyptians are mainly slow acetylators (44). Serum paraoxinase activity also shows a bimodal distribution in the human population, there being a 25-fold activity range between extreme cases (31).

Table I

Range of Inter-individual Differences in the Half-lives of Various Drugs in Man (64)

Drug	Range of half-lives
Acetylsalicylic acid	13-20 min
Acetylsulphisoxazole	8-32 hr
Amobarbitone	14-42 hr
Amphetamine	18-34 hr
Antipyrine	7-34 hr
Cephalexin	10-30 min
Chlorpropamide	25-42 hr
Diazepam	1.1-2.2 days
Digoxin	1.3-5.5 days
Diisopyramide phosphate	3.8-10.8 hr
Doxycycline	4-20 hr
Flucytosine	3-6 hr
Glutethimide	5-22 hr
Haloperidol	13-36 hr
Lithium	14-24 hr
Methaqualone	10-43 hr
Paracetamol	0.9-2.9 hr
Phenylbutazone	2.5-4.9 days
Phenytoin	19-28 hr
Quinidine	3-16 hr
Theophylline	2.9-7.1 hr
Warfarin	0.6-2.4 days

Other Factors Causing Human Variation

Among the other factors that influence drug metabolism, certain environmental factors are to some extent predictable from animal studies. These factors include diet, exposure to other chemicals, stress and climate. For example, compounds that induce drug-metabolising enzymes in animals at relatively low doses generally do so in humans (45). However, except in a few cases, such as epileptics receiving certain types of anti-convulsant therapy or during treatment with anti-coagulants, or overdose situations, it is unlikely that enzyme induction in man is of much clinical importance. Of greater consequence is enzyme inhibition, which can be predicted from studies in animals, e.g. inhibition of pesticide metabolism by piperonyl butoxide (46) or inhibition of a number of P-450 mediated xenobiotic oxidation reactions by cimetidine.

Certain diseases are likely to have a profound effect on drug disposition in man, but valid animal models of human diseases are surprisingly few. This has made the search for pharmacologically active drugs difficult, and as a result many of the pharmacological screening tests are "indirect". However, the effect of liver or kidney disease on drug disposition can be anticipated because of the role of these organs in drug elimination. Consideration of the disposition of the drug should indicate whether liver or kidney disease is likely to be important in its toxicity, and further evidence can be obtained from appropriate studies in animals (47) and during carefully controlled clinical pharmacokinetic studies.

Sex differences in drug metabolism are often observed in the rat and mouse, but not in many other mammalian species (47), humans are infrequently reported, and when observed are generally of doubtful significance.

In most species, drug metabolism pathways appear to be less active in the fetus, early neonate or elderly than in the young adult (48). The inferior ability of the elderly to metabolise drugs needs to be considered during clinical trials in patients, since the early developmental studies of a new drug in man (Phase 1) are usually conducted in young healthy subjects and pharmacokinetic parameters determined in those subjects may not be directly relevant to the "elderly patient". The importance of this aspect has been highlighted by the problems encountered with the anti-inflammatory drug, benoxaprofen (Opren).

Monitoring of Human Biological Fluids for Evidence of Reactive Metabolite Formation

A number of human tissue fluids may be monitored to indicate that a xenobiotic has been converted to an active metabolite e.g. blood, urine, saliva, semen. Evidence is often indirect. Urine may be screened for conjugates which have arisen from the reaction of reactive metabolites with endogenous molecules such as glutathione; e.g. the excretion of paracetamol mercapturic acid is indicative of the level of the reactive metabolites of paracetamol in the liver. The urine, either before or after treatment with deconjugating enzymes, may also be tested for mutagenic activity in the absence of liver 9000g supernatant (49).

Increasing attention is being devoted to the monitoring of haemoglobin as an indication of the concentration of reactive metabolites generated *in vivo*. This method, pioneered by Ehrenberg and co-workers (50), depends on the release of reactive metabolites from the cell or tissue where they were generated and their subsequent covalent binding to haemoglobin. The half-life of haemoglobin is about 120 days, so a particular advantage of this method is that it enables an assessment to be made of exposure of an individual over a period of months. Other circulating proteins could also be used for this purpose. Monitoring of alkylated purine and pyrimidine bases in urine may also be used as an index of the formation of alkylating metabolites. Changes in sperm counts or increases in sperm abnormalities may indicate exposure to a toxic chemical. Sperm may also be monitored for the presence of alkylated nucleic acids.

Use of Human Tissues

Metabolic studies using a variety of different human tissues can provide a valuable complementary approach to the very limited *in vivo* studies which can be carried out. Studies on the metabolic fate and effects of chemicals in different human tissues should aid our understanding both of the mechanisms of toxicity of chemicals and also the predisposition of certain target organs to toxicity.

Studies utilising human tissues may be divided into two broad categories, namely, the use of isolated enzymes and subcellular fractions and the use of systems with intact cellular integrity, such as organ culture, freshly isolated cells, and cell lines. Methods which utilise subcellular fractions are generally relatively simple and can give a good indication of reactive metabolite formation from a particular chemical. Methods, such as organ culture, which by maintaining cellular integrity preserve the normal balance of activating and deactivating enzymes, should give a more realistic assessment of the possible generation of reactive metabolites in the intact tissue and thus *in vivo*.

Whilst there are many complications in the use of human tissues, these should not deter appropriate scientific investigations of the full metabolic potential of such tissues. Recent advances in culture techniques now permit organ culture together with the maintenance of normal morphology of various human tissues, such as lung, bronchus, colon, breast, prostate, pancreas, oesophagus, urinary bladder, and endometrium. Many of these tissues have been shown to possess drug metabolising capability and the ability to activate carcinogens to reactive metabolites which bind to DNA (51). It is of interest that in such studies a large inter-individual variation occurs, both in metabolism and binding to DNA (51-53). A similarly large inter-individual variation occurs in the *in vivo* metabolism of compounds in man. Such large inter-individual variations naturally pose particular problems with regard to extrapolation. More-detailed investigation is needed to characterise those differences. Much basic work will also be required in the establishment of storage banks of human tissues. In this respect the work of Von Bahr et al. (35) is noteworthy. They have established in Sweden a "human liver bank" obtained from cadavers who were kidney transplant donors. Subcellular fractions were prepared immediately, partly used for immediate assay and the remainder stored. Similar work needs to be carried out on other human tissues and methods need to be developed for storing intact cells and tissues in a viable state.

PHARMACOKINETICS AND THE SELECTION OF ANIMAL SPECIES FOR TOXICITY TESTING

The selection of animals for toxicity testing is at present largely determined by animal husbandry considerations, cost and familiarity, in particular the availability of background information on the pathology of the chosen species. In order to take into account the wide extent of variability in biological response that may occur following exposure to a xenobiotic, it is common to use both sexes and to use a rodent and a non-rodent species. In practice, this means generally the use of the rat or mouse and dog or non-human primate. The practice of using albino rodents in safety evaluation is questionable in view of the knowledge that a relatively large number of xenobiotics are sequestered in melanin-containing tissues.

However, there is no surety that such species selection will enable the wide variability in human response to be spanned. If major differences in toxic effect are observed between rodent and non-rodent species, it is usually very informative to obtain pharmacokinetic data in both species and in man, in order to identify which, if either, species is the most relevant model for man. While pharmacokinetic data in man are readily obtained for most pharmaceuticals, ethical considerations make such data difficult to obtain for pesticides or industrial chemicals. Pharmacokinetic data are also very important to toxicological studies in situations where:

a. the exposure dose is not reproducibly related to the toxicological effects in one or more animal species;
b. the relationship between dose and toxicity is very steep and/or non-linear or changes significantly between single and multiple dosing at levels close to those at which human exposure may occur;
c. structural considerations or toxicological properties indicate that the xenobiotic may exert its effects via an active metabolite;

d. the xenobiotic structure indicates that it may be metabolised by a metabolic reaction in which marked genetic variations are known to occur (e.g. N-acetylation);
e. the xenobiotic is highly lipophilic;
f. exposure to the xenobiotic is likely to involve high dose-levels compared to those to which man is likely to be exposed;
g. the route of exposure is dermal or by inhalation (because large variations between species may be expected using these routes).

A suitable scheme for integration of in vivo and in vitro pharmacokinetic studies in toxicity testing is presented in Fig. 3.

It is nearly always valuable to determine the relationship between the extent of absorption and the chosen dose-levels using pharmacokinetic procedures. It should also be established whether the pharmacokinetics of the xenobiotic is altered during the multiple dosing regimen employed in toxicity testing.

THE ROLE OF PHARMACOKINETIC STUDIES IN THE ASSESSMENT OF ENVIRONMENTAL HAZARDS OF CHEMICALS

Environmental pollutants raise certain specialised problems in toxicity testing over and above those normally encountered with drugs, food additives, and other chemicals to which man is directly exposed. Apart from risks to man, there is concern about the effects of pollutants upon a wide range of beneficial organisms, including domestic and farm animals, wildlife, fish and game, as well as beneficial insects, such as bees, and parasites and predators of pests. Environmental studies must consider the question of transfer and bioaccumulation of a xenobiotic, for it is known that the concentrations of some persistent pollutants increase dramatically with passage through food webs. Amongst pollutants, pesticides raise particular issues because they are deliberately applied to the environment to control harmful organisms.

The Significance of Metabolism

Most of the metabolic changes which pollutants undergo bring about a loss of biological activity, and so have a protective function both for the organism performing the change and for the general ecosystem. First, as mentioned previously, some metabolic changes lead to activation, e.g. a number of organophosphate insecticides, such as disyston, diazinon and primiphos-methyl, are converted from inactive thions to active oxons by the oxidases of mammals, insects and plants. Secondly, certain fat-soluble pollutants are converted from inactive

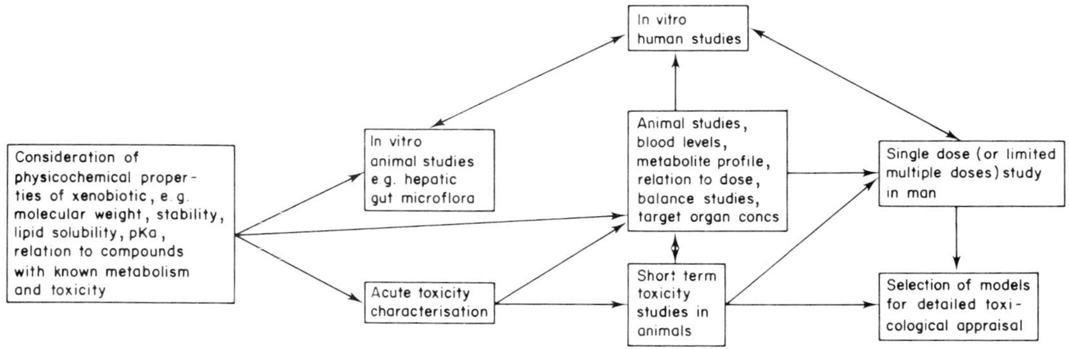

Figure 3 Scheme for the Integration of Pharmacokinetic Studies with a Toxicity Testing Programme

thions to active oxons by the oxidases of mammals, insects and plants. Secondly, certain fat-soluble pollutants are converted to metabolites which are more stable and persistent than the original compounds, with consequent problems of bioaccumulation. For example, pollutants such as DDE (a metabolite of DDT), dieldrin (a metabolite of aldrin as well as an insecticide in its own right), and the higher chlorinated isomers of PCB mixtures have very long half-lives in vertebrates, sometimes exceeding 100 days (5). Two properties are associated with this marked persistence: (i) very low water solubility, which encourages storage in fat depots, and largely precludes excretion, and (ii) very slow rates of enzymic degradation to water-soluble metabolites which are readily excreted. For example, hens accumulate PCB levels in their food over a period of 37 weeks (32,54).

Various studies in the field and in the laboratory indicate that fish-eating birds can bioaccumulate dieldrin, DDE or PCB by factors of 50 or more when continually exposed to low levels of these substances in their food.

The Significance of Species and Strain Differences in Enzymes

In the wider ecological context, species differences are very important in determining the distribution and bioaccumulation of pesticides in ecosystems. Where pollutants are fat-soluble and not readily metabolised, particular interest centres upon those species which are deficient in enzymes which can achieve degradation. The important monooxygenase system is often at very low levels in aquatic organisms such as fish, fish-eating birds, crustaceans and molluscs. Organisms such as these represent points in ecosystems where marked bioaccumulation can occur. Thus, key species of this kind should be given special attention in testing programmes for xenobiotics. Laboratory animals, such as rats, mice and rabbits, have much higher monooxygenase activities than many other species, and their use may therefore greatly underestimate the tendency for bioaccumulation in the environment. It should be emphasised that species which efficiently accumulate pollutants are not necessarily harmed by the pollutant. The species most at risk are sometimes predators which exist at or near the top of food webs and which achieve the highest concentration of certain pollutants.

One particular aspect of selective toxicity should be mentioned in the present context. When living organisms are exposed to a pesticide in the field, resistant populations often develop as a consequence of selection in favour of individuals with the lowest susceptibility to the chemical. There are many examples of insect pests developing resistance to organo-chlorine, organophosphate and carbamate insecticides, where the mechanism of resistance is largely due to an enhancement of detoxifying enzymes which is generally determined (i.e. not simply due to enzyme induction). Such resistance has also been demonstrated in vertebrates; for example, pine mice (*Microtus pinetorum*) in the USA have developed resistance to endrin (55).

Methods for Testing Metabolism of Wild Vertebrates and Invertebrates

A number of studies have been concerned with investigating the fate of pollutants in natural ecosystems. Such studies are necessary in certain cases, but are difficult and expensive to conduct and have the disadvantage of being under very limited control by the experimenter. Attempts have been made to construct simple model ecosystems which can be operated in the laboratory to study patterns of metabolism and bioaccumulation in "food chains". Unfortunately, the value of these systems is limited because they are highly artificial and do not bear a very close resemblance to natural ecosystems (5,56).

There are certain advantages in detailed investigation of the biotransformation of a xenobiotic by key species and attempting to develop pharmacokinetic models for pollutants, to enable the prediction of half-lives and bioaccumulation factors. It is possible to study the major metabolites of pollutants in a wider range of species by using *in vitro* systems. Such investigations can ascertain the rates of biodegradation in species with such low levels of xenobiotic metabolising enzymes that the biotransformation is difficult to detect *in vivo*. Information of this type may be more useful than that derived from biotransformation studies upon laboratory mammals, which are not at all representative of those species which are liable to bioaccumulate pollutants in the natural environment.

As a wider knowledge of the phylogenetic distribution of enzymes responsible for metabolising xenobiotics develops, together with some understanding of the physiological reasons for it (e.g. the influence of compounds in food and in the environment), a sounder basis for testing programmes on new pesticides and other potential pollutants will be achieved.

PREDICTABILITY OF PHARMACOKINETICS FROM PHYSICAL AND CHEMICAL PROPERTIES ALONE

Few systematic investigations have been made on the relationship between physical and chemical properties and pharmacokinetic behaviour, and those which have been carried out have been confined to a small number of xenobiotics. At present, prediction of pharmacokinetic behaviour is at the qualitative level rather than the quantitative one. Lipophilicity appears to be an important determinant of a number of pharmacokinetic processes, including membrane permeability (57-59), substrate interaction with cytochrome P-450, and binding to major sites of serum albumin (3,60,61). There is an approximate inverse relationship between lipophilicity and excretion of xenobiotics in urine and bile.

It has been shown that the presence of ionised groups in a xenobiotic tends to reduce the likelihood of effective absorption (except for very lipophilic xenobiotics) and encourage urinary and/or biliary excretion. Whether a xenobiotic and/or its metabolites is cleared in the urine or bile is also dependent on its molecular weight. High molecular weight (>500) tends to favour biliary excretion in most mammalian species. However, there are marked species differences in the molecular weight/biliary excretion threshold for anions, e.g. in the rat; the relevant molecular weight is approximately 300, whereas in man it is approximately 500 (9).

Hydrogen bonding and steric factors have also been demonstrated in certain circumstances to markedly affect intestinal absorption and tissue and xenobiotic metabolising enzyme binding (62). However, in our present state of knowledge, these effects are only predictable for a few structurally closely related species.

It is usually possible to predict which metabolites will be formed from a particular xenobiotic (although present knowledge of the metabolic fate of heterocyclic rings of compounds is still poor), but not the relative amounts which will be produced. Knowledge is particularly deficient on the influence of physicochemical properties on the tissue binding of xenobiotics.

If we are to move to a situation where reliable quantitative prediction of the pharmacokinetic fate of a xenobiotic in a particular species is possible from consideration of physicochemical properties, a careful systematic investigation of the influence of physicochemical properties on each pharmacokinetic process will be necessary, using a range of xenobiotic structures and dose-levels. Many of these studies should be carried out in vitro.

Bioaccumulation of organochlorine pesticides by marine organisms with very low biotransformation capacity (e.g. mussels) can be related to water solubility (63).

SUMMARY

1. Toxic responses may vary both between species and between individuals of the same species. The principal cause of this variation can often be ascribed to differences in the pharmacokinetic phase. Hence, proper characterisation of the pharmacokinetic phase is often essential for the prediction of likely toxic effects in one organism from the known toxic response in another.

2. Direct sampling of the target cell type or tissue component is the most relevant approach for determining the concentration of a xenobiotic and its metabolites at the site of action, although it is generally not possible for practical and ethical reasons to take such samples. The best alternative is to sample the blood which perfuses these tissues. Blood levels of unbound xenobiotic are usually more directly related to the magnitude of the toxic effect than is the dose administered.

3. Although the routes of biotransformation can usually be predicted from the structure of a xenobiotic, it is rarely possible to predict the relative rates of formation of particular metabolites or the rate of formation of an individual metabolite in different species. Thus, it is usually important to obtain some information on the pharmacokinetics of each xenobiotic in the species concerned, especially on the extent and rate of absorption and biotransformation.

4. In vitro preparations can be used to:

a. identify the metabolites of a xenobiotic which may be formed, including reactive metabolites;
b. obtain information on species differences in biotransformation or tissue binding which may explain differences in toxicity;
c. identify likely human variability in the biotransformation or tissue binding of the xenobiotic which may result in human differences in toxicity.

5. In vivo pharmacokinetic studies may be used to design more-relevant models for toxicity testing and thereby avoid the excessive use of animals. It is not possible to entirely replace in vivo pharmacokinetic studies by in vitro studies, because at present it is not possible to mimic all in vivo rate-controlling processes in vitro. However, judicious use of in vitro studies may reduce the number of in vivo pharmacokinetic studies which are required.

RECOMMENDATIONS

1. More studies on the absorption, distribution, biotransformation and excretion of drugs and other xenobiotics in man should be carried out. These must be thorough, utilising suitable sampling and analytical methods, and reported with relevant details on the exact dose, subject characteristics, etc. In the case of new drugs and other new products, the pressing need is for very early information in man in order to select the most relevant animal toxicity studies for identifying possible toxic risk to man. Such early information may also

result in a drug being discarded (e.g. for lack of efficacy, lack of tolerance, unsuitable pharmacokinetics) before extensive toxicity studies in animals have been conducted. For existing industrial chemicals, the need is to obtain reliable human data on their pharmacokinetics in order to set relevant safety standards for their use. This will require a considerable change in attitudes to human experimentation.

2. Pharmacokinetic investigations must become an integral part of toxicological testing procedures. At present they are often regarded as quite separate to investigations of the biological properties of a xenobiotic. This would reduce the number of inappropriate toxicological studies which are conducted and facilitate more-reliable extrapolation of animal findings to the likely human situation.

3. Methodology for preparing and storing in vitro preparations of human and animal tissues and of conditions for using such preparations for investigations of biotransformations, tissue binding, etc. should be standardised. This would enable ready comparison of data between laboratories to be made and would greatly facilitate the establishment of a data-bank, but would require interlaboratory collaborative studies. FRAME should undertake the co-ordination of such studies and should serve as an information source on in vitro methodology.

4. Banks of properly characterised preparations of human and animal tissues should be established in several centres in the UK to serve as reference laboratories for drug metabolism and toxicological research.

5. Meticulous, systematic comparisons should be made between the in vivo and the in vitro biotransformation of xenobiotics. Initially, the work should concentrate particularly on the relationship between the apparent in vivo and in vitro (hepatic) K_m and V_{max} values for elimination of xenobiotics by metabolism.

6. Studies aimed at understanding the relationship between the physicochemical properties of xenobiotics and their absorption, distribution, biotransformation and excretion should be given special encouragement.

7. Ready access to pharmacokinetic and other unpublished data relevant to toxicological investigations of xenobiotics should be permitted. Perhaps a time limit should be set on the maintenance of confidentiality of results obtained from safety evaluation studies.

8. The relevance of early biochemical changes in vitro resulting from exposure to a xenobiotic to the toxic events observed in

vivo should be evaluated, so that the relationship between *in vitro* biotransformation, tissue binding and toxicity can be established.

GLOSSARY OF TERMS

XENOBIOTIC. A low molecular weight chemical (<1000), not endogenous to the animal species under consideration; for example, pollutants, industrial chemicals, pesticides, food additives. Other terms: foreign compound, drug, anutrient, exogenous material.

BIOTRANSFORMATION. Biologically mediated conversion of a xenobiotic to other products. Other term: drug metabolism. (N.B. The term "drug metabolism" is also widely used to cover the processes of absorption, distribution, and excretion as well as biotransformation.)

PHARMACOKINETICS. The kinetics of the absorption, distribution, excretion and biotransformation of a xenobiotic. Other term: toxicokinetics.

PHASE 1 METABOLISM. The biotransformation of a xenobiotic by oxidation, reduction, hydrolysis, hydration or dehydrochlorination.

PHASE 2 METABOLISM. The biotransformation of a xenobiotic by conjugation, e.g. with glucuronic acid, glutathione, sulphate, acetate and glycine.

DISTRIBUTION. Reversible transfer of an absorbed xenobiotic and its metabolites throughout the body; this includes a consideration of tissue binding. Other term: disposition.

FIRST-PASS EFFECT. Biotransformation of an absorbed xenobiotic by an elimination organ before it reaches the systemic circulation, e.g. hepatic first-pass effect relates to the removal of an intestinally absorbed xenobiotic by the liver.

AREA UNDER THE CURVE (AUC). The area under a blood xenobiotic concentration/time curve (calculated to infinite time). It is usually proportional to the amount of that xenobiotic reaching the systemic circulation unchanged.

HALF-LIFE ($t\frac{1}{2}$). The time taken for the concentration of a xenobiotic in a body fluid or tissue to diminish by one half by a first-order process.

CLEARANCE. The volume of blood cleared of xenobiotic per unit time.

K_m. Michaelis constant. This reflects the affinity of an enzyme for its substrate.

V_{max} . Velocity maximum.

FIRST-ORDER KINETICS. The kinetics of a process (involving a xenobiotic) wherein its rate is proportional to the amount of xenobiotic present.

ZERO-ORDER KINETICS. The kinetics of a process (involving a xenobiotic) wherein its rate is apparently independent of the amount of that xenobiotic present.

VOLUME OF DISTRIBUTION. This parameter, which only rarely corresponds to a real volume, is a proportionality constant relating the amount of xenobiotic in the body to its concentration in the blood.

REFERENCES

1. Evans, W.E., Schentag, J.J. & Jusko, W.J. (eds.) (1980). "Applied Pharmacokinetics and Principles of Therapeutic Drug Monitoring". San Francisco: Applied Therapeutics Inc.
2. Waites, G.M.H. (1977). Fluid excretion in the testis. In "Advances in Physiology, Biochemistry and Function" (ed. A.D. Johnson & W.R. Gomes), pp. 91-123. New York: Academic Press.
3. Bridges, J.W. & Wilson A.G.E. (1976). Drug-serum protein interactions and their biological significance. In "Progress in Drug Metabolism" (ed. J.W. Bridges & L.F. Chasseaud), vol. I, pp. 193-247. Chichester: Wiley
4. Sturman, J.A. & Smith, M.A.H. (1967). The binding of salicyclate to plasma proteins in different species. Journal of Pharmacy and Pharmacology 19, 621-622.
5. Moriarty, F. (1975). Exposure and residue. In "Organochlorine Insecticides: Persistent Organic Pollutants" (ed. F. Moriarty), pp. 29-72. London: Academic Press.
6. Lutz, R.J., Dedrick, R.L., Matthews, H.B., Eling, T.E. & Anderson, M.W. (1971). A preliminary pharmacokinetic model for several chlorinated biphenyls in the rat. Drug Metabolism and Disposition 5, 386-396.
7. Brown, V.K., Robinson, J. & Richardson, A. (1967). Preliminary studies on the acute and subacute toxicities of photoisomerization product of HEOD. Food and Cosmetics Toxicology 5, 771-779.
8. Robinson, J., Richardson, A. & Brown, V.K. (1967). Pharmacodynamics of dieldrin in pigeons. Nature, London 213, 734-736.
9. Smith, R.L. (1973). "The Excretory Function of Bile: Elimin-

ation of Drugs and Toxic Substances in Bile" London: Chapman & Hall.

10. Chipman, J.K. & Walker, C.H. (1979). The metabolism of dieldrin and two of its analogues: the relationship between rates of microsomal metabolism and rates of excretion of metabolites in the male rat. Biochemistry & Pharmacology 28, 1337-1345.
11. Aldridge, W.N. & Reiner, E. (1972). Enzyme inhibitors as substrates: interactions of esterases with esters of organophosphorous and carbamate acids. In "Frontiers of Biology", North-Holland Research Monographs (ed. A. Neuberger & A.L. Tatum), vol. XXVI, pp. 328-359. Amsterdam: Elsevier/North-Holland.
12. Bridges, J.W. & Fry, J.R. (1979). The use of cultured hepatocytes in biochemical toxicology. In "Reviews in Biochemical Toxicology" (ed. E. Hodgson & R. Philpot), vol. I, pp. 201-248. Amsterdam: Elsevier/North-Holland.
13. Bridges, J.W. & Hubbard, S.A. (1981). Problems of providing an appropriate drug metabolising system for short-term screening tests. In "Predictive Value of Short-term Screening Tests for Carcinogenicity Evaluation" (ed. G.M. Williams, R. Kroes, H.W. Waaijers & K.W. can de Poll), pp. 69-88. Amsterdam: Elsevier/North-Holland.
14. Connelly, J. & Bridges, J.W. (1980). The distribution and role of cytochrome P-450 in extra-hepatic organs. In "Progress in Drug Metabolism" (ed. J.W. Bridges & L.F. Chasseaud), vol. V, pp. 1-112. Chichester: Wiley.
15. Watanabe, P.G., Ramsey, J.C. & Gehring, P.J. (1980). Pharmacokinetics and metabolism of industrial chemicals. In "Progress in Drug Metabolism" (ed. J.W. Bridges & L.F. Chasseaud), vol. V, pp. 311-343. Chichester: Wiley.
16. Wolf, P.J. (1980). Effect of overloading pathways in toxicology. Journal of Environmental Pathology and Toxicology 3, 113-134.
17. Levy, G. (1968). Dose-dependent effects in pharmacokinetics, in importance of fundamental principles. In "Drug Evaluation" (ed. D.H. Tedeschi & R.E. Tedeschi), pp. 141-172. New York: Raven Press.
18. Gehring, P.J., Watanabe, P.G. & Young, J.D. (1977). The relevance of dose-dependent pharmacokinetics in the assessment of carcinogenic hazards of chemicals. In "Origins of Human Cancer" (ed. H.H. Hiatt, J.D. Watson & J.A. Winstein), vol. A, pp. 187-203. New York: Cold Spring Harbor Laboratory.
19. Anderson, M.E. (1981). Saturable metabolism and its relationship to toxicity. CRC Critical Reviews of Toxicology 9, 105-150.
20. Hucker, H.B., Kwan, K.C. & Duggan, D.E. (1980). Pharmacokinetics and metabolism of non-steroidal anti-inflammatory agents. In "Progress in Drug Metabolism" (ed. J.W. Bridges

& L.F. Chasseaud), vol. V, pp. 165-253. Chichester: Wiley.
21. Glazko, A.J., Dill, W.A. & Wolf, L.M. (1952). The metabolic disposition of chloramphenicol in rat. Journal of Pharmacology and Experimental Therapeutics 104, 452-458.
22. Williams, R.T. (1971). Species variations in drug biotransformations. In "Fundamentals of Drug Metabolism and Drug Disposition" (ed. B.N. la Du, H.G. Mandel & E.L. Way), pp. 187-205. Baltimore: Williams & Wilkins.
23. Parke, D.V. (1972). The biochemistry of carbenoxolone. In "Carbenoxolone in Gastroenterology" (ed. F.A. Jones & F.M. Sullivan), pp. 19-32. London: Butterworths.
24. Bridges, J.W. (1980). The role of the drug metabolising enzymes. In "Environmental Chemicals, Enzyme Function and Human Disease" (ed. G. Lawrenson), pp. 5-24. Amsterdam: Elsevier/North-Holland.
25. Kato, R. (1979). Characteristics and differences in the hepatic mixed function oxidases of different species. Pharmacology & Therapeutics 6, 41-98.
26. Walker, C.H. (1980). Species variations in some hepatic microsomal enzymes. In "Progress in Drug Metabolism" (ed. J. W. Bridges & L.F. Chasseaud), vol. V, pp.113-164. Chichester: Wiley.
27. Walker, C.H. (1978). Species differences in microsomal monooxygenase activity and their relationship to biological half-lives. Drug Metabolism Reviews 7, 295-323.
28. Brealey, C.J., Walker, C.H. & Baldwin, B.C. (1980). 'A' esterase activities in relation to the differential toxicity of primiphos-methyl to birds and mammals. Pesticide Science 11, 546-554.
29. Benford, D.J., Boobis, A.R., Bridges, J.W., Kohn, G.C. & Davies, D.S. (1981). The selective activation of P-450 dependent microsomal hydroxylases in human and rat liver microsomes. Biochemical Pharmacology 30, 1702-1703.
30. Machin, A.F., Rogers, H., Cross, A.J., Quick, M.P. & Howells L.J. (1975). Metabolic aspects of the toxicology of diazinon I. Hepatic metabolism in the sheep, cow, pig, rat, turkey, chicken and duck. Pesticide Science 6, 461-473.
31. Zech, R. & Zurcher, K. (1974). Organophosphate splitting serum enzymes in different mammals. Comparative Biochemistry and Physiology 48B, 427-433.
32. Walker, C.H. (1982). Pesticides and birds: mechanisms of selective toxicity. Agriculture, Ecosystems and Environment 9, 211-226.
33. Chipman, J.K., Kurukgy, M. & Walker, C.H. (1979). Comparative metabolism of a dieldrin analogue: hepatic microsomal systems as models for metabolism in the whole animal. Biochemical Pharmacology 28, 69-75.
34. Mitchell, J.R., Potter, W.Z., Hinson, J.A., Snodgrass, W.R. Timbrell, J.A. & Gillette, J.R. (1975). Toxic drug reactions In "Handbuch der Experimentellen Pharmakologie" (ed. D.

Eichler, A. Farah, H. Herken, & A.D. Welch), pp. 348-419. Berlin: Springer.

35. Von Bahr, C., Groth, C.G., Jansson, H., Lundgren, C., Lind, M. & Glaumann, H. (1980). Drug metabolism in human liver in vitro: establishment of a human liver bank. Clinical Pharmacology & Therapeutics 27, 711-725.
36. Weisburger, J.H. & Weisburger, E.K. (1973). Biochemical formation and pharmacological, toxicological and pathological properties of hydroxylamines and hydroxamic acids. Pharmacological Reviews 25, 1-66.
37. Jusko, W.J. (1980). Guidelines for collection and pharmacokinetic analysis of drug disposition data. In "Principles of Therapeutic Drug Monitoring" (ed. W.E. Evans, J.J. Schentag & W.J. Jusko), pp. 639-680. San Francisco: Applied Therapeutics Inc.
38. Dedrick, R.L. & Bischoff, K.B. (1980). Species similarities in pharmacokinetics. Federation Proceedings 39, 54-59.
39. Boxenbaum, H. (1982). Interspecies scaling, allometry, physiological time, and the ground plan of pharmacokinetics. Journal of Pharmacokinetics and Biopharmacology 10, 201-227.
40. Vesell, E., Passananti, G.T., Greene, F.E. & Page, J.G. (1971). Genetic control of drug levels and of the induction of drug-metabolising enzymes in man: individual variability in the extent of allopurinol and nortriptyline inhibition of drug metabolism. Annals of the New York Academy of Sciences 179, 752-773.
41. Sjoqvist, F., Hammer, W., Idestrom, C.M., Lind, M., Tuck, E. & Asberg, M. (1968). Plasma level of monomethylated tricyclic antidepressants and side-effects in man. Proceedings of the European Society for the Study of Drug Toxicity 9, 246-257.
42. George, C.F., Shand, D.G. & Renwick, A.G. (eds.) (1982). "Presystemic Drug Elimination". London: Butterworths.
43. Idle, G. & Smith, R.L. (1979). Polymorphisms of oxidation at carbon centres of drugs and their clinical significance. Drug Metabolism Reviews 9, 301-317.
44. Uetrecht, J.P. & Woosely, R.L. (1981). Acetylator phenotype and lupus erythematosus. Clinical Pharmacokinetics 6, 118-134.
45. Hunter, J. & Chasseaud, L.F. (1976). Clinical aspects of microsomal enzyme induction. In "Progress in Drug Metabolism" (ed. J.W. Bridges & L.F. Chasseaud), vol. I, pp. 129-191. Chichester: Wiley.
46. Brooks, G.T. (1979). The metabolism of xenobiotics in insects. In "Progress in Drug Metabolism" (ed. J.W. Bridges & L.F. Chasseaud), vol. III, pp. 151-214. Chichester: Wiley.
47. Kato, R. (1977). Drug metabolism under pathological and abnormal physiological states in animals and man. Xenobiotica 7, 25-92.
48. Pelkinen, O. (1977). Transplacental transfer of foreign

compounds and their metabolism by the foetus. In "Progress in Drug Metabolism" (ed. J.W. Bridges & L.F. Chasseaud), vol. II, pp. 119-161. Chichester: Wiley.

49. Yamasaki, E. & Ames, B.N. (1977). Concentration of mutagens from urine adsorption with the non-polar resin XAD-2: cigarette smokers have mutagenic urine. Proceedings of the National Academy of Sciences, USA 74, 3555-3559.
50. Osterman-Golkare, S. & Ehrenberg, L. (1982). Covalent binding of reactive intermediates to haemoglobin as an approach for determining the metabolic activation of chemicals: ethylene. Drug Metabolism Reviews 13, 647-1069.
51. Harris, C.C., Autrup, H., Connor, R., Barrett, L.A., McDowell, E.M. & Trump, B.F. (1976). Inter-individual variation in binding of benzo[a]pyrene to DNA in cultured human bronchi. Science, New York 194, 1067-1069.
52. Cohen, G.M., Mehta, R. & Meredith-Brown, M. (1979). Large interindividual variations in metabolism of benzo[a]pyrene by peripheral binding tissue from lung cancer patients. International Journal of Cancer 24, 129-133.
53. Autrup, H. (1982). Carcinogen metabolism in human tissues and cells. Drug Metabolism Reviews 13, 603-646.
54. Davison, K.L. (1973). Dieldrin-^{14}C balance in rats, sheep and chickens. Bulletin of Environmental Contamination Toxicology 10, 11-24.
55. Webb, R.E., Randolph, W.C. & Horsfall, F. (1972). Hepatic benzopyrene hydroxylase activity in endrin-sensitive susceptible and resistant pine mice. Life Sciences 11, 477-483.
56. Metcalf, R.L., Sangha, G.K. & Kapoon, I.P. (1971). Model ecosystem for evaluation of pesticide biodegradability and ecological magnification. Environmental Science and Technology 5, 709-713.
57. Hansch, C. (1976). On the structure of medicinal chemistry. Journal of Medicinal Chemistry 19, 1-6.
58. Houston, J.B. & Wood, S.G. (1979). Gastrointestinal absorption of drugs and other xenobiotics. In "Progress in Drug Metabolism" (ed. J.W. Bridges & L.F. Chasseaud), vol. IV, pp. 57-129. Chichester: Wiley.
59. Sargent, N.S.E., Wood, S.G., Upsall, D.J. & Bridges, J.W. (1982). The relationship between chemical structure and the in vivo metabolism of an homologous series of n-alkyl carbamates. Journal of Pharmacy and Pharmacology 34, 367-372.
60. Al-Gailany, K.A.S., Houston, J.B. & Bridges, J.W. (1978). The role of substrate lipophilicity in determining its type I microsomal P-450 binding characteristics. Biochemical Pharmacology 27, 783-788.
61. Sargent, N.S.E., Upshall, D.J. & Bridges, J.W. (1981). The relationship between binding to cytochrome P-450 and

metabolism of n-alkyl carbamates by isolated rat hepatocytes. Biochemical Pharmacology 31, 1309-1313.
62. Houston, J.B., Upshall, D.G. & Bridges, J.W. (1975). Further studies on the role of lipophilicity in the gastrointestinal absorption of anutrients. Journal of Pharmacology and Experimental Therapeutics 195, 67-72.
63. Ernst, W. (1977). Determination of the concentration potential of marine organisms - a steady state approach: bio-concentration data for 7 chlorinated pesticides in mussels (Mytilus edulis) and their relation to solubility data. Chemosphere 11, 731-740.
64. Pagliaro, L.A. & Benet, L.Z. (1975). Critical compilation of terminal half-lives, per cent excreted unchanged, and changes of half-life in renal and hepatic dysfunction for studies in humans with references. Journal of Pharmacokinetics and Biopharmacology 3, 333-383.

Immunology in Safety Evaluation

KLARA MILLER

Whilst hypersensitivity and adverse reactions to certain drugs and food additives have been known for many years, it is only recently that other xenobiotics have been demonstrated to affect the immune system. As a consequence, there has been an increasing interest in the immune system as a target for toxic effects. Advances in immunology have provided techniques for more-sensitive and more-specific identification of toxic lesions, as well as increasing our understanding of immune regulatory mechanisms. There is little doubt that alterations in the immune response can represent an important indicator of cellular toxicity in the safety evaluation of xenobiotics.

The immune system in vertebrates is complex (Fig. 1), with several populations of cells acting independently and in concert to maintain surveillance mechanisms that protect the host from pathogenic microorganisms such as bacteria and viruses, and from cancer cells (1). The main cell lines involved in immune defence mechanisms are mononuclear phagocytes (macrophages) and two populations of morphologically indistinguishable lymphoid cells, the T and B lymphocytes. Macrophages recognise, phagocytose and process antigenic material for presentation to lymphocytes, and cellular interactions between lymphocytes and macrophages result in the activation of lymphocytes (2). The specifically activated lymphocytes proliferate and differentiate to express humoral or cell-mediated effector mechanisms, manifested either as the production of specific antibody by mature B lymphocytes or by the sensitised T lymphocytes themselves. Regulation and feedback control of immune responses depend on pharmacological mediators such as the interleukins, leukotrienes and prostaglandins. Abrogation of feedback control may lead to the development of autoimmune disease or other immunopathological disorders (3). On the other hand, an imbalance caused by cellular injury or dysfunction leads to reduced immune competence, and evidence for increased bacteria, viral, fungal and parasitic diseases in patients on chronic immunosuppressive chemicals is well documented.

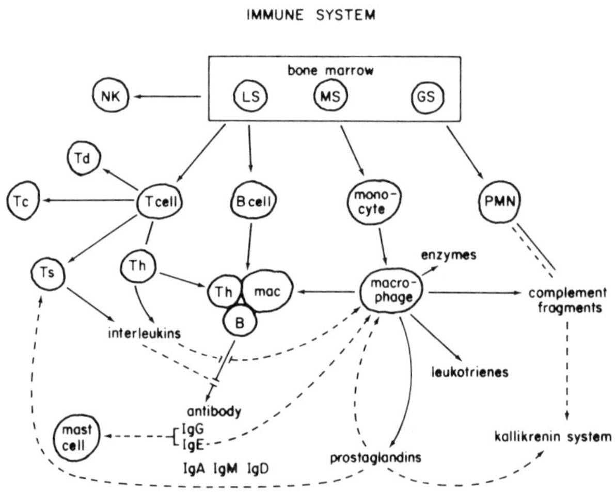

Figure 1 The Immune System

LS = lymphoid stem cell; MS = monocyte stem cell; GS = granulocyte stem cell; NK = natural killer cell; B = activated B lymphocyte (synthesises immunoglobulin - Ig); Tc = cytotoxic T cell (able to kill foreign and virus-infected cells); Td = lymphokine-secreting T cell (initiator of delayed hypersensitivity); Th = helper T cell (recognising antigen and inducing antibody responses); Ts = suppressor T cell (acting to diminish effect of helper T cells); PMN = polymorphonuclear leucocyte.

Several recent reviews (4,5) have provided proof that a number of xenobiotics cause immune alterations in experimental animals, and that the immune system is a very sensitive and perhaps early indicator of cellular toxicity. Polychlorinated biphenyls, for example, have been shown to cause macrophage dysfunction at levels where little evidence of pathological change was observed (6).

The thymus, which is the site of T lymphocyte maturation and specialises into different functional subsets of T lymphocytes, appears to be a particularly sensitive target for toxic effects. A wide range of compounds, with differing modes of action, have been shown to induce thymic atrophy and cause impairment of cell-mediated immune responses.

2,3,7,8-tetrachlorodibenzo-p-dioxin (TCDD)
2,3,7,8-tetrachlorodibenzofuran (TCDF)
polychlorinated biphenyls (PCB)
di-n-butyltin dichloride (DBTC)
di-n-octyltin dichloride (DOTC)
trichothecene mycotoxins
theobromine
glucocorticoid hormones

Discernment of the mechanisms by which a xenobiotic acts on the thymus would greatly aid understanding of how toxicological effects may be influenced by alterations in immune responses.

There are several factors that might explain the apparent sensitivity of the immune system to toxic injury. These include the rapid proliferation and differentiation that many cells undergo, as well as the intricate regulatory network involved in maintaining immunocompetence. It would be appropriate, therefore, to develop test systems for the early assessment of the potential immunotoxicity of xenobiotics, and several laboratories are in the process of evaluating such systems (7).

It is possible to expose in vitro cells involved in a particular phase of the immune response directly to the compound, and then to examine various immunologically-related parameters. Effects on mononuclear phagocytes, in particular, have been evaluated under these conditions, although such systems may not take into account the metabolism and pharmacokinetics of the xenobiotic. The inclusion of microsomal enzyme preparations may evaluate the reactivity of metabolites derived from a compound in an in vitro system. Another widely used approach in immunotoxicity studies is the in vitro testing of cell populations involved in immune responses obtained from animals during safety evaluation studies (8).

Lymphocyte proliferation assays and graft-versus-host reactions are examples of test systems currently in use to monitor immune alterations. Stimulation of blastogenesis of mononuclear cells in vitro with mitogens such as phyto-haemagglutinin, concanavalin A or lipopolysaccharide can be a measure of the functional competence of T and B lymphocyte populations. The graft-versus-host reaction, where lymphoid cells from a donor animal are injected into histocompatible recipients, provides the means for assessing the functional status of the recognition, activation and effector phases of the immune response of the donor. These immunological assays, which complement morphological changes with determinations of functional alterations, are in keeping with the present direction in toxicological testing.

There are many areas where investigations are still needed. In vitro stem cell analysis may be a useful indicator of toxicity in the early stages of immune cell maturation. Simple molecules such as drugs or some industrial products can have immunological effects by becoming haptens, and research efforts are needed to evaluate chemicals for the induction of hypersensitivity reactions. Studies directed toward elucidating the relationship between the chemical structure and immunological activity of compounds should prove useful in predicting the possible toxicological consequences of chemicals present in man's environment.

REFERENCES

1. Burnet, F.M. (1970). Relationship of diversity in histocompatability antigens to immunological surveillance mechanisms for the control of cancer. Nature, London 226, 123-126.
2. Bellanti, J.A. & Dayton, D.H. (1975). "The Phagocyte Cells in Host Resistance". New York: Raven Press.
3. Nicklin, S. & Shand, F.L. (1982). Abrogation of suppressor cell function by inhibitors of prostaglandin synthesis. International Journal of Immunopharmacology 4, 407-414.
4. Vos, J.G. (1977). Immune suppression as related to toxicology. CRC Critical Reviews of Toxicology 5, 67-101.
5. Faith, R.E., Luster, M.I. & Vos, J.G. (1980). Effects on immunocompetence by chemicals of environmental concern. In "Reviews in Biochemical Toxicology" (ed. E. Hodgson, J.R. Bend & R.M. Philpot), pp. 173-211. Oxford: Pergamon.
6. Loose, L.D., Silkworth, J.P., Pittman, K.A., Benitz, K.F. & Mueller, W. (1978). Impaired host resistance to endrilin and analaria in polychlorinated biphenyl and hexachlorobenzene-treated mice. Infection and Immunology 20, 30-35.
7. Dean, J.H., Luster, M.I., Boorman, G.A., Leubke, R.W. & Lauer, L.D. (1982). Application of tumour, bacterial and parasite susceptibility assays to study immune reactions induced by environmental chemicals. Environmental Health Perspectives 43, 81-88.
8. Archer, D.L. (1982). New approaches to immunotoxicity testing. Environmental Health Perspectives 43, 109-113.

Pharmacokinetics and Pesticides

G. T. BROOKS

Demographic projections indicate that by the year 2000 the world population will reach 6-7000 million (1). The need to feed this burgeoning population requires an intense effort to reduce the level of crop losses due to pest damage, which, considering both pre-harvest and post-harvest destruction, may render as much as half of the annual production useless. Against this background, it is apparent that there will be a need to use chemical pesticides in the foreseeable future, because they still provide the most efficient means of pest control.

In contrast to the situation with drugs in man, pesticides are intentionally applied at toxic levels to control the pests (insects, pathogens, weeds, certain birds, fish and mammals) that damage man's health or destroy his crops. Since there is inevitably the risk of incidental contact between pesticides and man or beneficial (non-target) organisms, the likely toxic hazards due to pesticide use have to be assessed in relation to environmental protection. Laboratory tests on animals have made a valuable contribution to such assessments (2). There is currently a demand for bioactive chemicals, which, when used in the field, will act selectively against a chosen pest or group of pests for a predetermined time, then rapidly disappear under the influence of the degradative processes of the biotic and abiotic elements of the environment.

The requirement for bioactive chemicals with low persistence, but high and selective toxicity toward pest (target) organisms is not easy to meet. When such chemicals are available, they will increasingly be used in integrated pest management programmes in combination with biological and other non-chemical methods of pest control. The full development of such methods designed to minimise the environmental burden of toxic chemicals and to delay the development of pest resistance to them, requires a very detailed knowledge of the biology, biochemistry and chemistry of pests and of the influence of local environment on their life processes. The necessary information can only come from appropriate research.

With regard to pharmacokinetic studies, the same general

principles that determine the efficiency of drugs used for human and animal health purposes also regulate the toxic effects of pesticides on both target pest species and any incidentally exposed non-target vertebrates or invertebrates. Consequently, studies of pesticide pharmacokinetics (henceforth called toxicokinetics) in the different species of concern, aid the design of environmentally acceptable pesticides by providing information important for:

a. the development of selective toxicants that kill pest species of vertebrates, insects, plants or fungi without harming incidentally exposed non-pest vertebrates;
b. the development of toxicants that select pest from non-pest invertebrates sharing the same environment;
c. the development of toxicants for the control of pests that have become resistant to other pesticide chemicals;
d. reducing environmental contamination due to pesticide chemicals by increasing the efficiency of contact between toxicant and target pest.

This last aspect involves research on the influence of pesticide formulations on the toxicokinetic behaviour of the bioactive ingredient on and within the pest organism, as well as research directed toward the improvement of practical application techniques.

Items a-c are closely related and of particular concern to this discussion, since quantitative differences between species in their rates of metabolic toxication or detoxication of pesticides are often the most important determinants of susceptibility, natural tolerance or acquired resistance to them. Such differences may therefore regulate the selectivity of toxicants for different species (interspecific selectivity). Herbicides and fungicides are not necessarily toxic to vertebrates or non-pest invertebrates, but this can only be determined by experimentation. The problem of selective toxicity is particularly severe in the case of insecticides, which have traditionally included rapidly acting nerve poisons with similar modes of action on both vertebrates and insects.

One way to avoid this difficulty is to search for other, non-nervous sites of toxicant action which are specific to insects. Thus, chemicals have recently been discovered which disrupt the deposition of insect cuticle, and there is much interest in the insect specific hormones that control their development and in the pheromones which regulate their mating and other types of behaviour (3). When new sites of action are discovered, toxicokinetic studies are an essential component in the elucidation of those differences between target and non-target species that can be used in the design of further chemicals with selective action. However, insecticides of the nerve poison class will continue to be used because of their outstanding efficiency. Within this class, the design of compounds exhibiting selective toxicity depends on a detailed knowledge of species differences both in the toxicokinetic behaviour of nerve poisons and in their interaction with the site of action. For example, the organophosphate and carbamate anti-cholinesterases kill both vertebrates and insects by inhibiting their acetylcholine hydrolysing enzymes (AChE). Nevertheless, much can be done towards reducing the vertebrate/insect toxicity ratio by altering chemical structure to take advantage of the known differences in insecticide metabolism and in the molecular structure of AChE between vertebrates and insects (4-7). A similar approach is involved in the search for the causes of insect resistance to insecticides, which is an example of intraspecific selectivity, the resistant strain(s) having arisen from the parent strain through extreme selection by the insecticide(s). Resistance has been described in more than 400 species of pests and is a serious economic problem (8).

For insecticides and other pesticides, as for drugs, motre information is required concerning the extent to which *in vitro* studies on pure enzyme preparations, subcellular fractions, cells in culture, tissue preparations, perfused organs, etc., can predict the differences in uptake, distribution, storage, excretion and especially metabolism, that are observed between species *in vivo* (9,10). Although the use of these preparations individually cannot be expected to reflect the behaviour of a pesticide in an intact animal, which has complex permeability barriers and control mechanisms, the summation of information from such experiments nevertheless contributes to the development of toxicokinetic models that in the long-term may have predictive value for pesticide behaviour and toxicity *in vivo*.

In some cases, the study of pesticide metabolising enzymes can be very revealing. For example, the high susceptibility of some birds to certain organophophate insecticides correlates with their low plasma 'A' esterase activity measured *in vitro*; mammals generally are protected by high plasma 'A' esterase activities, but may be just as susceptible as birds to those organophosphates with chemical structures that cannot be hydrolysed by these 'A' esterases (11,12).

For a number of vertebrates, there appears to be an inverse relationship between hepatic microsomal mixed function oxidase enzyme (MFO) activity and both body weight and xenobiotic half-life (9,12-14). Comparing creatures of same body weight, birds tend to be intermediate between mammals and fish in their MFO activities, with fish on average having 10-25 times less activity than mammals; aquatic birds such as the shag, cormorant and Manx shearwater have similar activities to fish (13). The low MFO activity in the livers of fish and some birds *in vitro* appears to explain, at least in part, their high susceptibility compared with mammals, to poisoning by a variety of pesticide chemicals. This deficiency in the MFO system also accounts for the accumulation of the persistent chlorinated insecticides in the tissues of fish and some birds and for the tendency of such chemicals to become magnified through food chains involving these species. A better understanding of the influence of diet and other environmental factors on the phylogenetic distribution of pesticide (xenobiotic) metabolising enzymes should lead to improved testing programmes and a reduction in unnecessary experimentation.

Mention must be made of the other values of non-vertebrate studies, apart from their relevance to vertebrate/invertebrate selectivity and to resistance mechanisms. Non-vertebrate organisms (e.g. bacteria, insects) provide test systems for the possible mutagenic and/or carcinogenic effects of both pesticides and drugs. Furthermore, there is often a qualitative similarity of the phase I metabolic pathways of xenobiotic metabolism between vertebrates and insects, which makes insects useful for metabolite identification and for the study of phenomena such as enzyme induction and the synergistic or antagonistic interactions between xenobiotics _in vivo._

In summary, toxicokinetic studies are a vital component in the assessment of possible environmental hazards due to pesticides and other xenobiotics and in the evolution of improved techniques for toxicity assessment which should, in the longer term, reduce the need for elaborate toxicity tests using intact animals _in vivo._

REFERENCES

1. Gray, R.H. (1976). Population and food production. In "Pesticides and Human Welfare" (ed. D.L. Gunn & J.G.R. Stevens), pp. 13-27. Oxford: Oxford University Press.
2. Barnes, J.M. (1976). Hazards to people. In "Pesticides and Human Welfare" (ed. D.L. Gunn & J.G.R. Stevens), pp. 181-192. Oxford: Oxford University Press.
3. Brooks, G.T. & Johnson, A.W. (1979). Chemicals and insects. Interdisciplinary Science Reviews 4, 279-289.
4. Brooks, G.T. (1976). Selective toxicity of insectides. In "The Future for Insecticides, Needs and Prospects" (ed. R.L. Metcalf & J.J. McKelvey), pp. 97-139. New York: Wiley.
5. Brooks, G.T. (1979). The metabolism of xenobiotics in insects. In "Progress in Drug Metabolism" (ed. J.W. Bridges & L.F. Chasseaud), vol. III, pp. 151-214. Chichester: Wiley.
6. Brooks, G.T. (1983). Metabolism and pesticide design. In "Progress in Drug Metabolism" (ed. J.W. Bridges & L.F. Chasseaud), vol. VIII (in press).
7. Fukuto, T.R. (1976). Carbamate insecticides. In "The Future for Insecticides, Needs and Prospects" (ed. R.L. Metcalf & J.J. McKelvey), pp. 313-342. New York: Wiley.

8. Report of the Second Session of the FAO Panel of Experts on Pest Resistance to Pesticides and Crop Loss Assessment. (1981). Report AGP 1981/M/2, pp. 25. Rome: FAO.
9. Walker, C.H. (1978). Species differences in microsomal mono-oxygenase activity and their relationship to biological half-lives. Drug Metabolism Reviews 7, 295-323.
10. Brooks, G.T. (1980). Perspectives of the chemical fate and toxicity of pesticides. Journal of Environmental Science and Health 15, 755-793.
11. Brealey, C.J., Walker, C.H. & Baldwin, B.C. (1980). 'A' esterase activities in relation to the differential toxicity of pirimiphos-methyl to birds and mammals. Pesticide Science 11, 546-554.
12. Walker, C.H. (1983). Pesticides and birds - mechanisms of selective toxicity. Agriculture, Ecosystems and Environment 9, 211-226.
13. Walker, C.H. (1980). Species variations in some hepatic microsomal enzymes that metabolise xenobiotics. In "Progress in Drug Metabolism" (ed. J.W. Bridges & L.F. Chasseaud), vol. V, pp. 113-164. Chichester: Wiley.
14. Walker, C.H. (1981). The correlation between *in vivo* and *in vitro* metabolism of pesticides in vertebrates. Progress in Pesticide Biochemistry 1, 247-285.

General Discussion

C. H. WALKER

Rapporteur

Professor L. GOLBERG commented that no mention had been made of the problem of co-oxidation during prostaglandin synthesis; toxic effects in the kidney medulla following administration of analgesics have been attributed to the production of active metabolites by this means. Professor DAVIES said that co-oxidation was important in microsomal preparations. In intact cells, on the other hand, active oxygen forms, generated during prostaglandin metabolism, are effectively eliminated. Thus, as in the case of paraquat metabolism, it is dangerous to argue from microsomal studies to the situation *in vivo*. He commented that it would be interesting to study the effects of specific inhibitors of prostaglandin biosynthesis upon toxic action of compounds *in vivo*.

Dr I.F.H. PURCHASE said that the importance of metabolism in carcinogenicity testing had been stressed. He asked whether any cases were known where positive evidence for carcinogenicity had been disregarded on the grounds that the species used in the test was metabolically different from man. Professor D.V.W. PARKE referred to Professor Golberg's question, and stressed the importance of the conversion of oxygen to hydroxyl radicals during the course of prostaglandin metabolism. Hydroxyl radicals are of particular interest, because they can attack certain molecules in sterically-hindered positions. In response to Dr Purchase's question, he said that two cases were worth mentioning where evidence on carcinogenicity had been disregarded on the grounds that the species in question provided an inappropriate model for man. The first case was that of the progestogen, linostenol, which was shown to act as a breast carcinogen in the beagle dog, and, the second case was of certain pesticides showing carcinogenicity in the mouse, but not in other vertebrate species. In both cases the evidence was regarded as invalid by the regulatory authorities. In the second case, attention had been paid to the fact that the mouse was metabolically different from other species in which the compounds were not carcinogenic.

Professor A. GOLDBERG asked about the use of human samples obtained by surgical techniques or autopsy for metabolism studies. Dr Klara MILLER said that peripheral blood mononuclear cells have been successfully employed in immunofunction assays. Professor DAVIES added that his laboratory had been involved in setting up a liver bank containing approximately 160 samples, in collaboration with two other centres. There were difficulties in this, however: first, the problem that samples often became available outside normal working hours, and, secondly, that storage conditions needed to be carefully monitored. He also commented that he had abandoned the idea of seeking an animal "like man". Professor BRIDGES commented that the question was not of finding an animal that was an exact model for man, but rather of finding one that is broadly similar. Referring to Dr Purchase's question, he said that he did not know of any suitable examples of evidence being rejected on grounds of non-comparability to man with regard to metabolism. The problem was that there was a shortage of information on human metabolism of carcinogens. With regard to mutagenicity testing he questioned the value of the S9 mix. It would be interesting to compare results obtained using intact cells with those obtained with this preparation. With regard to the use of human cells, he referred to the general problem of storing cells in a viable condition - and not just liver cells.

Mr G. HEALEY asked Professor Bridges if he would like to comment on the value of studies on staturation kinetics, the normal practice *in vitro*. Professor BRIDGES replied that it was important that comparisons be made between *in vivo* and *in vitro* kinetics.

Dr GOULDING asked whether any cases were known of clinical syndromes with an immunological basis which were caused by xenobiotics. Dr MILLER replied that a number of compounds caused autoimmune manifestations such as haemolytic anaemia. Dr GOULDING further asked whether such effects were known in man as opposed to rats. Dr MILLER said that there was evidence of depressed skin reaction to recall antigens and increased production of non-organ-specific autoantibodies in workers suffering from asbestosis and silicosis. She thought that a similar situation had been found in dairy farmers in Michigan who had been exposed to PBB.

Dr GOULDING commented on the desirability of regulatory bodies taking more account of metabolic studies from the outset. In this way it should be possible to tailor animal experiments more neatly, so that fewer animals would be required in toxicity testing. He also foresaw a danger in too many new approaches becoming fashionable - this could lead to the regulatory authorities becoming swamped with data, making decision taking difficult or impossible.

Long-term Toxicity

RALPH HEYWOOD

INTRODUCTION

The purpose of toxicity testing is to decide whether a compound is safe. Safety, however, should be related to the conditions of use. The principle of safety evaluation studies is to define the potential of a compound to cause damage, and from this information to deduce the dose which causes no effect. Such studies are based on two assumptions: that there is an appropriate animal model, and that a dose-response relationship can be demonstrated.

Animal studies follow precepts that were developed in the late 1950's, and only minor modifications to basic study designs have been made. Advice on the experimental approach to toxicity testing was codified in 1955 with the appearance in the Food Drug Cosmetic Law Journal (1) of contributions by the combined staffs of the Divisions of Pharmacology of the Food and Drug Administration of the USA. Since then the preclinical safety requirements have been defined in many countries in drug safety regulations and toxicological guidelines. The requirements of the western industrialised countries have been reviewed (2), and it is apparent that considerable differences are to be found between requirements, and attitudes to these requirements, from one country to another.

Of the relevant forms of toxicity testing, the most expensive, time-consuming and controversial was, and still is, the long-term or chronic procedure. The length of these studies is dependent on the proposed duration of the use or exposure in man, but generally they are between three months and two years in duration.

The standard approach to these studies has been described in numerous publications (3,4). These non-clinical laboratory studies are now governed, particularly in the United States, by the Good Laboratory Practice Regulations (5). Studies are required in two species - a rodent and a non-rodent. The conventional procedure is to have one control group and at least three groups of dosed animals, so that spontaneous and induced pathological manifestations can be compared in control and test animals simultaneously. There are considerable technical problems in performing these studies and the conduct of the study has considerable bearing on the final results. The conditions under which animals are kept affect the outcome of many studies and contribute to intralaboratory and inter-laboratory variations. Factors that can affect the laboratory environment include temperature, humidity, light, season, extraneous chemicals, housing and, in particular, the diet fed to the animals. The method of administration of the test compound, both route and dosage form, is also of considerable importance. The design and objectives of the study should be clearly defined (6,7), with the study design being proper for the chemical under investigation. It is particularly important that these studies are performed to high technical standards. During the course of toxicity studies, animals should be observed for possible effects on behaviour, body weight, food and water consumption, general state of health, haematological and biochemical values, urine, eyes, terminal macropathology, organ weight and histopathology.

SENSITIVE CRITERIA OF TOXICITY

Two surveys of the toxicological profiles have been carried out (8,9). In the first survey on 50 compounds, 23 of the compounds were studied in the rat (Sprague-Dawley strain) and the Beagle dog: 27 compounds were studied in the rat (Sprague-Dawley strain) and the non-human primate. In the second survey, 37 compounds were compared in the rat (Sprague-Dawley or Wistar strain) and the Beagle dog. The percentage of compounds affecting the standard toxicological parameters is shown in Table I.

Clinical signs are more readily detected in the non-rodent species. Death is the least equivocal of all the clinical signs, but in cases of sudden death it is often difficult to determine the cause. The clinical signs are, in the main, indicative of digestive disturbances or alterations to CNS activity. In the rat, many of the signs are non-specific, such as reduced grooming activity, piloerection and ptosis.

Of all the characteristics measured during the course of a toxicological study, body weight is one of the most important. Body weight is an extraordinarily sensitive and objective

	Survey I	Survey II	Survey I	Survey II	Survey I
	Rat (50 compounds)	Rat (37 compounds)	Dog (23 compounds)	Dog (37 compounds)	Monkey (27 compounds)
CLINICAL SIGNS	56	51	78	70	86
Body weight	82	84	61	54	55
increased	8	3	9	3	11
decreased	74	81	52	51	44
Food intake	64	-	-	-	-
increased	24	-	-	-	-
decreased	40	-	-	-	-
Water consumption	14	-	7	-	4
increased	12	-	7	-	4
decreased	2	-	0	-	0
Haematology	16	30	22	30	7
Blood chemistry	34	30	44	35	34
liver function	18	-	26	-	19
kidney function	8	-	13	-	7
Urinalysis	24	-	13	-	4
TERMINAL STUDIES					
Macroscopic PM (positive findings)	42	-	39	-	11
Organ weight	82	73	61	24	37
liver	56	43	26	11	26
kidney	38	32	30	8	7
endocrine	26	22	17	5	0
gonad	22	24	17	8	4
other	12	22	4	5	0
Histopathology (positive findings)	62	65	74	49	37

Table I

Compounds Affecting Standard Toxicological Parameters (%)

measure of the health of groups of animals, because growth integrates all the influences acting on an animal day by day. In the rat, suppression of body-weight gain is often associated with decreased food intake. Suppression of body-weight gain can have considerable effect on other biological parameters (10-12). Sex and age, when retardation of body-weight gain occurs, have been found to be important variables (Heywood, in preparation). The suppression of body-weight gain subsequently affects the organ weights. The difference in response between males and females as far as liver weight is concerned is of interest: the relative liver weight of males shows a decrease; while that of females shows an increase. For the kidney, the data indicate that there is a proportionally larger reduction in kidney weight in males than in females. The effects on the adrenal weights appear to be greater in females than in males. Brain weight is shown to be related to body weight. Data concerning the testes indicate that the effect is greater after sexual maturity. Leucocyte counts are reduced, whereas the haematocrit is slightly increased. The concentrations of triglyceride and inorganic phosphate are lower, as are alanine transaminase and alkaline phosphatase levels. Sex, age and start of food restriction interact to affect the pituitary weight, and complex endocrine involvement occurs. Serum LH in adult males and females is reduced, and FSH levels in adult females is increased. Reduced prolactin values are found in adult animals. Corticosterone values are reduced in female rats (both weanling and adult) with food restriction, whereas in males slightly increased values are recorded.

In the dog, a marked suppression of body-weight gain is associated with increased liver weight, both actual and relative, variable effects on the thyroid and adrenal glands, and suppression of gonadal weights. Marked suppression of body-weight gain in the monkey is associated with lower weights of liver, kidney and testes.

Blood cytological and chemical investigations, together with urinalysis, are valuable diagnostic procedures in toxicity testing. When the haemopoietic system is affected, the common finding recorded in all species is a reduction in the values related to the red blood cells. Tests of blood chemistry, directed in the main to the investigation of liver function, are reliable, but depend on the appropriate test being applied to the right species. Tests for renal functions, such as blood urea and serum creatinine, are useful only when considerable renal damage has occurred. Urinalysis is helpful and urinary concentration tests such as urine volume, specific gravity and osmolality following water deprivation, though not specific, are sensitive indicators of kidney function. All tests on urine are dependent on samples being collected in the correct manner and at the right time. Tubular necrosis is an event likely to occur early in the study, and urine samples to diagnose this are best collected during the first week of compound administration: on the other hand, renal papillary necrosis is a long-term event, and samples taken late in the study are more likely to be diagnostic for this condition.

Terminal studies make a major contribution to the determination of target organ toxicity. Macroscopic *post-mortem* examination of animals that die, or are killed at the end of the study, provide limited information on studies of three to six months; the observations are generally restricted to descriptions of size, colour and texture of organs. In studies lasting for more than six months, many tumours are detected macroscopically. It has been shown that 70-76% of those neoplasms diagnosed microscopically in carcinogenicity bioassays in rats were visible to the naked eye; tumours of the endocrine tissues, liver and lung have the lowest correlation rates (13). Organ weight analysis is of great importance in these general toxicity studies, particularly in the rodent studies. The surveys (8,9) have shown that, in the rat, organ weights were affected in 82% and 73% of the studies, whereas in the dog the organ weights were affected in 61% and 24% of studies. This species difference can best be explained in terms of uniformity. The rodents used are of defined strains and show a considerable degree of uniformity, whereas Beagle dogs and monkeys are of variable size and age. Organ weight analyses show that the liver of the rat is affected by many compounds. The liver is the central organ in the detoxification of compounds, with the detoxifying mechanism in the microsomal enzyme systems. A large number of chemicals cause liver enlargement through an increase in the size of the cytoplasm of the hepatocytes, with an increased rate of microsomal enzyme synthesis. This is an adaptive physiological response: in the survey of 39 pharmacological compounds investigated in the rat, 40% of these compounds showed this feature.

The kidney is the next organ most frequently affected. The kidney mass relative to body weight is greater in the rodent (0.65% of body weight) than in the dog (0.45% of body weight), or the non-human primate (0.42% of body weight): this could be an important factor in species susceptibility to renal toxicants. Endocrine and gonadal weights are frequently affected in rats. Effects on the endocrine and reproductive system can be by direct effect on the glands, or can be mediated via feed-back mechanisms through the pituitary hypothalamic axis, or can be related to effects on body weight.

The two surveys have shown that histopathological examination of tissue at termination contributed positively to the assessment of the toxicological profiles in 62-65% of rodent studies, 49-74% of dog studies, but in only about 37% of non-human primate studies. Considerable emphasis has been placed on defining morphological change. Tissues are sampled, fixed and then prepared for examination: all these processes allow for the development of artefacts. Single sections from each tissue are then examined. There are obvious problems in making a histopathological diagnosis from a single section, particularly from organs as large as the liver or kidneys; there is no means of knowing whether the incidence of abnormalities obtained by such a procedure is correct or incorrect, particularly if the lesions are focal. There are problems in defining incidences of spontaneous disease in species and strains of laboratory animals (14). There is considerable divergence of opinion with regard to histological interpretation. Some pathologists (15) recognise this problem and suggest that histological assessment should be made by two pathologists, with submission to a referee where there is disagreement.

Sensitive criteria of toxicity have been shown to be the simple characteristics, such as clinical observation of the living animal, growth and organ weight analysis, liver and kidney function tests, and histological examination of selected tissues. Animal safety studies are no more than simple screening tests: any type of mass screening involves compromise and toxicological screens are no exception.

TARGET ORGAN TOXICITY

This system of testing identifies target organ systems: several target systems may be identified for a single compound. In the rat, the liver is the most common target system, but the nervous, endocrine and reproductive systems are often involved. In the dog, the liver is also the commonest target organ, and the CNS has frequently been identified as a target system. In non-human primates, the nervous system is one of the most frequently identified target organs, together with the liver and the digestive system.

Information on target systems on its own is of little interest, but it does stimulate further questions; for example, can some of the target systems be predicted with prior knowledge of the pharmacology of the compound? To answer this question, the rodent and dog data generated with pharmaceutical compounds have been investigated further: 39 drugs have been studied in the rat and in the dog; in the rat, 79 target systems were identified, whereas in the dog 59 target systems were identified; 33% of the target systems identified in the rat and 46% of those identified in the dog, were predictable on the basis of known pharmacology.

It is relevant to ask the question, how often can the same target system be identified in the rodent and non-rodent species? The best correlations are never greater than 20%, even when considering hepatotoxicity. Compound correlations of target systems between the rodent and the non-rodent species are somewhat better; in the two surveys, positive correlations for primary and secondary target organ systems between the rat and the dog were 54% and 57% respectively.

Much of this target organ toxicity is identified at very high dose-levels. There are quantitative differences between those dose-levels that induce toxicity in different species: a higher dose-level can usually be given to rodents before causing system toxicity. The present practice results in dose-levels of up to, and even greater than, one hundred times the anticipated human exposure dose being accepted as the high dose-level. Identification of target systems in animals at such dose-levels is unlikely to have predictive value for man. With present-day practices it is not necessary to establish blood levels associated with pharmacological and toxicological effects. Developments in the safety evaluation of new drugs are dependent on an integrated approach to metabolic studies and toxicology. Metabolic studies in animals attempt to elucidate the absorption of the compound into the body, its distribution and accumulation throughout the body, and its subsequent elimination. These aspects of metabolism tend to be similar across species; the greatest difficulty in projecting data from animals to man arises from species differences in biotransformation. Comparison of plasma half-lives in man and laboratory animals show definite species differences. Toxicology of pharmaceuticals which ignores pharmacokinetics is virtually useless. Interspecies comparison cannot be made without knowledge of equal blood levels for equal duration of time. The appropriateness of the high dose-level could also be judged if pharmacokinetic data were available. I am convinced that with currently accepted high dose-levels, there is an oversaturation of receptor sites and the toxicological effects induced are mere phenomena, the results being irrelevant for man and, in many cases, misleading. The toxicological evaluation of industrial and agrochemicals poses considerable problems, for it is not possible to establish pharmacokinetics in man.

NO-EFFECT LEVEL

The "no-effect" level is an important concept for the regulatory agencies, for it is the basis for assessing safety and establishing acceptable daily intakes. The "no-effect" level is, in fact, a not-detectable effect level as defined by conventional toxicological studies (16). The "no-effect" level is not a clearly definable figure: it is affected by the species and strain of animal used, and by other factors. I have suggested that, in 60% of compounds, the "no-effect" level in rodents is higher than that in non-rodent species, and it is often greater by at least a three-fold factor. Calculation of how many times higher the "no-effect" dosage level is in experimental animals than the actual human exposure level gives the safety factor.

This safety factor is a purely arbitrary number. There are uncertainties associated with estimates of "no-effect" levels and admissible daily intakes: acceptable exposure cannot be related to simple numbers, but must be accepted as a fluid situation (17).

DURATION OF STUDY

The duration of the studies depends on the proposed duration of treatment or exposure. The generally accepted rule is that, for a single-dose administration, toxicity studies for 1-2 weeks are required; for administration for 1 week in man, 4 weeks are required in animals; 1-4 weeks in man calls for 3 months in animals; and over 4 weeks in man requires 6 months in animals. There are exceptions, in that the United States requires 12-month studies in non-rodents and 24-month studies in rodents for all drugs other than those intended for short-term use, and other regulatory authorities, such as those in West Germany, Sweden and Eire, have requested long-term studies for drugs intended for long-term use. Long-term studies (i.e. for 24 months) are also required for many agricultural chemicals and for food additives.

McNamara (18) has reviewed the available data and concludes that there is good evidence that satisfactory long-term "no-effect" doses can be established by toxicity tests of about 4 months duration. It is generally accepted by most toxicologists that there is little information to be gained from continuing animal studies beyond 6 months, and that there is considerable merit in restricting studies to 3-6 months. Salsburg (19) argues that, in these short-term studies, the control animals are usually "clean", and the highest dose animals show trends of well-defined patterns, many of which could have been predicted by the pharmacology of the compound. With life-time studies, random variation begins to mask the issues, so the interpretation of a long-term study, particularly in rodents, is extremely difficult. The occurrence of some lesions is often confounded with that of other lesions, and Salsburg (20) suggests that it may be impossible to test whether a treatment is toxic, and, in particular, carcinogenic, in the presence of such biological confusion.

The occurrence of tumours is affected by the effects of other lesions. Correlations can be established between non-neoplastic spontaneous diseases and tumours in the rat (14). It has been shown that in female rats there is a positive association between the presence of pituitary adenomas and follicular cysts of the ovaries, and also between the presence of pituitary adenomas and fibroadenomas of the mammary gland. A negative association has been indicated between the presence of follicular cysts of ovary and any type of mammary tumour. These data suggest that pituitary adenomas are of at least two basic functional types. In male rats there was a positive association between pituitary adenomas and the development of gynecomastia, and a negative association between pituitary adenomas and galactoceles, again suggesting that the pituitary tumours are of two types.

Every biologically active compound influences the pattern of old-age lesions. Age affects the functioning of clearing organs. In the liver, the metabolising capacity may be impaired by age; this could lead to reduced drug clearance and a higher steady state of plasma concentration. Hepatic blood flow is decreased with age, partly because of reduced cardiac output. Liver weights, both absolute and relative, decrease. In the kidneys, glomerular filtration falls in old age, and in the rat further complications result from the incidence of chronic progressive nephropathy. At one year of age, 22% of males and 15% of female rats are showing morphological changes in the kidney, and at 80 weeks of age, 47% of males and 25% of females are showing considerable degenerative changes. Because of changes in body composition occurring with age, the distribution of the test compound may be affected.

The rate of body-weight gain has a profound effect on age-related pathology. It has been established that restricting food intake in rodents results in improved survival and a reduced incidence of spontaneous neoplasms (21,22). It has been suggested that there is a relationship between serum prolactin levels and tumour profiles, and that diet restriction affects serum prolactin release (23).

Salsburg (20) suggests that we rethink these long-term studies by cutting them short while the animals are still in reasonable health: alternatively, we should analyse the data differently, looking for statistical patterns and clustering of the data in considering whether the patterns have biological meaning. If the data-base generated from long-term studies is as complex and as difficult to interpret as I fear it is, we should attempt to devise shorter-term studies that might be more meaningful.

CHOICE OF DOSE-LEVEL

The choice of appropriate dose-levels is an essential first step. The current practice of selecting dose-levels as multiples of the human exposure level on the basis of mg/kg/body weight is far too simplistic. The practice of selecting massively high dose-levels without any reference to blood or plasma levels is to be deplored. Identification of target systems at such unphysiological levels is unlikely to have predictive value for man. The low dose-level should be a simple multiple of the human dose, but it should also take into consideration the rate of drug administration. In general, small animals metabolise and excrete compounds much more rapidly than does man. If a compound has a short half-life in an animal, the regimen of daily gavage or injection will cause a rapid absorption of drug to produce a high peak concentration followed by a rapid decline to low or undetectable levels. In actual fact, in many of our chronic toxicity studies we are studying a series of single dose administrations. We should attempt at this low level to approximate constant-rate regimens. This could be done by administering the doses frequently, or by giving the compound in a formulation which retards absorption, or by the use of rate-controlled osmotic pump implants. To carry out a 4-week study with this methodology would be more meaningful than a 12-month study by our old methods.

EXTRAPOLATION OF ANIMAL DATA TO MAN

Surprisingly, there has been little effort to examine the qualitative predictability of human side-effects from animal studies. Occasionally, general papers have suggested that qualitative predictions are not bad, although quantitative predictions are unreliable (24,25). The most substantial data refer to anti-cancer drugs. Owens (26) studied 21 anti-cancer drugs and found good agreement for most organ systems, such as bone-marrow, gastrointestinal tract, liver and kidney, but poor agreement for the nervous system and skin. Freireich et al. (27) reviewed the data from 34 toxicity studies on 18 anti-cancer drugs in rodents, non-rodents and man, and found that the toxic effects of the agents were similar amongst species when dosage was measured on the basis of surface area. Schein (28) studied 25 anti-cancer agents in dogs, monkeys and man and concluded that the dog and monkey provided effective prediction of organ-specific toxicity in man. It is important not to make generalisations from data generated from anti-cancer drugs to other drugs, environmental and industrial chemicals. An attempt has been made to recalculate the data of Schein and Freireich et al. (29) and to extend the extrapolation theoretically to the total population and to toxic chemicals in general. Such an approach is suspect, being based on anti-cancer drugs which are designed to induce cellular damage.

With regard to the general pharmaceutical compounds, only two papers appear to be relevant: these are those by Litchfield and Fletcher. Litchfield (30) selected six drugs - an antibiotic, a synthetic antibacterial agent, a tranquilliser, a CNS depressant, a chemical blocking alcohol oxidation, and a glucocorticoid - which had been studied in detail in rats, dogs and man. In both rats and dogs, each drug had been studied for acute toxicity and by subacute short-term feeding for 30-90 days. In addition, each drug had been given to dogs for at least 6 months, and to rats for 12 months. Clinical summaries were available on 500 or more human cases for each drug, and all 6 drugs had been studied in man within the 6-year period under closely comparable conditions. The data for each drug in the three species, including man, were examined and the incidences of 89 different effects caused by the drugs were evaluated, discarding those symptoms which could not, for specific physiological reasons, be common to all three species. From the data pertaining to the rat and dog, he predicted the occurrence or absence of each effect in man by following two rules: (i) if a sign was found in both rat and dog, it was predicted to occur in man; and (ii) if a sign was found in either the dog or the rat, but not in both, it was predicted that the sign would not occur in man. Since he already knew the effects of the drugs in man, he set up a table and tabulated the results. Of 86 predictions for the 6 drugs, 26 of 38 (68%) positive predictions, and 38 of 48 (79%) negative predictions were correct. Litchfield pointed out that the probability of obtaining 74% correct predictions is small if it is dependent only on chance.

Fletcher (31) correlated toxicity in animals and adverse effects in man for 45 drugs and concluded that, for an individual drug, 25% of the toxic effects observed in animal studies may be expected to occur as adverse reactions in man. Vomiting and gastrointestinal disturbance had greater predictive capacity than had CNS signs such as ataxia, convulsions, sedation, salivation or tremor.

In the absence of better data, it must be concluded from these limited studies attempting to extrapolate data between laboratory animal species, and between laboratory animals and man, that there is no reliable method for predicting what type of toxicity will develop in different species in response to the same compound. The same conclusion was reached in a review article on animal extrapolation and environmental health (32).

CONCLUSIONS

Safety of chemicals is a governmental responsibility and it is inevitable for toxicological studies to be subject to regulation. It is important that guidelines are treated as guidelines and not considered as law. We should work towards harmonising regulatory toxicology, although international agreement is all too often difficult to achieve. The regulatory offices of governments should be persuaded to adopt a more flexible approach. The recent modifications in data requirements for Stage 1 studies that are now becoming operative in the United Kingdom is an example of this more flexible approach, and one that we should encourage and applaud (33).

Simple extrapolation across the species is unrealistic. The implications in quantitative terms of virtually any tests done in animals are not known. It could be of value if we looked more into the problems of extrapolation across the species barriers.

The conventional toxicological procedures directed towards morphological change can be used to give only limited indications of safety. The complexities of many toxic reactions cannot be predicted by these studies.

It was Barnes & Denz (34) who said, many years ago, that chronic toxicity tests are always makeshift affairs to be replaced as soon as possible by a more permanent structure of knowledge built on the foundation of physiology, biochemistry and other fundamental sciences. Some toxicologists (35) recognise the scope and limitations of animal models for the prediction of human toxicity. Formal toxicity studies in two species is not the best method of assessing safety. A tier system based on the biological activity of the compound might provide more-meaningful data. This could be achieved by carrying out a standard study in the rat for 3-6 months and supplementing this study with other studies in different species designed to answer specific questions about the compound's biological activity and toxic potential. New techniques should be developed to take into account the pharmacokinetics and metabolism of the compound within the toxicologically-tested species. If we progressed along these lines, the numbers of animals used in toxicity studies would be reduced; if we studied more-appropriate dose-levels, the incidence of dramatic and unacceptable manifestations of toxicity would be reduced; but what is equally important, we should have performed more-meaningful studies.

REFERENCES

1. Lehman, A.J., Patterson, W.I., Davidow, B., Hagan, E.C., Woodard, G., Laug, E.P., Frawley, J.P., Fitzhugh, O.G., Bourke, A.R., Draize, J.H., Nelson, A.A. & Vos, B.J. (1955). Procedures for the appraisal of the toxicity of chemicals in foods, drugs and cosmetics. Food Drug Cosmetic Law Journal <u>10</u>, 679-748.
2. Adler, S., Janton, C. & Zbinden, G. (1981). "Preclinical Safety Requirements in 1980". pp. 89. Zurich: Institute of Toxicology, Swiss Federal Institute of Technology and University of Zurich.
3. Food Safety Council, USA (1978). "Proposed System for Food Safety Assessment". Washington: Food Safety Council.
4. National Academy of Science, USA (1975). "Principles for Evaluating Chemicals in the Environment". A Report for the Working Conference on Principles of Protocols for Evaluating Chemicals in the Environment. Washington: NAS.
5. Food and Drug Administration (1978). Non-clinical laboratory studies. Good Laboratory Practice Regulations. Federal

Register 43 (247), 59986-60025.

6. Gralla, E.J. (1981). Protocol preparation: design and objectives. In "Scientific Considerations in Monitoring and Evaluating Toxicological Research" (ed. E.J. Gralla), pp. 1-26. New York: Hemisphere Publishing Corporation.
7. Baron, R.L. (1980). Chronic studies. In "Principles and Methods in Modern Toxicology" (ed. C.L. Galli, S.D. Murphy & R. Paoletti), pp. 191-206. Amsterdam: Elsevier/North-Holland.
8. Heywood, R.L. (1981). Target organ toxicity I. Toxicology Letters 8, 349-358.
9. Heywood, R.L. (1983). Target organ toxicity II. Toxicology Letters (in press).
10. Schärer, K. (1977). The effect of chronic underfeeding on organ weights of rats. How to interpret organ weight changes in cases of marked growth retardation on toxicity tests. Toxicology 7, 45-56.
11. Schwartz, E., Tornaben, J.A. & Boxill, G.C. (1973). The effects of food restriction on hematology, clinical chemistry and pathology in the albino rat. Toxicology & Applied Pharmacology 25, 515-524.
12. Oishi, S., Oishi, H., Hiraga K. (1979). The effect of food restriction for 4 weeks on common toxicity parameters in male rats. Toxicology & Applied Pharmacology 47, 15-22.
13. Kulwich, B.A., Hardistry, J.F. & Gilmore, C.E. (1980). Correlation between gross observations of tumors and neoplasms diagnosed microscopically in carcinogenesis bioassays in rats. Journal of Environmental Pathology and Toxicology 3, 281-287.
14. Thompson, S.W. & Vladislava, S.R. (1981). Some thoughts on attempts to correlate the occurrence of neoplastic and non-neoplastic spontaneous diseases in laboratory animals. Toxicological Pathology 9, 1-18.
15. Newberne, P.M. & McConnell, R.G. (1980). Toxicologic pathology: issues and uncertainties. In "Principles and Methods in Modern Toxicology" (ed. C.L. Galli, S.D. Murphy & R. Paoletti), pp. 223-258. Amsterdam: Elsevier/North-Holland.
16. Zbinden, G. (1979). The no-effect level, an old bone of contention in toxicology. Archives of Toxicology 43, 3-7.
17. Sharratt, M. (1976). Uncertainties associated with the evaluation of the health hazards of environmental chemicals from toxicological data. In "The Evaluation of Toxicological Data for the Protection of Public Health", Proceedings of the International Colloquium, pp. 105-122. Oxford: Pergamon Press.
18. McNamara, B.P. (1976). Concepts in health evaluation of commercial and industrial chemicals. In "New Concepts in Safety Evaluation" (ed. M.A. Mehlman, R.E. Shapiro & H. Blumenthal), pp. 61-115. New York: Wiley.

19. Salsburg, D.S. (1981). Statistics and Toxicology: an overview. In "Scientific Considerations in Monitoring and Evaluating Toxicological Research" (ed. E.J. Gralla), pp. 123-136. New York: Hemisphere Publishing Corporation.
20. Salsburg, D. (1980). The effects of lifetime feeding studies on patterns of senile lesions in mice and rats. Drug and Chemical Toxicology 3, 1-33.
21. Ross, M.H. & Bras, G. (1971). Lasting influence of early caloric restriction on prevalence of neoplasm in the rat. Journal of the National Cancer Institute 47, 1095-1113.
22. Tucker, M.J. (1979). The effect of long-term food restriction on tumours in rodents. International Journal of Cancer 23, 803-807.
23. Rose, F.J.C. (1981). Are nutritionists worried about the epidemic of tumours in laboratory animals? Proceedings of the Nutrition Society 40, 57-65.
24. Frohberg, H. (1977). What may be learnt from short- and long-term tests and from studies on carcinogenicity, teratogenicity and mutagenicity. Arzneimittel-Forschung 27, 228-241.
25. Peck, H.M. (1968). An appraisal of drug safety evaluation in animals and the extrapolation of results to man. In "Importance of Fundamental Principles in Drug Evaluation" (ed. D.H. Tedeschi & R.E. Tedeschi), pp. 450-471. New York: Raven Press.
26. Owens, A.H. (1962). Predicting anti-cancer drug effects in man from laboratory animal studies. Journal of Chronic Diseases 15, 223-228.
27. Freireich, E.J., Deham, E.A., Rall, D.P., Schmidt, L.H., & Skipper, H.E. (1966). Quantitative comparison of toxicity of anti-cancer agents in mouse, rat, hamster, dog, monkey and man. Cancer Chemotherapy Reports 50, 219-244.
28. Schein, P.S., Davis, R.D., Carter, S., Newman, J., Schein, D.R. & Rall, D.P. (1970). The evaluation of anti-cancer drugs in dogs and monkeys for the prediction of qualitative toxicities in man. Clinical Pharmacology and Therapeutics 11, 3-40.
29. Dixon, R.L. (1976). Problems in extrapolating toxicity data for laboratory animals to man. Environmental Health Perspectives 13, 43-50.
30. Litchfield, J.T. (1962). Evaluation of the safety of new drugs by means of tests in animals. Clinical Pharmacology and Therapeutics 3, 665-672.
31. Fletcher, A.P. (1978). Drug safety tests and subsequent clinical experience. Journal of the Royal Society of Medicine 71, 693-696.
32. Reichsman, F.P. & Calabrese, E.J. (1978). Animal extrapolation in environmental health: its theoretical basis and practical applications. Review on Environmental Health III, 59-78.

33. Mail 32, (Nov. 1981). Issued by Department of Health and Social Security, London.
34. Barnes, J.M. & Denz, F.A. (1954). Experimental methods used in determining chronic toxicity. Pharmacological Reviews 6, 191-242.
35. Z̄binden, G. (1981). Scope and limitations of animal models for the prediction of human toxicity. In "Organ-directed Toxicity" (ed. S.S. Brown & D.S. Davies), pp. 3-7. Oxford: Pergamon Press.

Is There an Alternative?

S. R. WALKER

INTRODUCTION

The last 20 years have witnessed an escalation in the number of safety evaluation studies required for new medicines, together with a demand for the increased safety of drugs. These changes have been accompanied by a proliferation of guidelines detailing the requirements to be fulfilled before a drug is given approval for use in man. The guidelines applicable to compounds for projected long-term administration to man often differ, requiring long-term animal toxicology of 6, 12, 18 or 24 months' duration, leaving aside the carcinogenicity studies necessary in certain cases.

In contrast, there is an increasing demand to rationalise and, where possible, decrease the amount of animal toxicology required in connection with the process of drug development. But this understandable and legitimate aim can only be pursued if proposals to decrease animal studies are based on carefully evaluated facts. Therefore, it is necessary to determine the scientific rationale behind these requirements and to demonstrate whether there is any evidence that longer term testing produces:

a. additional information with respect to target organ toxicity;
b. "safer" drugs, with toxicological studies of 12, 18 or

24 months' duration being better predictors of adverse drug effects in man than those of 3 or 6 months.

There have been a number of attempts to determine the appropriate duration of toxicity studies. Barnes & Denz in their review of chronic toxicity testing (1) concluded that there was little value in testing beyond 3-6 months. In support of this statement, Bein (2) reported his findings on 46 compounds studied at two Ciba-Geigy research centres, with the investigations at one centre limited to one month in rats, while studies at the other centre were conducted in excess of 6 months in rodents and often in dogs and monkeys as well. Bein stated that in no instance did the prolonged tests of 6 months or more disclose any deleterious effects which had not already been observed in the course of experiments lasting 4 weeks or even a few days. Paget (3) expressed the viewpoint of the expert committee on drug toxicity established by The Association of British Pharmaceutical Industry and reported, "We have been unable to find any evidence that these considerably prolonged (two years) studies give any useful information whatsoever, apart from on carcinogenicity, that cannot be predicted from the results of shorter studies".

Peck (4) described toxicology studies of varying duration from 1-24 months for each of 11 compounds. With one exception, extending the experiments beyond 3 or 6 months did not reveal any additional toxicity. The one exception was methyl-dopa, and this may have been due to the fact that the short-term tests lasted 6 weeks and the next autopsy was at 12 months. The additional effects seen at 12 months consisted of granular precipitate in the kidneys and bladders of rats, but this was not seen in dogs or monkeys. The precipitate occurred at high dose-levels, and was due to the saturation of urine with a metabolite of methyl-dopa. At therapeutic dose-levels such a precipitate would not be expected because the solubility of the metabolite would not be exceeded. It is important to note that this one exception out of 11 compounds is explained on the basis of dose, metabolism and species-specificity.

McCollister (5), reporting for the Committee of the Society of Toxicology, stated that, "With the exception of carcinogenesis and certain rare neurological defects there is little, if any, additional information obtained on the character of toxic effects that are not detected within three months of testing with animals". Therefore, it is still reasonable to ask what has been learned from tests lasting 12 months or more that could not have been observed from tests of only 3 months duration. Is there a rational basis for requiring toxicity tests of 12 months in the United States, whereas only 6 months is necessary in Europe for drugs used long-term in man? While it is appreciated that regulatory authorities are privy to data which may seem to support their positions on long-term studies, the data need to be examined and the case proved to the satisfaction of all concerned with the safety evaluation of medicines. This information is within the archives of pharmaceutical companies, but up to the present time has not been made available in a format that would allow these comparisons to be made.

METHODOLOGY

In view of the paucity of data in the literature on the comparative toxic response of any given chemical in which comparable biochemical, pathological and other criteria have been examined at varying periods of time under similar conditions in the same laboratory, the Centre for Medicines Research is carrying out a study to investigate the informational value of repeated-dose toxicity studies of different durations. The objective is to compare animal toxicity studies carried out over a period of one or 3 months with data from investigations of 6 or 12 months in order to determine the minimum period necessary to observe all the significant toxicological effects of the drug being evaluated. For this study the Centre is dependent on the provision by pharmaceutical companies in the UK of toxicological information on the compounds they have investigated during the last 20 years. These include companies in the UK responsible for setting up their own in-house toxicological studies, as well as those contracting out such investigations.

The data provided have included details of therapeutic class, the animal species investigated, route of administration, elimination half-life, LD50, the dose-levels used, and the duration of the studies. Details are recorded of clinical signs related to various body systems, including the criteria of body weight and food consumption; laboratory findings, including haematology, clinical chemistry and urinalysis; and pathological changes. The times and dose at which these effects occur, i.e. after one, 3, 6, or 12 months, are noted and in some instances the proportions of the animals affected are recorded. From these data it is possible to assess the minimum time to observe all effects. Subsequently, in conjunction with the company toxicologists who have carried out these studies, the time required to determine significant toxicological effects is identified. Further information can also be derived from the data, including the "no toxic effect" during short-term and long-term studies.

As this information will, in due course, be used for investigating the predictive value of these long-term animal studies for man, we have also identified whether there is extensive clinical experience, whether the drug is marketed and, if not, the reason for failure (i.e. animal toxicology, clinical efficacy, limited market potential, etc.).

RESULTS

It is only possible at this stage to report interim results, since a significant amount of the data has yet to be analysed. However, to date, information on 122 case studies involving 75 compounds has been received. A case study is here defined as the investigation of one compound in one species for an appropriate period of time which would allow the comparison of events occurring within at least two time periods.

A number of studies have been excluded fom this total database because they did not fulfil the criteria which would allow a comparison of short-term and long-term investigations. Twelve studies have been excluded because the maximum period of investigation was only 3 months, and for a further three studies the duration was 18 or 24 months. Eleven studies were excluded as no pathology was available for the shorter period of investigation. In addition, a further 43 studies are not included in the analysis as there were no abnormalities during the periods of study (8 studies), or we are awaiting further data (2 studies), or the studies have not yet been discussed with the companies providing the information (33 studies). Therefore, at this time, only 53 studies on 40 compounds are available for analysis.

An analysis of the number of studies relating the maximum period of testing to the species investigated identified 22 studies in the rat, 19 in the dog and 12 in primates. There are 29 studies which have been carried out for a maximum period of 6 months, thus allowing a comparison of either 3 and 6 months or one and 6 months. There are 24 studies carried out for a maximum period of 12 months, which allow a comparison between 3 and 12 months or 6 and 12 months.

CONCLUSION

The findings from these investigations, in the final analysis, will provide a basis for assessing the limited additional value of long-term studies compared with the conventional 3- or 6-month investigations. However, the true significance of these observations may only become apparent when a comparison is made between the animal toxicology and clinical experience, to determine whether the toxicological effects in animals were predictive of the adverse drug reactions occurring in man.

Long-term animal studies require a significant proportion of the total time, cost and animals utilised in the safety evaluation of new medicines. It is now essential to review retrospectively the informational value of these studies in comparison with short-term investigations, if we are ever to reduce the number of animals required without compromising the predicted safety of these drugs in man. The alternative is the unacceptable one of continuing to carry out existing tests uncritically and, in certain circumstances, of adding new ones without adequate validation.

ACKNOWLEDGEMENTS

The following companies have kindly provided data without which these studies would not have been possible: Beecham Pharmaceuticals, The Boots Company PLC, Ciba-Geigy Pharmaceuticals Division, Fisons Ltd., Glaxo Group Research Ltd., May & Baker Ltd., Laboratories Pfizer, Roche Products Ltd., Smith Kline & French Research Ltd., The Wellcome Foundation Ltd.

REFERENCES

1. Barnes, J.M. & Denz, F.A. (1954). Experimental methods used in determining chronic toxicity. Pharmacological Reviews 6, 191-242.
2. Bein, H.J. (1963). Time to appearance of toxic signs in Ciba studies of 46 compounds at Basel, Switzerland and Summit, New Jersey. Proceedings of the European Societies for Drug Toxicity 11, 15-24.
3. Paget, G.E. (1963). Standards for the laboratory evaluation of the toxicity of a drug - viewpoint of the expert committee on drug toxicity of The Association of the British Pharmaceutical Industry. Proceedings of the European Societies Study of Drug Toxicity 11, 7-12.
4. Peck, H.M. (1968). An appraisal of drug safety evaluation in animals and the extrapolation of results to man. In "Importance of Fundamental Principles in Drug Evaluation" (ed. D.H. Tedeschi & R.E. Tedeschi), pp. 449-471. New York: Raven Press.
5. McCollister, D.D. (1974). Society of Toxicology Ad Hoc Committee Comments on Health Research Group Petitions. Society of Toxicology Newsletter pp. 2 (cited from McNamara, B.P. (1976). Concepts in health evaluation of commercial and industrial chemicals. In "New Concepts in Safety Evaluation" (ed. M.A. Mehlman, R.E. Shapiro & H. Blumenthal), pp. 61-115. New York: Wiley.

Repeat-dose Long-term Toxicity Studies

J. P. GRIFFIN

As a discussant on conduct of repeat-dose toxicity studies, my contribution must of essence be short. I should therefore like to touch upon only three points, namely, design of studies, duration of studies, and predictability.

DESIGN OF STUDIES

It is necessary in the conduct of any study involving animals or human subjects to obtain the maximum amount of unbiased information concerning the principal action and side-effects of a drug or procedure from the minimum number of animals or human subjects in the shortest time with the least inconvenience to them.

It is, therefore, disconcerting as a person who regularly examines data derived from animal studies to find that some toxicity studies are:

a. defective in protocol design;
b. inappropriate or irrelevant;
c. conducted in a slovenly manner so that the maximum amount of useful data is not generated.

Such studies are a waste of money, a useless expenditure of valuable time, and an unjustifiable use of animals. Detailed criticisms of the shortcomings of animal toxicology studies conducted in support of applications for clinical trial approval or product licences have been made elsewhere (1,2).

Another point of justifiable criticism in this area can be levelled at national regulatory authorities who require studies to be conducted according to incompatible protocols which must of necessity lead to unnecessary duplication of studies. I am pleased to say that the European Community's Committee on Proprietary Medicinal Products Working Party on Safety Requirements has produced a set of seven guidelines [COM.(80) 789 (final)] which should lead not only to harmonisation of requirements for safety studies, but set standards for well conducted studies.

Dr Heywood has stressed that there should always be pharmacokinetic studies conducted under the umbrella of long-term toxicity studies in order to ascertain the relevance of the toxicity studies to man. This can be illustrated by the following example which relates to a drug whose pharmacokinetics were studied in the rat. Plasma levels of the drug were measured on days 3, 10, 17 and 24, and the drug was administered daily at 3, 10 and 20mg/kg. At 3mg/kg, the plasma levels ranged from 1.35 to 3.23μg/ml; at 10mg/kg, the plasma levels ranged from 2.30 to 7.46μg/ml; and at 30mg/kg, the plasma levels ranged from 33.21 to 40.48μg/ml. There was no evidence of accumulation with repeated dosing, although there was indication of non-linear kinetics.

In 10 and 6 male volunteers, respectively, doses of 0.3 mg/kg/day and 0.5mg/kg/day were administered for 35 days. The plasma concentrations on the first day were of the order of 2.0μg/ml and 3.0μg/ml, respectively, but on the 35th day were 6.0 to 16.0μg/ml at daily doses of 0.3mg/kg, and 19.9 to 36.2μg/ml at daily doses of 0.5mg/kg.

In the rat toxicity studies, centrilobular hepatic necrosis had occurred in rats dosed at 15.0, 30.0 and 60.0mg/kg. The toxicologist would have envisaged that the doses being studied were 30, 60 and 120 times the therapeutic dose, but because of cumulation in man the dose that was shown to be therapeutically effective was giving plasma levels in excess of that producing toxicity in the rat.

This example is a case where reliance on the differential between dose-levels administered in the animal studies and the therapeutic dose given to man would, without the accompanying metabolic investigation, have given rise to a false sense of security about the safety of the drug.

A further point that has been mentioned is that the use of extremely high doses of a drug in toxicological studies can give misleading results. Williams et al. (3) described the metabolism of a new selective β_2-adrenergic agent, rimiterol, in six species, administered at different dose-levels by the intravenous route. It was clearly demonstrated that there were considerable species-differences in the plasma half-life of rimiterol. It was also shown in the rat that the urinary pattern of metabolites differed qualitatively at different dose-levels. This was eventually shown to be because the β_2-adrenergic actions of rimiterol at high doses caused splanchnic vascular shut-down with consequent reduction in liver blood flow and therefore almost complete elimination of the hepatic phases of drug metabolism.

The CPMP Guidelines specifically deal with the need for pharmacokinetic studies in toxicity evaluation.

A toxicity study must be designed to reveal target organ

toxicity and not a demonstration of "nil-effect" for an enthusiatic marketing organisation.

DURATION OF STUDIES

The duration of repeated-dose toxicity studies should be appropriate to the expected duration of human use. As a rule of thumb, the guidelines drawn up by the CPMP Safety Working Party recommend:

Proposed duration of human treatment	Suggested duration of repeated-dose toxicity studies
One or several doses within one day	2 weeks
Repeated-doses for up to 7 days	4 weeks
Repeated-doses for up to 30 days	3 months
Repeated-doses beyond 30 days	6 months

In my experience, it is not of value other than in carcinogenicity studies to demand repeated-dose toxicity studies for longer than 6 months. In debate on the necessity for longer duration of exposure, the only justification advanced by proponents for longer exposure appears to be that the complications of the toxic effect should be allowed time to develop. For example, if a substance is diabetogenic, this will show up in the first few months, but, if it is given for long enough, it is to be expected that the complications of this condition (e.g. cataracts, renal problems, etc.), which may not be present at 3 or 6 months, will appear at 12 or 18 months. Can this not be inferred from the basic toxic effect?

PREDICTABILITY

As a working hypothesis, it has to be assumed that a toxicological screen using a range of tests as indicated above has predictive value. In accepting the predictive value of such tests, a substance that was markedly toxic in the animal studies would be unlikely to be administered to man. In fact, the administration to man of such a substance would probably not be countenanced ethically unless some unique advantage in terms of efficacy was envisaged. Therefore, substances which are markedly toxic in animals are seldom administered therapeutically and therefore whether these substances are equally toxic for man is not evaluated.

The converse is not true, since substances which do not show marked toxicity in animal studies in the usual range of tests may be administered to man and subsequently reveal a hitherto unexpected spectrum of adverse reactions. This situation may arise: first, because the syndrome of toxicity experienced in man cannot be reproduced in animal models (e.g. the practolol syndrome); secondly, the appropriate animal model may not have been devised or utilised in the safety screening programme; or, thirdly, one aspect of the drug's toxicity in animals may have become a limiting factor, in that this aspect of toxicity appeared and limited the study in either duration or dosage so that another relevant aspect to man of the drug's toxicity could not be revealed. This is a common problem with non-steroidal anti-inflammatory drugs, where gastrointestinal side-effects tend to be the most apparent toxic effect for the whole class.

It must, therefore, be apparent that, when looking at the spectrum of clinical adverse reactions to therapeutic substances and then comparing these with the toxic effects seen in the animal studies to see if they were predictive, there are limitations on what can be expected. We can only expect to find prediction in terms of mild to moderate animal toxicity in those organs which prove to be the human target organ, since if there was flagrant toxicity in the animal models, the drug would not have been used therapeutically in man.

Animal toxicity studies are useful in predicting adverse reactions which are due to the primary pharmacological action or to direct toxic actions of the drug. Animal studies are not of so much value in predicting purely subjective adverse reactions, such as hallucinations, hypersensitivity reactions (e.g. skin rashes), and cases of agranulocytosis due to hypersensitivity.

In a study on seven anti-arrhythmic agents ((4), Table I), it was found for some products that almost the whole spectrum of adverse drug reactions was predicted in the animal toxicity studies; at the other end of the spectrum there were cases of much less predictability from the animal studies for the human spectrum of adverse drug reactions (e.g. perhexilene neuropathy, which is related to genetic differences in mixed oxidase function; this affects the metabolism of the drug in man, and slow metabolisers are more susceptible to this adverse effect). However, it must again be stressed that such a study excludes exposure of man to drugs which are overtly toxic in animals and is therefore biased against the predictability of animal studies. Nevertheless, it is worthy of note that even in such a study a predictive value of animal studies can be demonstrated.

DRUG	REPORTED HUMAN ADVERSE REACTIONS			EVIDENCE OF ANIMAL TOXICITY
Amiodarone				
Indication	Myocardial depression	(L)	(YC)	+
	Thyroid gland changes	(L)	(YC)	+
Wolff Parkinson	Corneal changes	(L)	(YC)	-
White Syndrome	Hepatitis	(L)	(YC)	+
resistant	Peripheral Neuropathy	(L)	(YC)	(±)*
arrhythmias	Fibrosing alveolitis	(L)	(YC)	-
	Nausea and vomiting	(L)	(YC)	+
	Photosensitivity reactions	(L)	(YC)	-

* ataxia and reduced muscle tone observed.

DRUG	REPORTED HUMAN ADVERSE REACTIONS			EVIDENCE OF ANIMAL TOXICITY
Disophyramide				
Indication	Anticholinergic effects	(L)	(YC)	+
Ventricular arrhythmias	Myocardial depression and hypotension	(L)	(YC)	+
	Hepatitis, jaundice	(L)	(YC)	+
	Gastric irritation	(L)	(YC)	+
	Skin rashes	-	(YC)	-
	Agranulocytosis	(L)	-	-
	Renal damage, mild inflammatory effects	-	-	(+)
Mexiletine				
Indication	Convulsions	-	(YC)	+
	Tremor	(L)	-	+
Ventricular	Ataxia	(L)	-	+
arrhythmias	Nausea and vomiting	(L)	(YC)	+
	Hepatic damage	(-)	(YC)	+
	Rashes	(-)	(YC)	-
Nifedipine				
Indication	Precipitation of angina	(L)	(YC)	-
	Lower limb oedema	(L)	(YC)	-
Anti-anginal	Gastrointestinal intolerance	(L)	(YC)	+
	Headache, tremor, paraesthesia	(L)	(YC)	-
	Rashes	(L)	(YC)	-

Table I

DRUG	REPORTED HUMAN ADVERSE REACTIONS		EVIDENCE OF ANIMAL TOXICITY
Perihexilene			
Indication	Peripheral neuropathy	(L) (YC)	-
	Papilloedema	(L) (YC)	-
Anti-anginal	Ataxia	(L) (YC)	+
	Hepatitis and jaundice	(L) (YC)	-
	Hypoglycaemia	(L) (YC)	-
	Rashes	(L) (YC)	-
	Nausea, vomiting, anorexia	(L) (YC)	+
Verapamil			
Indication	A-V block	(L) (YC)	+
	Cataracts and lens opacities	(-) (-)	(+)
Supraventricular arrhythmias	Gingival hyperplasia	(-) (-)	(+)
	Hepatic damage, hepatitis or enzyme changes	(L) (YC)	(+)
Anti-anginal	Nausea, vomiting	(L) (YC)	(+)
Tocainide			
Indication	A-V block	(L) (-)	(-)
Ventricular arrhythmias	CNS effects tremor nystagmus, paraesthesia, cerebellar signs	(L) (-)	(+)
	Rash + fever	(L) (YC)	(-)
	Bone marrow depression	(Data Sheet?)	(-)
	LE Syndrome, fibrosing alveolitis	(Data Sheet?)	( )

YC = yellow card (adverse reactions)

L = literature (reported)

Table I (continued)

CONCLUSION

Despite the many criticisms that can be made of long-term animal toxicity studies in terms of their design and conduct and, even when well conducted, of their predictability, they remain, in the current absence of any reasonable alternative, the best predictors of risk to man that we have.

REFERENCES

1. Griffin, J.P. (1977). The seven deadly sins. In "Quality Control in Toxicology" (ed. G.E. Paget), pp. 25-33. Lancaster, M.T.P. Press.
2. Griffin, J.P. (1979). Animal toxicological studies in the safety evaluation of new drug substances. In "Drug Assessment Criteria and Methods" (ed. J.Z. Bowes & G.P. Velo), pp. 107-119. Amsterdam: Elsevier/North-Holland.
3. Williams, J.R.B., Griffin, J.P. & Maughan, E. (1977). The influence of species, dose and route on the metabolism of rimiterol. In "Current Approaches in Toxicology" (ed. B. Ballantyne), pp. 249-260. Bristol: J. Wright & Son.
4. Griffin, J.P. (1982). Toxicological evaluation of cardiac drugs. In "Symposium on Chronic Anti-arrhythmic Therapy" (ed. J.P. Bandurme, M.G. Bogaert, D.G. Julian, H. Kulbertus); sponsored by the European Society of Cardiology, Gent, Belgium (in press).

General Discussion

A. N. WORDEN

Rapporteur

Dr F. ROE enquired whether those who considered that 6 months was long enough for a toxicity test would consider it unnecessary to record anything but the incidence and nature of the tumours in a carcinogenicity study. Dr J.P. GRIFFIN replied that it was morally obligatory to try to obtain as much information as possible from any study that had been undertaken, even if only on the basis that something may have been missed the first time round, or that a different strain of animals was being used.

Several contributors to the discussion queried the suggestion that the no-effect level, rather than the target organ toxicity, was of primary importance. Dr GRIFFIN felt that one handicap lay in the search for only one target organ, whereas several organs might show up in a well-conducted toxicity study. However, he accepted Dr Heywood's point that dosing may be pushed so high that it reveals one aspect of toxicity early and masks the manifestation of the others. Dr R. HEYWOOD said that he, too, believed in defining target organ toxicity, but it was the massive dose-level at which it was defined in many current studies with which he disagreed.

Dr Rosemary HAWKINS asked Dr Griffin whether he felt that the introduction of Good Laboratory Practice (GLP) requirements in the UK would reduce the number of wasted studies to which he had alluded. Dr GRIFFIN replied that this really depended on where the toxicity study was being conducted. He had no way of predicting what might happen in the future, but he was convinced that in the USA, where GLP was in force, and in those laboratories in the UK where GLP was being put into effect, there had been a considerable improvement in the quality of the studies and in the way in which they were being carried out. He could not say, however, that any improvement was visible on the logic that was being put into the study itself: the logic behind toxicity studies was still equally lacking.

Dr J. FOWLER queried whether Dr Heywood was being consistent in his argument over the no-effect level by using blood levels, and whether he was referring to the area under the curve or the peak blood level. How, in fact, did the no-effect level operate? Dr HEYWOOD replied that in talking of no-effect level he was implying an absence of effect, with no target organ toxicity detected at the dose-levels employed, and that currently he was not concerned with blood levels, either peak levels or areas under the curve. He and his colleagues were just putting in compounds at a simple multiple of the human dose at the low level and at intermediate levels, in order to define safety factors. He agreed with the need to make testing procedures more sophisticated and, as Dr R. Goulding, Chairman of the Acute Toxicity session had phrased it, to make them more elegant. Toxicologists should be looking at the parameters that Dr Fowler was suggesting.

Dr GOULDING asked Dr Griffin whether, in view of the devastating adverse criticisms of industrial toxicity testing, he would advocate that all firms should put the design and the whole scheme of investigation before the collective wisdom of the regulatory body in advance. Dr GRIFFIN replied that the scheme should certainly be seen by somebody. There were members of Section 4 Committees present, and though he very much doubted that they would want to be overburdened by being asked to comment on all the studies to be undertaken, somebody should see proposed schemes. He wished to state that the licensing authority officers were very pleased to discuss any design of studies with those who were drawing up a programme for evaluation of a drug. This point was received with warm approval.

Dr D. CHANTER discussed the need to do away with empiricism in toxicity testing and to move more into science. He regarded the no-effect level as highly empirical, but, since this point had already been picked up, he wished to address the remark in the context of the way in which the dose-level of a compound was incorporated in the treatment, particularly in the long-term feeding study in which the animal was growing all the time: the proportion of the diet used for maintenance and the proportion used for growth were changing all the time. In the young animal, much was being utilised for growth, and in the adult it was all for maintenance. This must surely affect the fate of the compound which was eaten, and it would seem to be more scientific to find some method of changing the dose as the animal grew in order to reflect this. In acute studies, it would seem more logical to give the dose as a proportion of the metabolic rate rather than as a proportion of body weight. Dr GRIFFIN replied that toxicity testing was a crude business in which refinement seemed to have little place. What was being looked for was the potential of a substance to cause harm when it was let loose on an enormously variable human population, much of it sick or old or young or growing or pregnant. The best that could be hoped for was to gauge the extent to which the potential of a substance came up in toxicity studies.

Ms Sheila SILCOCK said that Dr Heywood's criticisms had been levelled at the long-term toxicity testing of substances intended for administration to man: would he use similar criteria for industrial substances which posed a hazard but were not intended for administration, and what were his views on the no-effect level in such cases? Dr HEYWOOD replied that he did not work with environmental chemicals. Professor A. McLEAN said that they posed a very different problem in that the risk and the benefit, which involved the same person in the case of a drug, could go to very different people for environmental chemicals, industrial chemicals and pesticides - and, to some extent, food additives.

Dr A. FLETCHER suggested that, if reasonable standards of hygiene and safety were adopted and efforts were concentrated on these aspects, it would be interesting to speculate how much increase in poisoning would result if no long-term toxicity testing whatsoever were carried out. A member of the audience asked if any testing at all was necessary for non-drugs. Professor McLEAN doubted whether anyone would dare to answer such a question, since the reasons for testing were social and ones of justice - and of justice being seen to be done - as much as the avoidance of risk, especially when one considered that historically injustices had been done. Dr A. COHEN made a specific response: acetylaminofluorine, a classic chemical carcinogen used in numerous carcinogenicity tests, had been going to be introduced as an insecticide. The carcinogenicity test was positive and all subsequent metabolic data suggested that the same pathways in terms of N-hydroxylation would occur in man. It had therefore not been introduced.

Dr CALVIN enquired of Dr Griffin what proportion of protocols relating to industrial organisations were regarded as deficient and whether the DHSS preferred to be able to inform these organisations that their work was deficient. Professor McLEAN said that before Dr Griffin answered this question he would like to say that, in looking back at all the experiments conducted in his own laboratory, not in the context of testing, he could not think of any with which in retrospect he was totally satisfied. He hoped the same was true of industrial testing, so it was not surprising that every experiment that had been reported had its deficiencies. However, could these deficiencies be reduced by discussion and by better education of toxicologists? Dr GRIFFIN replied by referring to a chapter he had written on "Seven Deadly Sins" in "Quality Control in Toxicology" (ed. G.E. Paget). Deficient testing was less common now than 5 years ago, when it was well over 50%; today it was of the order of 15-20%. He implied that this scale of deficiency was unacceptable, and beyond the general dissatisfaction with hindsight referred to by Professor McLean.

Carcinogenicity

I. F. H. PURCHASE

INTRODUCTION

The primary method of identifying carcinogens has been based on the use of animal studies since the observations of Yamagiwa & Ichikawa in 1918 (1). Their experiments demonstrated for the first time that skin cancer could be produced by the repeated application of chemicals to the skin of rabbits. Until recently, such animal carcinogenicity studies were the only test systems with any degree of reliability. Even now, in vivo studies form the most reliable basis on which the carcinogenicity of chemicals can be determined. Such studies are also invaluable in identifying those factors which influence the incidence of cancer in an untreated population and in understanding the mechanisms of action of chemical carcinogens. Nevertheless, there is growing concern about the use of animals in toxicity testing, and the value and role of alternatives in an assessment of toxic hazard should be examined in this light. This paper examines the justification for conducting laboratory studies to detect carcinogens, and reviews the utility of short-term and long-term tests and the design, conduct and reporting of animal carcinogenicity studies.

CANCER - ITS IMPORTANCE AS A CAUSE OF DEATH

There is no doubt about the high incidence of cancer in man. In 1980, there were 130,073 deaths from cancer in England and Wales, representing over 20% of all deaths occurring during that period. After cardiovascular disease, cancer is the second most common cause of death amongst the populations of England and Wales (2). Cancer is the leading cause of death in all age groups between 35 and 54, and the second most common cause of death in the age groups 5-34 and 55-74. These figures demonstrate the importance of cancer as a cause of death, both from the point of view of public health and of perceptions of members of the public, most of whom know of relatives and friends who have suffered from the disease.

The proportion of deaths due to cancer has increased during this century with the reduction in competing causes of deaths, such as infectious diseases. As cancer is predominantly a disease of middle and older age groups, the number of deaths due to cancer will increase as the average age of the population increases. There has been little change in the age-adjusted rates of cancer over the last few decades in those countries in which statistics are sufficiently accurate for such comparisons to be made. There are a few individual exceptions to this general rule; for example, respiratory tract cancer has increased dramatically over the last few decades in association with the increase in cigarette smoking. There has also been a decrease in the incidence of stomach cancer in most Western societies, although the reason for this is not known.

CANCER - EVIDENCE FOR ITS CAUSATION

As cancer is such a common cause of death, identification of the main reasons for this high incidence is of great importance. There are four main lines of evidence which suggest that extrinsic factors are the predominant causes of cancer (3):

Variation in Incidence Between Communities

There are substantial variations in the incidence of cancer of all types between various communities. For some cancers, these differences can be as large as 300-fold. For example, skin cancer, which is known to be caused by exposure of fair-skinned people to UV light, is extremely common in Caucasians living in sunny climates. Incidence rates in Australian Caucasians can be as high as 20%, whereas in Indians living in India or in Caucasians in temperate climates, the incidence may be up to 200-fold lower. Another example is the high incidence of liver cancer in Mozambique, which is 100 times higher than that observed in England.

Although there are differences in the completeness of registration of cancers in different communities, this does not explain the differences in incidence between population groups. For example, in the USA, Mormons and Seventh Day Adventists have exceptionally low incidences of gastrointestinal, respiratory and genital tract cancers when compared with other groups. In this case, the cancer registries are the same for all the population groups being studied. The high incidence of cancer in some countries in which cancer registries are poorly developed in comparison with the low incidence in the same type of cancer in countries where the registries are well developed is further evidence that inadequacies of registration are not overriding.

These differences in cancer incidences are seen for virtually all types of cancer and lead to the conclusion that either genetic differences in populations or extrinsic or environmental factors must be contributing to the incidence of cancer in high incidence areas.

Cancer Incidence in Migrants

There is good evidence that migrants carry the cancer risk pattern with them to the countries to which they migrate, but eventually, after several generations, their cancer risk pattern is the same as that in the local population, but different from the population from which they have descended. This phenomenon is illustrated by a comparison of the cancer incidence of black and white people in the United States with that of black people in Nigeria. For cancer of the rectum amongst males, the incidence in blacks and whites in the United States is high (approximately 200 per million per annum), while in Nigeria the incidence is low (34 per million per annum). For all cancers studied there is a difference in incidence between the United States and Nigeria, and incidences within various parts of the United States are similar but different from those in Nigeria. Similar observations have been made amongst Japanese migrants to Hawaii, where the incidence of cancer of the migrants is similar to that of Caucasians living in Hawaii and different from that of Japanese living in Japan.

These observations led to the conclusion that genetic factors play only a secondary role in the causation of most types of cancer, although it is recognised that certain genetic sub-groups may be particularly susceptible. The major factors resulting in high incidences of cancer can be attributed to social and life-style factors which influence environments within which people live.

Changes in Incidence with Time

As mentioned earlier, there has been a rapidly increasing incidence of lung cancer in England and Wales and the USA over the last few decades. This increase is generally attributed to the increase in the number of people smoking which occurred 10 to 20 years earlier. Lung cancer is now the commonest form of cancer in England and Wales. On the other hand, stomach cancer incidence has been decreasing over the last 25 years in virtually every country in which accurate records have been kept, although the reason for this is unknown. Incidence rates in England and Wales, for example, are now 49% lower than they were in 1950.

These changes in incidences observed in stable populations over a period of time provide convincing evidence that environmental or extrinsic factors are responsible for the incidence of cancer.

Identifiable Causes of Cancer

On the basis of careful examination of epidemiological studies, approximately 40 causes of cancer have been identified. Eighteen of these are associated with occupation, such as exposure to aromatic amines, asbestos, benzene, and other industrial chemicals. A further 13 are iatrogenic in origin, and 12 are associated with particular social or life-style factors, such as smoking, chewing of betel nuts or exposure to UV radiation in sunlight. All of these causes can be considered as environmental, although their total contribution to human cancer incidence is relatively small.

By a careful analysis of differences in incidence rates and incidence of cancer, Doll & Peto (3) have estimated the proportions of cancer deaths which can be attributed to various different factors. About 35% of the total incidence of cancer can be attributed to factors associated with diet, such as fat intake or meat consumption.

A further 30% are associated with tobacco usage. Infection from such parasites as Schistosoma and Chlonorchis could contribute up to 10% of cancers in certain populations. Reproductive and sexual behaviour, alcohol consumption, and occupation are associated with smaller percentages of cancer deaths. This suggests that between 40% and 50% of cancers can be attributed to causes likely to be identifiable by laboratory experiments aimed at detecting carcinogenic chemicals.

When all of the above evidence is taken together, it provides overwhelming support for the view that the majority of cancers are caused by environmental or extrinsic factors. These factors vary from one community to another, producing different patterns of cancer incidence in those communities.

STRATEGIES FOR REDUCING MORBIDITY AND MORTALITY FROM CANCER

There have been substantial improvements in the early diagnosis and treatment of certain cancers. It is not the purpose of this paper to review these improvements, but merely to note that although improvements in the treatment of, for example, leukaemia and the diagnosis of, for example, bladder and cervical cancer have taken place, this has had little overall effect on mortality from cancer. There seems to be little prospect for an easy or simple cure for cancer. Early diagnosis and effective treatment do form an essential component of our armoury for tackling the problems of cancer, but they are insufficiently developed to be relied on in isolation.

In the absence of universally effective treatment, and because treatment is ineffective in preventing human suffering, prevention should play an important role in tackling this problem. A key feature of any strategy of prevention must be the accurate identification of the cause of the disease which will allow the development of strategies for its control. It is for this task that laboratory experimentation, which may use animals, is an essential component.

THE IDENTIFICATION OF CARCINOGENIC HAZARDS

There are three basic methodologies available for the identification of carcinogenic hazards, namely, epidemiology, short-term tests, and in vivo tests. In addition to these methods, a variety of ancillary information, such as chemical structure analysis and toxicological information, can be used to assist in establishing the carcinogenicity of a chemical. The ancillary data are, however, insufficient in themselves to define a carcinogenic hazard.

Epidemiology

The study of cancer incidence in human populations is the only method which provides the ultimate proof of human carcinogenic risk. Epidemiological studies are, therefore, indispensible in the identification of carcinogens, particularly where a risk factor can be identified with some precision. Nevertheless, the difficulties of conducting adequate epidemiological studies have resulted in only about 40 risk factors being identified with reasonable certainty (4).

In spite of their importance, epidemiological studies do suffer from major strategic and operational shortcomings. The successful identification of a carcinogenic hazard using epidemiological techniques requires that a high incidence of cancer has occurred in an exposed population. Hence, the risk is already present and prevention can only be directed towards limiting further exposure with the likelihood that this will take several years to produce a reduction in morbidity. There are also significant practical and operational problems associated with the conduct and interpretation of epidemiological studies. The commonest of these is the difficulty of adequately defining exposure levels, particularly in situations of mixed exposure. In addition, a relatively small number of people may be exposed in occupational settings, often for brief periods of time, a number of people may be lost to follow-up, and finally, it is difficult to define with precision the normal population with which to compare cancer incidence in the exposed populations. There are also a variety of factors which confound the interpretation of results; these include social and geographic differences in incidences, problems with the accuracy of diagnoses, particularly on Death Certificates, and the problem of the "healthy worker effect" due to careful selection of healthy people for a particular work-force.

In spite of these difficulties, epidemiological studies play an important role in identifying carcinogenic hazards and in monitoring the effectiveness of control procedures, but are inadequate in preventing the introduction of new chemicals with carcinogenic properties.

Short-term or *In Vitro* Tests for Carcinogens

The main drawbacks to animal carcinogenicity studies are the large resources required to carry out such studies and the long time taken before results are available. Following the report by Ames and co-workers (5) that a *Salmonella*-based mutation assay was capable of identifying a large proportion of carcinogens accurately, over a hundred short-term assay systems have been developed (6).

Most of the short-term tests are based on mutagenesis assays and thus identify chemicals with mutagenic potential. There is strong circumstantial evidence to support the contention that mutation is an important initial step in the carcinogenic process, and hence the identification of mutagens using these short-term tests also identifies chemicals which have carcinogenic potential. Now that more extensive experience has been obtained in the use of these assays, it is clear that not all mutagens are carcinogens, nor are all carcinogens mutagens, and mutagens may not be active in all genetic assays (7). The mechanisms of chemical carcinogenesis remain largely unknown and, although there is circumstantial evidence supporting mutations as an integral event in carcinogenesis, this cannot be considered to be proven.

Even the simplest two-stage model of carcinogenesis, involving a single application of an initiator and repeated applications of a promoter, cannot be totally explained on the basis of mutation. In this model only the initiators are regularly identified as mutagenic and in general the promoters are not mutagenic. The consequence of this lack of knowledge of mechanisms of carcinogenesis, or of its relationship to the mechanisms involved in short-term tests, makes it advisable to rely on validation of the short-term tests using historical carcinogenicity data. In these validation studies, chemicals classified as either carcinogenic or non-carcinogenic are submitted for testing in the short-term assay. On the basis of the results obtained, the sensitivity, specificity and accuracy of the short-term test using the test chemicals can be defined.

There are many assay systems available, not all of which are equal in terms of their performance nor in terms of the degree to which they have been validated. A recent review has identified those tests which have reached various levels of validation and divides them into three classes (8):

1. The developing test. At this stage it is believed that the predictive test is of some value, and usually some mechanistic link with the chemical induction of cancer can be deduced. During this stage, relatively few chemicals will have been tested, often as few as 10, and usually less than 100.

2. The developed test. The test will have been submitted to a formal validation study where more than 100 chemicals of diverse chemical classes have been studied. It may be ready to use as a predictive test for carcinogenicity, depending on the outcome of validation studies. A successful test will have been demonstrated to have substantial advantages over an existing test or to complement it.

3. An established predictive test. By this stage, the test is in use in a number of the laboratories and a large number of chemicals, ideally more than 1000, have been tested. As a consequence, it has been shown to be of value in a number of laboratories. An understanding of the extrapolative value of the test results is beginning to develop and some of the limitations of the test are understood.

Using the above classification, the only test which can be considered to be established is the *Salmonella typhimurium* microsome assay, though a similar assay in *Escherichia coli* was also included because of its similarity to the *Salmonella* test. Of the 9 tests which were considered to be developed, only three appeared to meet the criteria of having reliable validation results and complementing the *S. typhimurium* assay. *In vitro* transformation in hamster cells provided satisfactory results in validation studies, but suffered from the problem of inter-laboratory variability. The *Drosophila* sex-linked recessive lethal assay and the micronucleus test in mice were considered to be successfully developed tests.

These established and developed tests are now widely used in laboratories throughout the world. The initial enthusiasm and optimism which greeted the introduction of the *Salmonella* assay systems have given way to a more realistic acceptance of their usefulness and a recognition that there are a variety of problems which limit their utility. It is now a well established fact that results from certain chemicals can be considered to be false, in that either carcinogens are not detected in the assay system or non-carcinogens are shown to be positive. The main reasons for these false results appear to be related either to detailed technical problems which may be overcome by modification of protocols, or to substantive differences in the mechanisms of the assay systems when compared with the mechanisms known to operate for carcinogens, or, thirdly, because of the well recognised limitations of in vitro systems with respect to the activation and metabolism of organic chemicals. These problem areas are often associated with particular chemical classes, which leads directly to the view that all in vitro or short-term tests have chemical class specificity as one of their characteristics. It is for this reason that the use of sensitivity, specificity and accuracy figures derived from validation studies cannot be used to predict the likely outcome of test results in isolation. The sensitivity and specificity figures are themselves altered by the selection of chemicals submitted for validation. For example, the sensitivity and specificity values for the Ames test varied between 40% and 100% (8). It is for these reasons that the simple positive or negative result from a short-term test should not be considered in isolation in judging the potential carcinogenicity of a chemical.

A series of decision criteria have been developed to assist in judging the results of short-term tests (9). The first, and most important step, is to establish that the result from a short-term test is confirmed. For this confirmation, it must meet the following criteria:

a. The result should be derived from a test carried out to a protocol meeting minimum criteria - i.e. the protocol should be supported by a formal validation study - or the chemical class control pairs should have performed as expected in the same experiment. A chemical class control pair is defined as a pair of chemicals, both structurally related to the chemical under test, one of which is carcinogenic, whilst the other is non-carcinogenic.
b. The results should be the same in two test systems with unrelated end-points.
c. The result should be consistent with the experimental design: for example, there should be a clear dose-response relationship; where no increase in colonies is seen in the bacterial mutation test, it should be established that this is not due to high toxicity; in a bacterial mutation test an increase in colony counts should be confirmed by a replicate plating.
d. The positive control used to check the reliability of the test should be used in parallel with each experiment.

e. The result should be reproducible if performed at different times in separate laboratories.
f. Assessment should be made of the likely contribution of impurities to the test result. Impurities which are strongly positive in the test system or highly toxic to the test organism can lead to incorrect results.

A confirmed positive result is produced under conditions where there are a variety of specific controls and checks in the experiments. Thus, the result is the best possible indication of carcinogenicity, short of actually carrying out an animal carcinogenicity study, although it falls short of proof of potential carcinogenicity.

In conclusion, it can be said that in vitro or short-term tests for carcinogenicity have developed rapidly in recent years. The most widely used and best established is the S. typhimurium mutation assay (Ames Test) for organic chemicals. This, and other methods, have a correspondence with animal carcinogenicity studies of between 50% and 90%, depending on the type of chemical tested. They suffer from the disadvantages inherent in in vitro tests for toxicity evaluation, particularly the unrepresentative metabolic system and the absence of complex immunological and physiological processes present in the whole animal. Their use is most beneficial for:

a. testing of chemicals used on a small scale;
b. selecting new chemicals for development, thereby giving a higher probability that animal carcinogenicity studies will be negative;
c. providing a better selection of existing natural and synthetic chemicals for submission to animal studies;
d. providing information on mechanisms of action.

These in vitro assays are not substitutes for carcinogenicity studies, as they provide data of a different nature, but they do improve the usefulness of conventional animal studies.

In Vivo Tests for Carcinogenicity

In spite of the strong humanitarian grounds for wishing to use in vitro tests to detect chemical carcinogens, the preceding discussion has indicated the limitations that these test systems have. The shortcomings of epidemiological studies, particularly in terms of their lack of sensitivity and their inability to detect carcinogenic activity of new chemicals, lead us inexorably to the conclusion that in vivo animal carcinogenicity studies must be used to detect potential human chemical carcinogens. The techniques used for animal carcinogenicity studies rely heavily upon observations made in the early part of the century and subsequently on the biology of cancer in experimental animals and man. The work of Yamagiwa & Ichikawa (1) demonstrated two key features of the carcinogenic process, namely, that repeated administration of carcinogens was required to produce an effect and that there was a considerable latency period before the occurrence of cancer.

Animal carcinogenicity studies have several advantages. Biologically, both naturally-occurring and chemically-induced cancers seen in experimental animals are equivalent to cancer in man. The long period of latency and the fact that for most carcinogens repeated treatment is required are common, both to experimental animals and man. Of more importance is the patterns of metastasis and organ specificity among the mammalian species. The experience of the intervening years has demonstrated that for the majority of human carcinogens which can be identified as specific chemical entities, there are experimental animal models which demonstrate an equivalent carcinogenic effect. In fact, apart from benzene and arsenic, both of which are human carcinogens for which no good animal model is available, all known human carcinogens are carcinogenic in one or other animal species. Of course the converse is not true; there are many hundreds of animal carcinogens for which there are insufficient data from epidemiological studies to determine whether they are carcinogenic in man or not. It is possibly worth mentioning within the context of the humane treatment of animals, that the majority of animals used in long-term carcinogenicity studies live out their normal lifespan. Indeed, survival of a large proportion of the animals to late in their lifespan is a prerequisite for accurate estimation of carcinogenic potential.

The main practical disadvantage of animal carcinogenicity studies is the enormous resource and extended time period which is required for the completion of a successful study. Depending on the protocol used, between 500 and 1000 animals may be required, and costs in excess of £200,000 may be incurred. From the initiation of a study to the final completion of a report can take between 3 and 4 years. A major disadvantage is the relatively large number of animals which are used for this type of study. Further disadvantages include the large number of unknown factors involved in the process of carcinogenicity, and poor understanding of the precise mechanisms of chemical induction of cancer. Also, the fact that the latency of carcinogenic effect appears to be proportional to the lifespan of the animal being studied is a paradox which is not yet understood. A further practical problem is that the shape of the dose-response curve at the low doses which might be incurred for environmental chemicals cannot be determined.

In general, the advantages of animal carcinogenicity studies override the disadvantages. There are no suitable alternatives which give the same amount of information which is relevant to the human situation. In particular, animal carcinogenicity studies provide the only data which can be used, other than those derived from epidemiology studies, to determine the potency of a chemical carcinogenic effect. Thus, if we wish to identify mammalian carcinogens and estimate the potency of their effect, and hence identify potential human carcinogens, we must rely on animal carcinogenicity studies at this stage of the development of the subject.

Although the principle of animal carcinogenicity studies is simple, namely, the application of a chemical to a group of animals and the determination of the cancer incidence in that group, in practice the conduct of these experiments is amongst the most complex in the field of toxicology. In a single study for regulatory purposes, 500,000 data points are accumulated. These must be tabulated and analysed accurately in order for the study to be completed satisfactorily. It is, therefore, not surprising that difficulties occur in the design and conduct of these studies.

The International Agency for Research into Cancer publishes a series of Monographs on "The Assessment of Carcinogenic Risk of Chemicals to Man". The Agency calls together expert groups who examine the published data on the carcinogenicity of a series of chemicals. These groups critically evaluate the published reports and in the process of their evaluation identify deficiencies. From a survey of volumes 26 and 27 of the monograph series, 76 reports with deficiencies were identified:

Inadequate reporting		33	(53%)
Inadequate design		25	(40%)
No controls	9		
Dose too low	5		
Test substance	4		
Duration too short	3		
General	2		
Supply of animals	1		
Numbers of animals	1		
Inadequate conduct		18	(29%)
Survival	10		
General	4		
Histology	3		
Inconclusive	1		

In the section that follows, an attempt has been made to highlight a few of the more pertinent issues with respect to the humanitarian aspects of carcinogenicity studies. The guiding principle is that, if animals are to be used for these types of studies, great care should be taken in their use so that the maximum amount of information is obtained from the minimum acceptable number of animals. The issue of individual care of animals has not been addressed, since it is common to the whole field of toxicology.

Experimental Design

The numbers of animals used have a direct influence on the statistical power of the experiment. An illustration of the number of animals per group required to give a 90% chance of detecting certain increases in incidence is given in Table I. For many chemicals which are being tested for carcinogenicity there is a potentially large human population which may be exposed. For such populations, increases of as little as 5% would provide a devasting epidemic of cancer; however, it can be seen that extremely large group sizes would be necessary to detect increased incidences of this magnitude. Experience from larger-sized studies has demonstrated that there are severe logistic problems in the conduct of studies with large numbers of animals. These logistic problems may lead to increased variability which would nullify the increased power resulting from the larger number of animals. Hence, a compromise must be struck between the desire to provide a statistically powerful study and the practical and resource constraints which will tend to limit the size of the study. For most regulatory purposes, between 50 and 100 animals of each sex are used for each group.

Table I

The Number of Animals Per Group Required to Give a 90% Chance of Detecting Certain Increases in Incidence When the Control Group Has a 10% Incidence and Using a Significance Level of <0.05

Increase in incidence to	Number of animals per group
80%	12
60%	21
40%	46
20%	255
15%	826

In the past, control groups were frequently omitted from carcinogenicity studies, on the basis that the background incidence of cancer was well characterised within the colony. Recent evidence suggests that there is a wide variability in the cancer incidence in control groups, so it is essential to provide data for concurrent and historical controls (10). In fact, many laboratories are now using two control groups in studies with three treatment groups, in order to reduce the chances of natural variability confounding the outcome of the study.

The test material should be characterised accurately. Knowledge of impurities and, ideally, stability, absorption and distribution are essential prerequisites for accurate interpretation of studies. For some chemicals, for example short-lived reactive molecules, the design of carcinogenicity studies is very difficult. For others with high proportions of impurities, identifying the chemical which causes the carcinogenic response may present problems.

The accurate setting of dose-levels is one of the most difficult features of experimental design. Because of the relatively small number of animals used in carcinogenicity studies, higher doses are frequently incorporated in experimental design to compensate. For chemicals with low systemic toxicity, there are occasions when heroic doses have been used in order to achieve the so-called "maximum tolerated dose". These doses frequently disrupt the normal metabolism and physiology of the animal to the extent that interpretation of the study becomes impossible. The aim should be to determine the highest dose in the study on the basis of a careful study of metabolism and disposition and organ toxicity, with the requirement that this dose produces no major derangement in the physiology of the animal being tested.

The duration of carcinogenicity studies has to approach the normal lifespan of the species under test, because of the long latency of the induction of cancer. However, if studies are allowed to carry on too long, the background incidence of tumours becomes so high that interpretation becomes difficult. Once again, a compromise must be achieved. The great advantage of applying a finite limit to the duration of a study is that the spontaneous cancer incidence is reduced, providing clearer criteria for judging the outcome of the study. From a humanitarian point of view, animals should be examined sufficiently frequently so that they may be killed before they suffer pain from any cancers that develop.

The strain of animals should be selected on the basis of avoiding the complicating effects of a high incidence of spontaneous tumours. The lower the spontaneous incidence of tumours the greater is the statistical power of the experiment. Ideally, an understanding of the metabolism and disposition of the chemical in the strain to be used should be determined prior to the use of that strain.

Randomisation is another vitally important aspect of the experimental design. Animals should be randomised with respect to litter, treatment group and location within the animal room. A block design is generally considered to be superior to complete randomisation. An illustration of this effect on body weights is given in Table II. For the majority of treatment weeks, there is a substantial reduction in error variance due to the blocking effects. Although there are no data to demonstrate that the same reduction occurs with respect to tumour incidence, there is a relationship between body weight and tumour incidence for both liver and pituitary tumours.

The macroscopic and microscopic pathology gives the majority of the information on which the carcinogenicity is judged. It follows, therefore, that attention should be directed at reducing errors in the collection and reporting of pathology data. One of the major errors in this field is the sampling error which arises as a consequence of selection of organs and parts of organs for histopathological examination. Standardised techniques which are used across all groups help to reduce these errors.

Table II

Percentage Reduction in Coefficient of Variation in Body-weight Gain Due to the Blocking Effect of Randomised Block Design in Comparison to Complete Randomisation

	Mouse		Rat	
Week	Male	Female	Male	Female
1	45	25	34	33
2	42	16	a	21
3	58	27	a	15
4	48	23	a	21
5	46	22	a	-
6	44	11	a	23
8	39	11	a	25
10	39	4	a	21
12	34	8	a	24
16	16	3	a	20
20	15	7	6	17

It is worth noting that the blocking effect was not observed in this study in male rats after week 24, and was also not observed when organ weights were considered. (a = data not available)

Experimental Conduct

Intercurrent disease is one of the most frequent confounding factors in long-term animal studies. The identification of limited duration as one of the problems in the conduct of studies reviewed by IARC points to the importance of disease-free animals. In general, facilities and procedures should be such as to control disease, so that early mortality is avoided and intercurrent disease does not confuse the interpretation of the histopathology. Various forms of specific pathogen-free and barrier-contained facilities are generally used for this purpose. In spite of this, early mortality from respiratory disease is a common problem in long-term studies.

The meticulous recording of data should be a feature of all experimental toxicology laboratories. The internationally-accepted Good Laboratory Practice procedures, which provide for the collection and recording of data in such a way that the study may be reconstructed from its records, form the standard which should be aimed at. Within the context of obtaining the maximum use of data from animals used, this principle should receive the support of all who are interested in the humane use of animals in carcinogenicity testing.

Reporting

The largest single factor which has led to inadequate studies is reporting. Because of the large amount of information now being reported in scientific journals, there is a drive towards reducing the length of reports. This impetus is leading to the publication of a number of reports which are inadequate for evaluation by the critical reader. This problem particularly involves methods and results sections, where critical events are too often omitted from descriptions of the experiments carried out. The essential features of an adequate report of a carcinogenicity study are:

Methods:
- Numbers, sex, strain and origin of animals
- Origins and purity of test material
- Duration
- Observations made including identity of organs examined by gross and histopathological techniques and the methods of selecting samples for study
- Method of randomisation with respect to identifiable confounding factors (e.g. litter, location, group)
- Statistical techniques selected
- Quality controlled diet

Results:
- Incidence, diagnosis and location of tumours
- Ancillary information on chronic toxicity to aid interpretation (especially histopathological data)
- Survival and time-to-tumour should be reported or specifically included in statistical analyses
- Statistical analysis which corrects for survival or incorporates time-to-tumour in the analysis

STRATEGY FOR TESTING AND EVALUATION

There are both scientific and humanitarian reasons for making the maximum use of the information available in assessing the carcinogenicity of a chemical. In particular, it should be recognised that data from animal carcinogenicity studies should not be taken in isolation, nor should such studies be conducted without reference to other valuable information on the chemical and biological properties of the compound concerned.

A good deal of information can be obtained by an initial examination of the structural, physical and chemical properties of the substance to be tested. Comparison of the structure and physical properties with known carcinogens and non-carcinogens, together with an appreciation of the likely metabolic pathways, can give valuable information for use in the assessment of carcinogenicity. The second obvious step is that an extensive literature search should be carried out to establish whether there is already any information available on the biological properties of the chemical under test. Even if long-term carcinogenicity studies are not available, other information on acute and subacute toxicity may well provide critical data for the design of longer-term studies. The third step which should always be carried out before embarking on longer-term studies is an examination of the action of the test substance in *in vitro* short-term tests. The appropriate tests should be selected on the basis of existing knowledge of chemical structure and activity. A thorough evaluation of all data accumulated from these first three steps should be carried out before the chronic animal study is planned. It should then be possible to identify the critical factors which determine the precise design and conduct of the carcinogenicity study.

In the evaluation of the data from both short-term and long-term carcinogenicity studies, it should be remembered that there is not complete correspondence between the biological effects of chemicals in the various systems and species under consideration. For short-term tests, such as the Ames test, sensitivity and specificity values of approximately 90% are frequently quoted. This is not the same as saying that the result from a short-term test has a 90% chance of being accurate. Such a statement can only be made in terms of general populations of chemicals which are being tested on the basis of the assumption that the chemicals to be tested have the same proportions of carcinogens and non-carcinogens as those used in the validation studies. This provides a paradox to the experimenter, who will only know retrospectively whether the chemicals under test are carcinogenic or not. Thus, the application of structure/function information and the careful evaluation of other toxicological data are necessary safeguards for the accurate interpretation of data from short-term tests.

Even data from long-term animal carcinogenicity studies cannot be considered to provide equivocal evidence of human carcinogenicity. The two exceptions of arsenic and benzene have already been mentioned. A comparison of the carcinogenicity of 250 chemicals in rats and mice demonstrated that for each species there was a sensitivity and specificity of about 85% for predicting carcinogenicity in the second species (11). Although little is known about the mechanisms of induction, there are examples of chemicals which produce cancer by indirect mechanisms. For example, diethylene glycol when administered to rats produces bladder cancer. In an elegant series of experiments, Weil and co-workers (12) demonstrated that the production of urinary bladder calculi was an essential prerequisite to the induction of bladder cancer. Doses of diethylene gylcol which did not induce calculi did not produce cancer. The examples of kidney cancers induced by nitrilotriacetic acid and local sarcomas produced by the subcutaneous injection of hypertonic solutions give further emphasis to the need for careful interpretation of the results of chronic animal studies.

In recent years there have been particular problems associated with the extremely high and variable incidence of certain neoplasms, particularly liver and lung cancer, in some strains of mice. The problems created by these variable incidences make the interpretation of studies extremely difficult. In addition, factors which can modulate a high incidence of cancer without themselves being carcinogenic have been identified. For regulatory purposes, it is frequently a requirement that carcinogenicity studies should be carried out in two species. The reasons for this are not entirely clear, but may relate to the intuitive judgement that the data from carcinogenicity studies from one species are not completely coincident with those from a second species. The perceived need for conservatism has then led to the requirement for a second carcinogenicity study. If it is accepted that the rat forms the basis of the first carcinogenicity study, the mouse is the most frequently selected second species. However, the difficulties in interpretation of mouse studies have led many to question whether this is a suitable strategy. The use of longer-lived and larger species, such as dogs or primates, for carcinogenicity tests should be limited for both humanitarian and logistic reasons. The need for a second species may be eliminated by the careful selection of data from a variety of short-term tests which are complementary to one another and to the results from the rat carcinogenicity study.

ACKNOWLEDGEMENTS

I thank Mr M. Godley and Mrs J.D. Wade for their assistance in preparing data for this study.

REFERENCES

1. Yamagiwa, J. & Ichikawa, K. (1918). Experimental study of the pathogenesis of carcinoma. Journal of Cancer Research 3, 1-29.
2. OPCS Monitor. (1981). Deaths by cause. Ref. DH2/81/4, 1/9/81. London: Office of Population Census and Surveys.
3. Doll, R. & Peto, R. (1981). The causes of cancer. Journal of the National Cancer Institute 66, 1191-1308.
4. International Agency for Research on Cancer. (1979). Chemicals and industrial processes associated with cancer in humans. IARC Monographs, supplement 1. Lyon: IARC.
5. Ames, B.N., Dursten, W.E., Yamasaki, E. & Lee, F.D. (1975). Carcinogens and mutagens: a simple test system combining liver homogenates for activation and bacteria for detection. Proceedings of the National Academy of Sciences, USA 70, 2281-2285.
6. Hollstein, M., McCann, J., Angelosanto, F.A. & Nichols, W. (1979). Short-term tests for carcinogens and mutagens. Mutation Research 65, 133-226.
7. Purchase, I.F.H. (1980). Appraisal of the merits and short-comings of tests of mutagenic potential. In "Mechanisms of Toxicity and Hazard Evaluation" (ed. B. Holmstedt, R. Lauwerys, M. Mercier, & M. Roberfroid), pp. 105-119. Amsterdam: Elsevier/North-Holland.
8. Purchase, I.F.H. (1982). An appraisal of predictive tests for carcinogenicity. Mutation Research 99, 53-71.
9. Anon (1980). A contribution to the strategy for the identification and control of occupational carcinogens. European Chemical Industry Ecology and Toxicology Centre, monograph 2, 1-22. Brussels: ECETOC.
10. Fears, T.R., Tarone, R.E. & Chu, K.C. (1977). False-positive and false-negative rates for carcinogenicity screens. Cancer Research 37, 1941-1945.
11. Purchase, I.F.H. (1980). Interspecies comparisons of carcinogenicity. British Journal of Cancer 41, 454-468.
12. Weil, C.S., Carpenter, C.P. & Smyth, H.F. (1967). Urinary bladder calculus and tumor response following either repeated feeding of diethylene glycol or calcium oxalate stone implantation. Industrial Medicine and Surgery 36, 55-57.

Carcinogenicity Testing

F. J. C. ROE

I need first to make clear that I fully associate myself with the aims of FRAME and greatly admire the efforts they are making, especially the organisation of this Meeting. However, I find that the sections of the FRAME Toxicity Committee's Report on long-term toxicity testing and on carcinogenicity testing inadequately recognise the extent to which present methods of testing are unsatisfactory. During the last few years I have been saying increasingly loudly that the way we keep and overfeed laboratory animals renders them exceedingly prone to laboratory artefacts, including very high incidences of neoplasms of various kinds and numerous manifestations of endocrine disturbance. These artefacts interfere with the interpretation of tests and frequently lead to their having to be repeated.

I disagree with conclusion 8 in the Summary of Conclusions and Recommendations section of the Report, "Except when carcinogenicity is being investigated, or where there is good scientific evidence to suggest to the contrary, the routine long-term toxicity test should not exceed 6 months duration". I am aware of many examples where non-predictable toxic effects have not become manifest in rats or mice until much later than this. A test which goes on for only 6 months covers only the rapid growth period of life plus a short part of early adult life, and would be irrelevant to the detection of effects on diseases which arise late in life or are the consequence of cumulative toxicity. It is sometimes possible to reduce the numbers of animals used by combining chronic toxicity testing with lifespan carcinogenicity testing and this is commonly done. In any case, it is in my view indefensible not to look as hard as possible for non-neoplastic pathological affects as well as neoplasms in the evaluation of carcinogenicity tests.

The Preliminary Report does not address adequately the distinction between carcinogens which initiate cancer by interacting with DNA and those which predispose to cancer by one of a wide variety of other mechanisms. In the present state of our knowledge, there are some grounds for hoping that *in vitro* methods might eventually be reliable enough largely to replace animal tests for the detection of genotoxic carcinogenicity. But the subject of non-genetic carcinogenesis is still in its infancy. All we know is that a wide variety of quite different mechanisms can be involved and that many of these entail the disturbance of homeostasis at the tissue level or whole animal level rather than at the cellular level. It is, therefore, in my view, premature to suggest that the search for in vitro methods for detecting non-genotoxic carcinogenicity should be encouraged.

In August of this year the DHSS published its "Guidelines for the Testing of Chemicals for Carcinogenicity", and I commend this document to all who are involved in the problem of carcinogenicity testing as the wisest official document on this subject so far published.

There are at this Meeting many notable experts on carcinogenicity, but only a few of them spend many hours every week looking down a microscope at sections of tissues from animals in carcinogenicity tests. It is one thing to think theoretically about carcinogenesis mechanisms, it is another to look at tumour incidence tables for significant differences between treated and control groups, and yet another still actually to look at the living animals and at their tissues after necropsy. Let me share this experience with you.

1. Here is a list of per cent incidences of certain lesions in control Sprague-Dawley male rats in a carcinogenicity study which I am presently reading:

Moderate to severe glomeronephritis	67
Parathyroid hyperplasia	67
Calcification of aorta	34
Adrenal medullary	
- hyperplasia/neoplasia	32
- neoplasia	20
Chronic fibrosing myocarditis	83

Does anyone know a human population for which these untreated rats would be an obvious model? These animals would, on the basis of these figures, be useless for assessing renal toxicity, cardiovascular toxicity, and disturbance of calcium metabolism.

2. The following hormone-associated neoplasms (%) were found by Kociba et al. (1) in ad libitum fed Sprague-Dawley rats (86 of each sex) observed for up to 26 months:

		Male	Female
Pituitary		31	63
Adrenal	- cortex	2	7
	- medulla	51	8
Thyroid	- C-cell	8	8
Parathyroid		0	1
Pancreas	- exocrine	33	0
	- endocrine	16	9
Testis		7	-
Ovary		-	5
Mammary	- fibroadenoma	-	76
gland	- adenoma	5	12
	- other	-	29

Could one have any confidence that an experiment conducted in such rats would be of any value for detecting a carcinogen acting on the female breast, or on the pancreas? In such rats one does not think in terms of percentage of animals with cancer, but in terms of mean numbers of, say, 3-10 tumours per rat.

3. At least six unnatural aspects of a laboratory rat's life clearly predispose it to a wide variety of disturbances of endocrine status, including the development of benign and malignant tumours of endocrine glands and of hormone-influenced tissues:

Food available 24 hours per day
Excessively nutritious diet
No need to forage
No need to avoid predators
Enforced celibacy despite sexual stimulation
General boredom

4. Consider the serum prolactin levels (ng/ml) in <u>ad libitum</u> fed Sprague-Dawley rats:

Age (months)	Male	Female
2	26	21
3	27	37
4	28	34
7	35	74
13	128	214
19	119	345

These and even higher figures in other experiments are secondary to hyperplasia and neoplasia of the pituitary gland - the tumours being prolactinomas. (N.B. The prolactin level in non-pregnant women is 20-40 ng/ml.)

5. The work of Tucker (2) illustrates the beneficial effect of controlled feeding, as distinct from *ad libitum* feeding, on the incidence of pituitary and mammary tumours:

	Male		Female	
Feeding regimen	*ad lib.*	restricted	*ad lib.*	restricted
Rats with pituitary tumours (%)	32	0	66	39
Rats with mammary tumours (%)	0	0	34	6

Conybeare (3), in an experiment involving groups of 160 male and 160 female mice, found that "controlled" feeding, as distinct from "uncontrolled", *ad libitum* feeding, reduced the incidences of a wide variety of tumours, including many of a non-endocrine nature:

	Male		Female	
Feeding regimen	*ad lib.*	75% of *ad lib.*	*ad lib.*	75% of *ad lib.*
Type of tumour				
Lung	30	19	24	8
Liver	47	12	7	1
Lymphoma	4	1	11	4
Other	8	4	12	4
Any tumour at any site	71	36	50	17
Any malignant tumour	17	7	23	7

6. Dietary fat can reduce liver tumour incidence dramatically in C57BL female mice (4):

	Mice with liver tumours (%)	
	Benign or malignant	Malignant
SS diet with 5% GNO	8	1
SS diet with 10% GNO	43 9	

(GNO = groundnut oil)

My plea is that if we want to cut down the numbers of animals used in long-term toxicity and carcinogencity testing, then we should fund and undertake research aimed at defining the conditions in which untreated laboratory animals can be maintained in good health until they are old. The research most needed relates to reducing the present astronomically high incidences of endocrine disturbances and tumours. Better control of the quality and quantity of diet is probably more than half the battle, but other aspects of animal husbandry need attention, particularly sexual frustration. In the long run, research of this kind will reduce the unnecessary use of animals by far more than pious hopes based on misconceptions of what carcinogenicity is all about.

REFERENCES

1. Kociba, R.J., Keyes, D.G., Lisowe, R.W., Calnins, R.P., Diffenber, D.D., Wade, C.E., Gorzinski, S.J., Mahle, N.H. & Schwetz, E.A. (1979). Results of a two year chronic toxicity and oncogenic study of rats ingesting diets containing 2,4,5-trichlorophenoxyacetic acid (2,4,5-T). Food and Cosmetic Toxicology 17, 205-221.
2. Tucker, M.J. (1979). The effect of long-term food restriction on tumours in rodents. International Journal of Cancer 23, 803-807.
3. Conybeare, G. (1980). Effect of quality and quantity of diet on survival and tumour incidence in outbred Swiss mice. Food and Cosmetic Toxicology 18, 65-70.
4. Gellatly, J.B. (1975). Natural history of hepatic parenchymal nodule formation in a colony of C-57 black mice with reference to the effect of diet. In "Hepatic Neoplasia" (ed. W.H. Butler & P.M. Newberne), pp. 77-108. Amsterdam: Elsevier.

New Approaches

J. W. WEISBURGER

The so-called "classic" procedures for the testing of potential carcinogens in animals have not changed fundamentally for the past fifty years. The standard bioassays for the detection of chemical carcinogens, as developed by the National Cancer Institute (NCI), require the use of male and female rats, mice, and occasionally, hamsters of strains selected for their sensitivity to carcinogenic agents. The standard test involves determination of the maximally tolerated dose (MTD) of a substance, after which groups of 50 males and 50 females are given the MTD and the half-MTD for two years. Other organisations, including the Food and Drug Administration, the Environmental Protection Agency, the Consumer Protection Safety Commission and the Occupational Safety and Health Administration of the National Toxicology Program, have come to require specific additional tests and expanded data. When the NCI began its carcinogen-screening programmes in 1962, a study of a given chemical compound undertaken in one species took as little as 8 months and its cost was of the order of $10,000 to $15,000. By 1972, a more extensive test in two species with larger numbers of animals took about 30 months and cost about $72,000. Today, after a further 10 years, tests on a chemical for multiple observational end-points takes up to 64 months and may cost from $300,000 to $500,000. The authors point out that animal bioassays by themselves can yield ambiguous results, especially in relation to human risk assessment.

When a test compound has yielded a statistically-significant excess of tumours compared with the control animals, it has been labelled a carcinogen, and the regulatory agencies have had to take appropriate steps to remove such a product, or otherwise to protect potentially exposed individuals. Most known human carcinogens yield a high incidence of cancer at a given site in several species in a relatively short period of time. In order to define human risk, relatively little additional information may be needed for such compounds.

Many other chemicals, however, yield less definitive evidence upon testing, but have nevertheless been represented as human cancer risks. An example is amaranth (FD & C Red Dye No.2), which appeared to produce a statistically-significant incidence of total tumours in female, but not male, rats in the absence of increases at any specific site. Nitrate was reported to cause slight increases in the incidence of spontaneous splenic sarcomas in rats. At very high levels, saccharin was reported as increasing the incidence of tumours in rats in a 2-generation test. As a result of these findings, amaranth was banned in the USA, but not in other countries, while regulatory actions were formulated, but not implemented, for nitrate and saccharin. Halogenated hydrocarbons appeared to increase even further the 20-40% spontaneous incidence of liver tumours in the mouse strains used, but were without any other evidence of carcinogenicity. On the other hand, false negative results appeared to have been obtained with vinylidene chloride.

During the last 20 years, however, there have been

considerable advances in our knowledge of mechanisms of carcinogenesis and, in particular, those related to the metabolic activation of chemicals to reactive electrophilic compounds: these can interact with nucleophilic cell components, including DNA. These developments appear to provide a framework for intergrating the determination of the genetic effects of chemicals into carcinogenicity testing, and a systematic decision-point approach has been evolved which entails a sequential decision-making process whereby specific tests are performed and evaluated prior to the initiation of higher-order, more complex tests (1):

Stage A. Structure of chemical

Stage B. Short-term tests <u>in vitro</u>

1. Bacterial mutagenesis
2. Mammalian mutagenesis
3. DNA repair
4. Chromosome tests
5. Cell transformation

<u>Decision-point 1</u>: Evaluation of all tests conducted in stages A and B

Stage C. Limited bioassays <u>in vivo</u>

1. Skin tumour induction in rats
2. Pulmonary tumour induction in mice
3. Breast cancer induction in female Sprague-Dawley rats
4. Altered foci induction in rodent liver
5. Assays for promoters

<u>Decision-point 2</u>: Evaluation of results from stage A through all the appropriate tests in stage C

Stage D. Long-term bioassay

<u>Decision-point 3</u>: Final evaluation of all the results. This evaluation must include data from stages A and B to provide a basis for mechanistic considerations

When compared with conventional bioassays in rodents, this approach provides knowledge based on mechanisms of carcinogenesis, yields a substantial amount of data at minimal cost and forms a solid base for eventual health risk assessment. The first six steps (stage A plus steps 1-5 in stage B) form the basis for decision-point 1. After definitive evidence of genotoxicity in more than one test is obtained, the chemical is regarded as highly suspect. By contrast, genotoxicity in only one test requires interpretation with caution. For decision-point 2, the presence of positive results in two or more of the rapid *in vitro* tests, together with a definite positive result in the limited *in vivo* bioassays, would render the substance highly suspect as a potential carcinogenic risk to man, especially if the results were obtained with moderate dosages. In addition, convincing evidence would be the finding of a good dose-response, particularly in respect of the multiplicity of lung or mammary gland tumours and positive results for mutagenicity and DNA damage. For decision-point 3, long-term bioassays should, as an end-point, yield definitive data on carcinogenicity, provided the bioassays have been properly conducted. Even so, results of the short-term *in vitro* tests should be taken into account in the assessment of the mechanisms of action and in the extrapolation of risk to man. Convincing positive results in the *in vitro* tests, together with documented carcinogenicity *in vivo*, permits classification of the substance as a genotoxic carcinogen. Such compounds, typically, are able (under some conditions) to be effective in a single dose, or they may show cumulative effects and potential additive or synergistic effects with other genotoxic carcinogens. If there is no convincing evidence of genotoxicity, but there are positive results in animal bioassays, the compound may be an epigenetic carcinogen. The fact that some stable organochloride pesticides do not show genotoxic properties in liver culture systems representing the target cell-type *in vivo*, may be regarded as providing substantial evidence for an epigenetic mechanism of action. Epigenetic mechanisms are poorly understood, and it is thought that they may involve long-term tissue injury, immunosuppression, hormonal imbalance, stimulation of cell proliferation, release of existing altered cells from growth control, or other processes not yet known. Most epigenetic carcinogens are active only at high, sustained doses and, up to a point, their effects are reversible. Such agents may represent only quantitative hazards in man and it may be possible to formulate safe levels of exposure after appropriate toxicological dose-response studies.

REFERENCES

1. Weisburger, J.H. & Williams, G.M. (1981). Carcinogen testing: current problems and new approaches. Science, New York **214**, 401-407.

General Discussion

PETER KNOX

Rapporteur

Professor David CONNING said that Dr Roe had explained how the apparent health of experimental animals could be improved by controlling diet and had asserted that this was the basis of a truly scientific approach. He would like to ask him if there was evidence that control of diet affected the sensitivity of animals to known carcinogens. Dr ROE replied that the carcinogenesis literature is confused in that artefacts cannot be distinguished from true effects; most carcinogens are compounds that increase the incidence of endocrine tumours in animals that have very abnormal endocrine status; this results in a confused literature. In one study carried out by Mary Tucker at ICI, using two carcinogens, there was a difference in tumour incidence in the groups of animals that were overfed, underfed or diet-controlled. This study, however, did not contain some necessary controls. For a given carcinogen, there should be treated and untreated animals in both dietary categories, namely, diet-restricted and fed ad libitum. FRAME could carry out a useful function in funding the experiments necessary to establish the effect of diet on carcinogenesis.

Professor CONNING recalled that Dr Purchase had indicated that the number of animals required for a statistically significant study is increased because of the "background noise" that occurs when the animals get older and reach the age at which tumours develop. He commented that epidemiological studies in man have also shown that there is an increased tumour incidence above the age of 35. He would therefore like to know if Dr Purchase, in order to reduce the background noise, would advocate terminating carcinogencity studies in the rat when they reached one year of age. Would it in fact be possible to design experiments to give accurate results at the one year stage? Dr PURCHASE replied that, while it is possible to design an experiment of one year's duration using the rat, it is anticipated that this would only detect the most potent of carcinogens. An experiment of longer duration would be necessary in order to detect most carcinogens. Dr PURCHASE added that he would like to raise some other points.

Dr Roe had pointed out that diet can affect tumour incidence, but he had oversimplified the situation. If one extrapolates to zero, i.e. if the rats are not fed at all, then of course they will not develop tumours. Therefore, in what way did Dr Roe suggest that the diet should be restricted? For instance, should the total intake be reduced or should the amount of protein or fibre be altered? He felt that there is so little data available that we should not at this time undertake carcinogenesis studies using diet-restricted animals. He agreed that it was true that if the noise is reduced then the statistical significance becomes better. However, there is always variability. Some studies use two separate control groups and it is not infrequent that there are different tumour incidences in the two control groups. Diet is not the only factor responsible for such variation. When he and his colleagues used animals and conditions similar to those used by Mary Tucker, they had not obtained the same results.

Mathematical Modelling

M. S. TUTE

OBJECTIVES OF MODELLING

The correlation of molecular structure with biological activity is fundamental both to our understanding of how drugs act and to the rational design of more-effective analogues. In recent years, considerable advances have been made in studies of structure-activity relationships, largely because of the trend towards expressing aspects either of "structure" or of "property" in quantitative terms. Quantitative expressions of structure-activity relationships have been used as mathematical models, and attempts made to fit biological data to these model equations, usually with the aid of a computer (1,2).

Frequently, models take the form of equation (i), where biological response (denoted by BR) is expressed on a logarithmic scale and correlated with indices (x_1, x_2,...x_n) of molecular structure or property. The indices usually relate to the degree of variation in a particular property among a series of related chemicals; they are then referred to as parameters.

$$\log BR = ax_1 + bx_2 + ...k \tag{i}$$

Suppose that x_1 and x_2 are measures of two physical properties, e.g. lipid solubility and ionisation constant. Such a relationship could be found to hold by using the computer to search for significant relationships between BR and a wide variety of physical properties; alternatively, such a relationship could be postulated to exist as a result of some theoretical model of drug action proposing that the drug should pass through lipid membranes and then act on its target (receptor) as the ionised form. In the former case, the computer has been used to derive a model. In the latter, the computer will be used to test a model.

Applications of statistical tests to equation (i) will reveal the overall significance of the relationship. The constant k in the equation relates to the sensitivity of the biological response being measured, and also to the activity of the invariant part of the structures being compared. The coefficients a, b.... of x_1, x_2.... reveal the sensitivity of response to the changes in properties parameterised by x_1, x_2 etc.

If the equation is found to be highly significant, then it is useful in two ways. First, a good correlation with physical or chemical properties can give insight into the mode of action of the compounds, and thus allow a more rational approach to be adopted to the synthesis of more effective, or perhaps less toxic, analogues. The equation thus has diagnostic value. Secondly, a good correlation with physical, chemical, or structural indices can be used to predict the biological response from other, related chemicals.

Models have been used to predict correctly the potency of analogues in many series of related compounds. They have been useful in providing insight into mechanism, and hence led to more rational compound design. They have also allowed an evaluation of the relationship between physical properties and pharmacokinetics (2).

RELEVANCE OF MODELS TO ANIMAL EXPERIMENTATION

An equation correlating biological response with various physicochemical or structural parameters is known as a "QSAR" (quantitative structure-activity relationship). As a QSAR may be of both diagnostic and predictive value, there are two ways in which a QSAR may be used to limit animal experiments. These are of particular importance in the context of the work of the FRAME Toxicity Committee.

1. The QSAR can suggest that it is no longer profitable to modify or extend a series of compounds in a particular way. As a result, no more compounds are made and resources - which include animals for biological screening - are not wasted.

2. The QSAR can allow the prediction that a compound which is available, but not yet tested, will elicit a particular response in an animal. Provided there is no regulatory body requirement for animal data, animals will not be used. The compound will be discarded without further testing (if the prediction is for an unfavourable or toxic response), or else be passed directly to a later phase of the development protocol. In this category, the response predicted may be either a beneficial one, or else be a

crude indication of overall toxicity (LD50, etc.), or of some specific toxic effect (convulsant, CNS depressant, nephrotoxicity, mutagenicity as measured in the Ames test, etc.).

Intelligent modelling, with derivation of a significant QSAR, is now an integral part of the research carried out in many laboratories, particularly in the pharmaceutical industry (3). Attention to the derivation of a QSAR can prevent a huge waste of effort and resources in the later phases. In a retrospective study, Kim et al. (4) analysed results from the testing of potential antimalarials. The Walter Reed Army Institute of Research had organised a huge programme of synthesis and testing; development of a QSAR for dialkylamino alkylcarbonols synthesised early in the investigation showed the futility of modification of the dialkylamino group in a search for more potent analogues, and yet many more such analogues were made and their activity assessed in mice. This was a retrospective study; what must be encouraged is more use of prospective QSAR in order to determine the direction of future synthesis and prevent much futile animal experimentation.

METHODS

Statistical Techniques

The technique most frequently used is linear multiple regression, and the least squares method is employed to find the equation of "best fit" between biological activity and a combination of parameters. Pitfalls to this technique have been discussed by Tute (5).

There are three common pitfalls. First, there must be a sufficient number of compounds included in developing the model to allow statistical significance to be reached despite the considerable error which usually exists in a biological - especially a whole animal - experiment. The more complex the model, i.e. the greater the number of independent variables x_1, $x_2 \ldots x_n$, the more compounds must be included. As a general, "rule of thumb", there should be at least four compounds per independent variable, but this will depend somewhat on the precision of the biological measurement.

Greater precision in the biological measurement (dependent variable, log BR) can to some extent be achieved by using more animals, but a better method is to ensure that the animals used are healthy and properly matched for age, sex, etc. The advice of a statistician is essential.

A second pitfall to avoid is that of including in the input data one extreme value of a particular parameter. Error in an extreme value (i.e. one lying well outside the range of values encompassed by all others) can seriously influence the result and lead to misinterpretation. A suitable "spread" but no extremes in any variable represents the ideal.

A third pitfall, very common in structure-activity models, is that some of the so-called "independent" variables x_1, x_2,.... x_n may be inter-related. This is best avoided by judicious choice of compounds for deriving the QSAR (6). A properly written computer program will test for covariance between all pairs of variables at the start of an analysis.

In the past ten years many other statistical techniques besides linear multiple regression have been applied to development of a QSAR. Thus, cluster (7), principal component (8), discriminant (9,10), pattern recognition (11,12) and non-linear regression analysis (13,14) are now routinely used (2). The choice of technique depends upon the quality and the quantity of data available (15).

Correlation with Property

Certain parallels, i.e. linear relationships between biological activity and physical property, had been noticed by the turn of the century. These relationships were between relatively non-specific and common activities such as narcotic activity, and properties such as solubility or oil-water partition co-efficient.

Only fragmentary progress was made until Hansch et al. (16) applied the linear free energy formalism of physical organic chemistry, using substituent constants rather than physical measurements on the whole molecule. An appropriate transformation of the biological activity data was made, to log BR = log 1/C where C stands for molar concentration of compound required to elicit a particular response. Substituent constants chosen for the parameters x_1, x_2.....x_n were quantitative descriptors of changes in hydrophobicity, electron effects, and steric effects. A particular triumph was the demonstration that incorporation of a squared term for the hydrophobic effect usually gave a correlation superior to that obtained by including only a linear term, rationalising the observation that an optimal hydrophobicity exists for all biological responses.

The Hansch approach has since been justified not only by many excellent correlations, of both diagnostic and predictive value, but also by giving chemists and biologists a physicochemical model of how drugs may act; in this way it has opened a new era of rational drug design (2,5,17).

Correlation with Structure

The classical Hansch approach strictly refers to the use of physicochemical descriptors for the right-hand side of the equation. This feature is generally regarded as an advantage, for it enables drug response to be visualised as the result of a series of physical and chemical interactions with body fluids, membranes, and receptors. But physicochemical property is not equivalent to structure. Many different structures can have the same partition coefficient between oil and water, i.e. property is a redundant parameter. This is not true of structure. If three-dimensional descriptors are used, structure can be expressed uniquely. Three-dimensional descriptors are essential to describe the difference between optical isomers (right and left handed forms) which can have identical physical properties but undergo quite different biochemical reactions. The ultimate goal is to express structure in numerical terms, such that significant correlations with biological activity may be achieved, and resulting QSARs decoded to predict structures rather than optimal properties.

As a result of the limitations of property correlations, there is growing interest in the application of pattern recognition methods. The main difficulty wth these methods, though, seems to be in "decoding" the QSAR in order to identify particular structural fragments responsible for the expression of a particular activity (18). And even if identified as "responsible" for activity, far harder questions for the model to answer are whether the structural fragment so identified is "sufficient" for activity, whether it is always "necessary" for activity, and to what extent its expression is modified by its molecular environmental.

Most pattern recognition methods use as numerical descriptors either the presence or absence of a particular fragment or feature (coded 1 or 0), or frequency of occurrence of a feature. They may be made more sophisticated by coding the spatial relationship between features. One interesting approach known as Molecular Connectivity has been pioneered by Kier & Hall (19). In their method, atom types and their connections are encoded in a set of descriptors at increasing levels of complexity. Molecular Connectivity descriptors seem able to express size and discriminate between structural isomers, e.g. between 1,2- and 1,3-dichlorobenzene, but they do not express shape or discriminate between optical isomers, e.g. D- and L-alanine. They can be used in conjunction with property descriptors (20).

Theoretical Calculations

Both structure and property of a molecule depend ultimately on two fundamental features: the position and the energy of all electrons. With the advent of quantum mechanics, the distribution and energy of electrons in molecules of biological interest can now be calculated, and such calculations are being applied to account for the affinities of drugs with their receptors (21-23).

The principal drawback to a quantum mechanical calculation is that one is forced, generally, to calculate properties of the isolated molecule. The influence of solvent, counterion, or receptor itself on the drug conformation is ignored, and of course, only certain facets of drug-response can begin to be treated by this method; complex phenomena such as drug transport cannot be modelled by quantum mechanics. Another drawback is that the calculations can be very expensive in terms of computer time. A trade-off is generally acheived between cost and precision: approximate values are obtained more cheaply using less sophisticated programs. Unfortunately, results of very high reliability and precision can only be obtained on relatively small molecules with the resources of most research groups. At present, quantum mechanics is being used as a sophisticated approach to obtaining physicochemical parameters by calculation rather than by measurement. The parameters that have been found useful in biological correlations are charge, electrostatic potential and the energy of the highest occupied and lowest empty molecular orbitals. Calculations are also applied to determine most likely conformation, ionic forms, and tautomeric forms.

RESULTS

Prediction of Acute Toxicity

The toxicity of a drug depends not only on its intrinsic activity at sensitive sites, but also on accumulation of toxic metabolites and loss of the drug to serum and tissue proteins. The prediction of toxic response is therefore not only one of the greatest challenges to modelling but probably also its most difficult objective. Nevertheless, a statistical method for prediction of acute toxicity has been reported (24). Enslein & Craig argued that the estimation of toxicity as reflected in the LD50 would appear to be a biological measure to which the QSAR technique can be applied. The expectation would be an equation that would give insight into those structural features which in general increase toxicity, and which could be used to predict the LD50 value of untested chemicals. Given sufficient confidence in the equation, perhaps the predicted LD50 may be used to categorise expected toxicity, and so avoid animal experimentation.

An initial equation was derived using data on 525 compounds selected from 549 in the Toxic Substances List (25). The selection procedure removed from consideration certain unique compounds which would have unfairly biased the equation, and contributed little to the analysis - a sound statistical method. Of the 525 selected, 100 were randomly set aside as a "testing" set, and the remaining 425 used as the "learning" set, or data-base to derive the equation.

The problem of choosing suitable parameters was next

addressed. This is particularly difficult in deriving a model to cover a wide diversity of structures, rather than a particular class of components. It was necessary to use many discontinuous variables, to code for the presence or absence of specified groups of atoms and structural features in addition to molecular weight (a crude indicator of size) and partition coefficient (often an indicator of transport through membranes). In all, 27 parameters were used in the first model to predict rat oral LD50.

A test of the equation with the 100 compounds not used in its design showed that 56% of the compounds were predicted with less than a three-fold difference between estimated and measured value. Enslein & Craig are currently recalculating the model, with a greatly enlarged training set (ca. 4000 compounds) and anticipate the standard error of the estimate eventually to fall below that obtainable experimentally from a single LD50 determination. Should this anticipation be realised, then the method could be used to predict the LD50 of compounds whose structures were "similar" to structures present in the training set. How similar they would have to be is a subjective judgement.

After publication of the preliminary model, members of the IUPAC (International Union for Pure and Applied Chemistry) working party on QSAR sought out comments from experts in QSAR on the merits of the approach. The working party produced a report, condensed into a publication by Rekker (26). This makes the observation that in order to develop a useful QSAR, i.e. to predict a biological end-point, three criteria should be met:

a. The mechanism by which the response occurs should involve a common rate-determining step.
b. The compounds considered should belong to a congeneric (closely related) series.
c. The active site in the biological system should be the same for each compound.

Clearly, since lethal toxicity can be the result of a great many mechanisms, involving different target organs or enzyme systems, neither criteria (a) nor (b) are likely to be met, unless the compounds are very closely related. In fact, the compounds are far from being closely related, and one can only conclude that none of these criteria for successful QSAR have been met, and that toxicity estimates from the model will frequently be very poor.

Another investigation into prediction of rat oral LD50 has been made by G.W. Adamson, D. Bawden & D. Saggers (personal communication). This study used data from one laboratory determined over a short time-span, and encompassing a wide range (1000-fold) in LD50 value. A relatively large, but more importantly for the study, a highly congeneric set (all 2-

trifluoromethylbenzimidazoles) was analysed. The high congenericity increases the likelihood that a common response-determining step, and common biological target, are involved in the lethal event.

Despite such criteria for successful modelling having been met, and after exploration of both discontinuous and continuous (i.e. structural and physicochemical) parameters, the best equations developed for the benzimidazoles still did not allow prediction with a precision higher than that obtained in the work of Enslein & Craig.

These studies would appear to establish that an oral LD50 value does not fulfil the requirement of representing a well-defined biological interaction for QSAR analysis. But, further studies are called for because it is still not clear from the published work whether the large standard deviation of the model is due to an inappropriate end-point for QSAR (LD50), or merely to experimental error in measurement.

We have come to the conclusion that any QSAR equation developed in this area should be viewed with extreme caution. It is not likely to replace animal experimentation, and at most can only be used for "range-finding" or to set priorities for testing. It may also be used to eliminate from consideration compounds likely to be highly toxic.

Prediction of Acute Toxicity of Hypnotics and Sedatives

Although the prognosis for development of a generally useful LD50 model is poor, modelling may help if the specific toxic interaction can be identified, and an appropriate biological measurement made. In the case of certain structurally non-specific CNS depressants, pharmacologically hypnotics, sedatives, and some anticonvulsants, the effect of the drug results from accumulation in the CNS. This effect may be directly correlated with physicochemical properties, though it is still complicated by blood flow and metabolism. King & Moffatt (27) refer to the fact that for a group of barbiturates, log P (P is the octanol-water partition coefficient) is highly correlated both with the LD50 for mice, and with the blood concentration associated with human fatalities.

Prediction of Mutagenicity

Much work has been undertaken to study the mutagenicity of organic compounds with the Ames test. Formulation of QSARs from the results can be helpful in diagnosing mechanism, and good QSARs can be useful for interpolative prediction.

In a study of the mutagenic potency of nitroimidazoles, nitrobenzenes, and nitrofurans Chin et al. (28) showed a correlation between electron affinity and mutagenic potency. Hansch et al. (29) developed a QSAR for triazenes and for platinum compounds, both important classes of antitumour drugs. The biological end-point used was the molar concentration producing 30 mutations/10^8 bacteria in Salmonella typhimurium (TA-92). For the triazenes, high hydrophobicity and electron-releasing substituents were found to increase mutagenicity. For the platinum complexes, hydrophobic effects were not found to be significant, and electron withdrawal promoted mutagenicity.

These results show that no generalisation can yet be made. Equations are useful only for interpolative prediction (prediction of a similar compound under identical test conditions). Moreover, to quote Hansch et al., "the equations apply only to especially sensitive bacteria in vitro. Whether the same compounds acting on mammalian cells in vivo will show the same sensitivity to substituent effects is an open question which urgently calls for investigation" (29).

Prediction of Carcinogenicity

Based on theories of the mechanism of carcinogenesis, there have been many attempts to correlate carcinogenic potency with reactivity indices. This endeavour started with the Pullmans (30) who used calculated electron density at the K-regions and L-regions of polycyclic aromatic hydrocarbons (PAH). Other attempts to explain PAH carcinogenicity were made by Hansch & Fujita (31) who used total K-region charge and hydrophobicity, and by Franke (32) who used K-region and L-region reactivity and protein binding.

Some unjustified assumptions in this early work, reviewed by Herndon (33) and Scribner (34) were:

a. that a reaction characteristic of homogeneous organic chemistry will be the rate-controlling reaction in a biological system;
b. that the carcinogen reacts directly with the target (rather than via a metabolite) to produce cancer.

In the last 5 years, models for carcinogenic activity have been refined. Attention has been paid to size and shape descriptors for the PAH (35,36) and on the theoretical side, calculations have been made at a much more sophisticated level. The Pullman K-region theory is now obsolete, since it failed to take into account the need for metabolic activation.

Many carcinogenic PAH contain a "bay-region", this being the region of the molecule between adjacent fused aromatic rings. After identification of the diol epoxide (A) as the ultimate carcinogenic metabolite of benz[a]pyrene (B), the "bay-region theory" was proposed: namely, that bay-region diol epoxides are the active forms of most carcinogenic PAH.

This theory received support from molecular orbital calculations of the energy differences between the diol expoxides and the carbocations that would be formed from them. There was a rough correlation between this energy, and carcinogenic activity of the parent PAH (37,38).

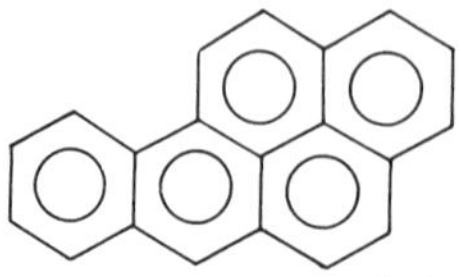

(A)

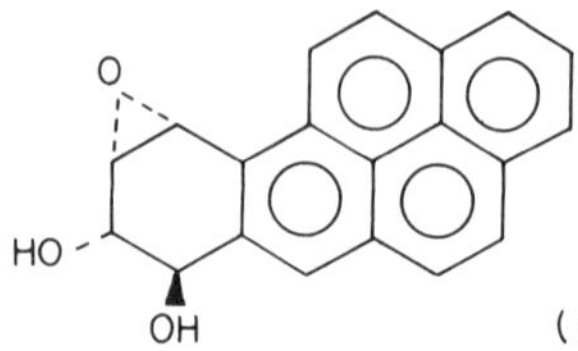

(B)

The bay-region theory was a major advance, but had to be modified to account for carcinogenic activity of PAH that are structurally incapable of forming bay-region diol epoxides, or indeed of PAH that have no bay-region. It is now believed that epoxides are formed from all PAH, and that carcinogenic potential is related to the stability of the electrophilic carbocation produced from the epoxide. Indeed, the concept of electrophilic attack on DNA, to induce heritable transformation, by some activated intermediate has proved to be a useful model to explain the activity of most classes of compounds which are carcinogenic (39,40).

In addition to quantum mechanical calculations, necessarily limited to in-depth study of a few key compounds, pattern recognition methods have been applied to correlation of structure with carcinogenic activity. Pattern recognition has been used by Chou & Jurs (41) to develop discriminant functions useful in predicting carcinogenicity of N-nitroso amides and amines. A set of 15 calculated molecular structure descriptors was used to develop a linear discriminant function able to separate successfully 116 carcinogens from 28 non-carcinogens, support a hypothesis as to mode of action, and allow high predictability.

LIMITATIONS OF MODELLING

All models of biological activity suffer from two types of limitation. A model is limited:

a. because of the simplifying assumptions inherent to it;
b. because of the approximations and/or lack of precision in the parameters chosen to represent biological, structural, or physicochemical effects (42).

Frequent assumptions of a mathematical model are:

a. that conformational changes in drug or receptor can be ignored;

b. that metabolism does not interfere;
c. that all compounds have the same rate(response)-determining step;
d. that linear free-energy parameters relevant to receptor affinity are additive;
e. that potency-hydrophobicity relationships will be linear or parabolic.

The clean separation of hydrophobic, electronic, and steric effects by use of relevant parameters is basic to the use of QSAR analysis as a diagnostic and predictive tool. Just as any biological screen is limited in its value by its relevance to a clinical objective, so parameters are limited by their relevance to the physicochemical effect being estimated. Particular difficulty is presently encountered in deriving relevant indices to represent intermolecular electronic effects, and all steric and conformational effects.

The limitations of mathematical modelling may appear to be overwhelming, but it should be emphasised that limitations are not inherent solely in a mathematical model, but are also present in any animal model used to predict a human response. The inherent assumptions and limitations of every alternative must be carefully assessed, and when this is done then the mathematical model will frequently be the method of choice.

SUMMARY

Over the last 20 years, models have been developed and refined in parallel with increasing knowledge of structure-activity relationships, and increasing availability of computers. The limitations of modelling heterogeneous, kinetically-determined biological actions using physicochemical parameters derived from homogeneous, thermodynamically-controlled experiments are clear. Despite these limitations, models have enabled us to gain considerable insight into the mechanisms involved in, e.g., carcinogenesis (43).

There is increasing use of structural data, and of theoretical indices derived from molecular orbital calculations. The problems of steric and conformational effects are now being tackled by interactive computer graphics (44,45).

Computer modelling has proved to be of some considerable value in rationalising and predicting biological data. This has not led directly to a reduction in use of animals to derive data, but has led to more careful experimental design with less wasteful use of animal resources. This trend will continue and must be encouraged.

PROSPECTS

The ultimate goal is an assessment of the biological reactivity, beneficial effects, toxic effects, or carcinogenic potentials of an unknown or untested substance simply from a knowledge of its structure. Given much more information, and an increased awareness of what is both relevant and reliable information to store in computer data-bases, this should one day be possible, and a marked reduction in animal usage will then be realised.

REFERENCES

1. Burger, A. (1971). Drug design and development. A realistic appraisal. Journal of Medicinal Chemistry 21, 1-4.
2. Martin, Y.C. (1981). A practitioner's perspective of the role of quantitative structure-activity analysis in medicinal chemistry. Journal of Medicinal Chemistry 24, 229-237.
3. Cramer, R.D., Snader, K.M., Willis, C.R., Chakrin, L.W., Thomas, J. & Sutton, B. (1979). Application of quantitative structure-activity relationships in the development of the antiallergic pyranenamines. Journal of Medicinal Chemistry 22, 714-725.
4. Kim, K.H., Hansch, C., Fukunaga, J.Y., Steller, E.E., Jow, P.Y.C., Craig, P.N. & Page, J. (1979). Quantitative structure-activity relationships in 1-aryl-2-(alkylamino) ethanol antimalarials. Journal of Medicinal Chemistry 22, 366-391.
5. Tute, M.S. (1971). Principles and practice of Hansch analysis: a guide to structure-activity correlation for the medicinal chemist. In "Advances in Drug Research" (ed. N.J. Harper & A.B. Simmonds), vol. VI, pp. 1-78. London: Academic Press.
6. Wooldridge, K.R.H. (1980). A rational substituent set for structure-activity studies. European Journal of Medicinal Chemistry 15, 63-66.
7. Hansch, C., Unger, S.H. & Forsyth, A.B. (1973). Strategy in drug design. Cluster analysis as an aid in the selection of substituents. Journal of Medicinal Chemistry 16, 1217-1222.
8. Streich, W.J., Dove, S. & Franke, R. (1980). On the rational selection of test series. Principal component method combined with multidimensional mapping. Journal of Medicinal Chemistry 23, 1452-1456.
9. Martin, Y.C., Holland, J.B., Jarboe, C.H. & Plotnikoff, N. (1974). Discriminant analysis of the relationship between physical properties and the inhibition of monoamine oxidase by aminotetralins and aminoindans. Journal of Medicinal Chemistry 17, 409-413.
10. Moriguchi, I., Komatsu, K. & Matsushi, Y. (1980). Adaptive least-squares method applied to structure-activity corre-

ation of hypotensive N-alkyl-N"-cyano-N'-pyridylguanidines. Journal of Medicinal Chemistry 23, 20-26.

11. Dunn, W.J. & Wold, S. (1978). A structure-carcinogenicity study of 4-nitroquinoline-1-oxides using the SIMCA method of pattern recognition. Journal of Medicinal Chemistry 21, 1001-1007.
12. Cammarata, A. & Menon, G.K. (1976). Pattern recognition. Classification of therapeutic agents according to pharmacophores. Journal of Medicinal Chemistry 19, 739-748.
13. Kubinyi, H. (1976). Quantitative structure-activity relationships. Arzneimittel Forschung 26, 1991-1997.
14. Martin, Y.C. (1980). The quantitative relationships between pKa, ionization, and drug potency. In "Physical Chemical Properties of Drugs" (ed. S. Yalkowsky, A. Sinkula & S.C. Valvani), pp. 49-110. New York: Marcel Dekker.
15. Tute, M.S. (1979). Correlation analysis as an aid to the diagnosis and prediction of drug activity. In "Recent Advances in Drug Research", pp. 95-120. London: Symposium Press.
16. Hansch, C., Muir, R.M., Fujita, T., Maloney, P.P., Geiger, F. & Streich, M. (1963). The correlation of biological activity of plant growth regulators and chloromycetin derivatives with Hammett constants and partition coefficients. Journal of the American Chemical Society 84, 2817-2824.
17. Hansch, C. (1973). Quantitative approaches to pharmacological structure-activity relationships. In "International Encyclopaedia of Pharmacology and Therapeutics" (ed. C.J. Cavallito), sect. 5.1, pp. 75-166. Oxford: Pergamon Press.
18. Golender, V.E. & Rozenblit, A.B. (1980). Logico-structural approach to computer-assisted drug design. Drug Design 9, 299-337.
19. Kier, L.B. & Hall, L.H. (1976). "Molecular Connectivity in Chemistry and Drug Research". 257 pp. New York: Academic Press.
20. Kier, L.B. & Hall, L.H. (1977). The nature of structure-activity relationships and their relation to molecular connectivity. European Journal of Medicinal Chemistry 12, 307-312.
21. Richards, W.G. (1977). "Quantum Pharmacology". 213 pp. London: Butterworths.
22. Green, J.P. & Weinstein, H. (1981). Recognition, response. The Sciences 21, 27-29.
23. Kier, L.B. (1971). "Molecular Orbital Theory in Drug Research". 258 pp. New York: Academic Press.
24. Enslein, K. & Craig, P.N. (1978). A toxicity prediction system. Journal of Environmental Pathology and Toxicology 2, 115-121.
25. Christensen, H.E. (1974). "The Toxic Substance List". HEW Publication No. (NIOSH) 73-134, 904 pp. Rockville, Maryland: NIOSH.

26. Rekker, R.F. (1980). LD50 values: are they about to become predictable? Trends in Pharmacological Sciences 1, 383-384.
27. King, L.A. & Moffatt, A.C. (1981). Hypnotics and sedatives: an index of fatal toxicity. Lancet ii, 387-388.
28. Chin, J.B., Sheinin, A.M. & Rauth, A.M. (1978). Screening for the mutagenicity of nitro-group containing hypoxic cell radiosensitizers. Mutation Research 58, 1-10.
29. Hansch, C., Venger, B.H. & Panthananickal, A. (1980). Mutagenicity of substituted (O-phenylenediamine) platinum dichloride in the Ames test. A quantitative structure-activity analysis. Journal of Medicinal Chemistry 23, 459-461.
30. Pullman, A. & Pullman, B. (1955). Electronic structure and carcinogenic activity of aromatic molecules: new developments. Advances in Cancer Research 3, 117-169.
31. Hansch, C. & Fujita, T. (1964). ρ-σ-π-Analysis. A method for the correlation of biological activity and chemical structure. Journal of the American Chemical Society 86, 1616-1626.
32. Franke, R. (1969). The possible role of hydrophobic interactions of polycyclic aromatic hydrocarbons with protein in chemical carcinogenesis. Molecular Pharmacology 5, 640-657.
33. Herndon, W.C. (1974). Theory of carcinogenic activity of aromatic hydrocarbons. Transactions of the New York Academy of Sciences 36, 200-217.
34. Scribner, J.D. (1975). Molecular orbital theory in carcinogenesis research. Journal of the National Cancer Institute 55, 1035-1038.
35. Kaliszan, R., Lamparczyk, H. & Radecki, A. (1979). A relationship between repression of dimethylnitrosamine-demethylase by polycyclic aromatic hydrocarbons and their shape. Biochemical Pharmacology 28, 123-125.
36. Arcos, J.C., Valle, R.T., Bryant, G.M., Buu-Hoi, N.P. & Argus M.F. (1976). Dimethylnitrosamine-demethylase: molecular size-dependence of repression by polynuclear hydrocarbons. Journal of Toxicology and Environmental Health 1, 395-408.
37. Jerina, D.M. & Daly, J.W. (1977). Oxidation at carbon. In "Drug Metabolism" (ed. D.V. Parker & R.L. Smith), pp. 13-32. London: Taylor & Francis.
38. Harvey, R.G. (1980). Carcinogenic hydrocarbons: metabolic activation and the mechanism of cancer induction. In "Safe Handling of Chemical Carcinogens, Mutagens, Teratogens and Highly Toxic Substances" (ed. D.B. Waters), vol. II, pp. 439-468. Michigan: Ann Arbor Science.
39. Lowe, J.P. & Silverman, B.D. (1981). Simple molecular orbital explanation for "bay-region" carcinogenic reactivity. Journal of the American Chemical Society 103, 2852-2855.
40. Ford, G.P. & Scribner, J.D. (1981). MNDO molecular orbital study of nitrenium ions derived from carcinogenic aromatic amines and amides. Journal of the American Chemical Society 103, 4281-4291.

41. Chou, J.T. & Jurs, P.C. (1979). Computer assisted structure-activity studies of chemical carcinogens. An N-nitroso compound data set. Journal of Medicinal Chemistry 22, 792-797.
42. Tute, M.S. (1980). Limitations and prospects for the Hansch approach to SAR. In "Physical Chemical Properties of Drugs", (ed. S. Yalkowsky, A. Sinkula & S.C. Valvani), pp. 141-162. New York: Marcel Dekker.
43. Walters, D.B. (ed.). (1980). "Safe Handling of Chemical Carcinogens, Mutagens, Teratogens and Highly Toxic Substances", vol. II, 278 pp. Michigan: Ann Arbor Science.
44. Gund, P., Andose, J.D., Rhodes, J.B. & Smith, G.M. (1980). Three-dimensional molecular modelling and drug design. Science, New York 208, 1425-1431.
45. Langridge, R., Ferrin, T.E., Kuntz, I.D. & Connolly, M.L. (1981). Real time color graphics in studies of molecular interactions. Science, New York 211, 661-666.

Structure-toxicity Studies

DAVID BAWDEN

The theme of this contribution is the increasing potential for rationalisation and prediction of toxic effects by statistical analysis of computerised collections of structure-toxicity data.

In recent years there has been a great expansion in the computerised storage and retrieval of chemical structures and associated property data. Such data-banks are maintained by both governmental and industrial organisations: some are generally available, while access to others is restricted. Data relating to toxicity, including carcinogenicity and mutagenicity, features in many such compilations. Associated with this has been the development of methods for retrieving, displaying and analysing the data, both structural and numeric, in the computerised collections. The facilities now exist for studying relationships between chemical structure and molecular properties, in this case toxic effects, rapidly, conveniently, and on a routine basis. One application is the examination of the inter-relationships between different test procedures (*in vivo/in vitro*, long-term/short-term, etc.) by means of multivariate statistics. Another, which is the main topic here, is the quantitative relation of chemical structure to toxicity. Chemical structure records may be automatically analysed to determine structural features present (ring systems, functional groups, etc.) and these may be directly related, by statistical analysis, to toxicity. Alternatively, numeric indices representing the chemical structure, or its physical properties, may be calculated from the computerised structure record, and these indices related to toxicity. This combination of a computerised data-bank, techniques for generating "descriptors" (structural features or numeric indices), and methods for multivariate statistical analysis, is a very powerful aid to the scientist in interpreting and extrapolating the results of toxicity testing. In some cases, this may amount to computerised assistance in the carrying out of "classical" quantitative structure-activity studies. Frequently, however, a different kind of analysis may be performed, characterised by analysis of large sets of diverse chemical structures, with descriptors based directly on structure rather than on physical properties. Such analyses may aim at prediction of some toxic effect, at the ranking of compounds according to toxic potential, or at indicating particular features of the chemical structure associated with toxicity.

Such analyses of toxicity-related data are being increasingly carried out by governmental organisations (e.g. the EPA's HEEDA system), by pharmaceutical and chemical companies working with their own data, and by certain commercial concerns on a contract basis. Doubt has been cast on the validity and appropriateness of some of these analyses, largely on the grounds of the poor data-sets used and the inadequacy of toxicological end-points, such as the LD50, for analyses of this sort. Dr Tute has echoed such doubts in his paper.

It is my view, however, that too hasty a condemnation of these approaches is a serious mistake, for two principle reasons. First, and rather negatively, there seems little doubt that such methods will continue to be used, and will indeed increase in scope. Given the proliferation of computer data-banks of structure-activity data, the availability of "packaged" computer programs to perform analyses rapidly, conveniently and at low cost, and the ethical and economic pressures for minimising the extent of experimental toxicology work, it seems inconceivable that such methods will not be used. Rather than adopting an attitude of indifference, or one of outright hostility, it is preferable to work for the improvement of such techniques, and for a well-informed assessment of their potential and their limitations. Justifiable criticism of current examples should not extend to a blanket condemnation of the whole area. Secondly, and more positively, we should remember that the material in our data-banks has been acquired at great cost in terms of human expertise, of economic resources, and not least, of numbers of animals used. It is therefore our duty to extract the maximum amount of information from this data, by whatever means possible. Structure-activity analyses are a powerful means for achieving this. If the data in our collections is really unanalysable, and must be used only for archival storage and retrieval, then the value of carrying out the experiments in the first place must be seriously questioned. If nothing else, structure-activity studies point out sharply the value, or otherwise, of compilation data, and of the toxicological end-points used.

It is, of course, of vital importance that the results of such analyses must be evaluated by appropriately experienced specialists, and that they be considered together with other structure-activity studies. Use of structural feature descriptions in analyses of diverse structures may well give insights complementary to those from "classical" QSAR studies, and I cannot therefore agree with Dr Tute's suggestion that future structure-toxicity studies should be concentrated solely on congeneric series and physicochemical properties. Since it is, in my view, both inevitable and desirable that such studies should continue, there are several areas which greatly need consideration and further research. First, the quality of data in computerised compilations must be constantly monitored, and improved: this may well necessitate improvements in the reporting of toxicology data in the primary literature. Secondly, much more work is required for improving the methodology of this area, in particular, investigating the optimal types of structural descriptors used, and the most appropriate statistical procedures. At present, virtually all such work in the UK is being conducted in industry, and it is desirable that there should be more involvement of academic and governmental bodies. Thirdly, there must be a wider appreciation of these methods, and of their limitations. Particular problems will arise for regulatory agencies and for the compilers of data-banks themselves, in knowing how to deal with "predicted" values for toxic effects.

REFERENCES

1. Craig, P.N. & Enslein, K. (1981). Structure-activity in hazard assessment. In "Hazard Assessment of Chemical" (ed. J. Saxena & F. Fisher), vol. 1, pp. 389-420. New York: Academic Press.
2. Hopfinger, A.J., Potenzone, R., Pearlstein, R. & Kikuchi, O. (1980). Structure-activity analyses in the classification of toxic chemicals. In "Safe Handling of Chemical Carcinogens, Mutagens, Teratogens and Highly Toxic Substances" (ed. D.B. Walters), vol. 11, pp. 385-409. Michigan: Ann Arbor.
3. Weir, B.R., Simmons, W.S., Fan, A.M., Livingston, D.L., Tesche, N.S. & Walton, A.H. (1981). Development of a format

for abstracting dose-response information from published studies for use in quantitative structure-activity relationships. Journal of Chemical Information and Computer Science 21, 14-18.

4. Lefkovitz, D., Rispin, A., Kulp, C. & Hill, H. (1981). EPA health and environmental effects data analysis system. Journal of Chemical Information and Computer Science. 21, 18-28.

Mathematical Models in Pharmacotoxicity

E. R. CARSON

INTRODUCTION

The role of mathematical modelling as an aid to the process of toxicity testing is assuming increasing significance. One facet of this has been highlighted by the previous contributions concerned with quantitative structure-activity relationships (QSAR), modelling the relation between chemical structure and biological response. There are, however, other facets of modelling which impinge upon toxicity testing. In particular, examining the overall research process within the pharmaceutical industry, it is clear that considerations of pharmacotoxicity are closely related to those of pharmacokinetics. To extract the maximum amount of information from pharmacokinetic studies it is necessary to make use of appropriate mathematical models. It is therefore appropriate to examine some of the key features of good mathematical modelling technique.

Modelling, if it is to be carried out successfully, should adopt a method such as that shown in Fig. 1. It can be clearly seen that overall modelling is an integrated and iterative process with components of model purpose, the relevant laws, theory and data, model formulation, model identification and model validation (1,2). In relation to obtaining model-based information which is to be used in connection with toxicity testing, the following features are particularly important.

THE PURPOSE OF MODELLING

The form of the mathematical model and the processes by which it is derived are principally determined by the purposes for which it is required. These include:

Estimation of physiological parameters which cannot be measured directly. Models can be used to make estimates of quantities such as fractional transfer rates, thereby enabling measures to be obtained for hepatic uptake of drugs and metabolites. Model-based parameter estimation can thus reduce the need for invasive animal experiments.

Enhancing experimental design. Models can be used in order to improve experimental design, for instance, where the dynamic response of a physiological system is being defined following the administration of a radioisotopic tracer. Since experimental data in such cases are often obtained by counting radioactivity in blood samples withdrawn over a period of time, there is a limit imposed on the information that can be extracted as a result of limitations on sample size and frequency. Using appropriate models, sampling patterns can be optimised so as to obtain the maximum of information about the system from the minimum of blood samples.

Dose-response models. Appropriate mathematical models can fulfill an important predictive role in relation to drug administration. Provided that they have been adequately validated, such models can be used to predict the response of the organism to varying doses of a particular drug or conversely can be used to determine the dose pattern required to bring about a particular metabolic effect.

MODEL FORMULATION

As can be seen from Fig. 1, there are three distinct components to the process of model formulation. The first involves the definition of its conceptual form. This requires specifying the variables to be included and the assumed nature of the relationships between them. In conceptualisation, assumptions of aggregation, abstraction and idealisation are necessary, consistent with the model's purpose in order that it shall be tractable. For instance, metabolic and pharmacokinetic/dynamic systems are often represented in terms of lumped compartments.

Having produced an appropriate conceptual model, equations are then constructed either describing the overall relations contained within the functional model or providing a detailed description of the physicochemical processes involved. Within the model, the relevant variables are commonly connected through

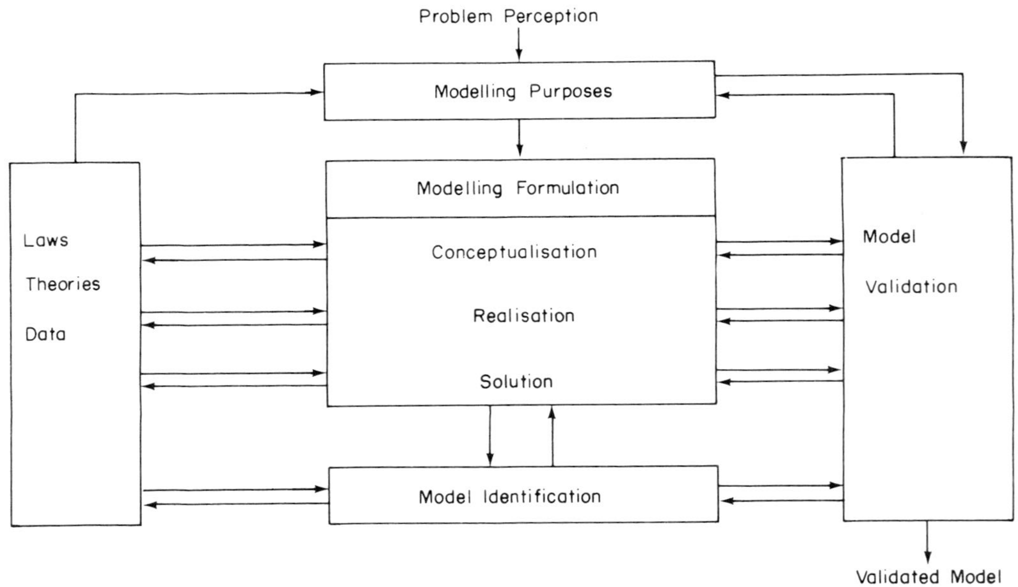

Figure 1 The Modelling Process (Carson et al. 1982a)

complex relationships, for example, differential equations. Model solution involves obtaining the required explicit relations between variables and/or parameters, often by computer implementation. In some cases, model structure and parameter values may be known a priori. Often, however, there is uncertainty in the structure of the model and/or its parameters. In this situation, solution is not possible directly and identification of the model from input/output data must be carried out. The two model forms most widely adopted in the pharmacokinetic context are compartmental and the so-called non-compartmental models which focus upon overall input/output relationships at the level of the intact organism. The only compartments explicitly considered are those, usually one or two, which are directly accessible to measurement. This approach, largely based on mathematical realisation using integral (convolution) equations, is particularly useful for studying systems where the parameters of interest relate to the one or two accessible compartments, for example, the blood-stream. Parameters estimated using this approach include distribution volumes, clearance rates and transit and residence times (1,2). Caution is needed however, since many non-compartmental models assume steady-state conditions. Whilst this results in easier analysis, it may not adequately reflect the underlying metabolic and pharmacokinetic processes, in which case a more complicated, but more valid, non-linear formulation should be used.

A more detailed description of processes involving chemical transformation and material transfer requires formulation as a compartmental model. Strictly, compartmental models represent metabolic processes in which the flow of material from one compartment to another can be assumed to depend, linearly or non linearly, upon the mass or concentration of material in the source compartment only. Such models offer the benefit of enabling estimates to be made of fractional transfer rates as well as compartmental sizes and other parameters which could also be obtained using non-compartmental approaches.

EXPERIMENTAL DESIGN

As previously stated, one important role of mathematical models is in relation to the design of experiments. This is particularly true in the case of dynamic studies including those involving the use of radioactive tracers, whether the experiments be carried out upon human subjects or upon animals. Where data for model identification are obtained from such dynamic studies there is often the requirement to minimise experimental effort, e.g. by minimising the number of blood samples collected. The principal experimental design features which then need to be considered include:

a. the form of the test signal (e.g. injection, infusion, or combinations of such signals);
b. the duration of the time over which output variables are measured, T;
c. the number of samples N obtained during T;
d. the sampling schedule SS - that is, where the N samples are located in T (i.e. the choice of t_1, t_2,..., t_k,... t_N).

It is now possible to design the experiment in such a way as to enhance the accuracy of the estimates of derived parameters, such as distribution volumes or transfer rate coefficients. Equally, it is possible to arrange a sampling schedule so that the number of samples required is reduced to a minimum. Details of the techniques whereby experimental designs can be improved in such ways can be found in DiStefano (3,4).

MODEL VALIDATION

Model validation involves assessing the extent to which a model is well-founded, tractable, and fulfils the purposes for which it is formulated. It is important to realise that it is an integral component of the modelling process, being firmly embedded within all its stages rather than merely being an activity which is carried out once model identification has been completed. The criteria in terms of which validity is assessed thus reflect the several stages of the modelling process. Validity is a multi-dimensional concept reflecting model purpose, current theories and experimental test data relating to the particular system of interest, together with other relevant knowledge. As new theories are developed and additional data become available, the requirements for a model to be deemed valid can change although its validity is still assessed in terms of the same criteria (2,5). The validity criteria involve first judging conditions within the model without external reference to purpose, theory or data. This involves examining the model's consistency - requiring that the model contains no logical, mathematical or conceptual contradictions (e.g. checking that the model equations do have a true steady state), and algorithmic validity - requiring that the algorithm for solution or simulation is appropriate and leads to accurate solutions. Having satisfied these preliminary tests, the model should then be assessed in terms of empirical validity, whereby the model should correspond to the available data and theoretical validity which requires the model to be consistent with accepted theories or models. Both empirical and theoretical validity criteria should be applied at any stage within the modelling process in a recursive manner. If at any stage the model fails to satisfy the appropriate criteria, it is necessary to return to theory and data, in some cases designing new experiments before entering the model formulation process.

The other validity criteria are pragmatic validity which is assessed by testing the extent to which the model satisfies the objectives of the use to which it is to be put (e.g. are the predictions of the model sufficiently accurate to be useful) and heuristic validity which assesses the potential of the model for scientific explanation, discovery and hypothesis testing.

Validation is carried out both within the modelling process as well as upon the completed model. For instance, within the modelling process the purpose for which the model is intended prescribes the condition of pragmatic validity which the model must meet together with any considerations of heuristic value. External validity criteria must also be considered in conceptual modelling and mathematical realisations, e.g. postulated compartmental structures must be in accord with available laws and data concerning physical and chemical effects occurring in the organism.

Dependent upon the model's testability, the final stages of validation involve performing tests and evaluating results obtained in terms of a number of criteria of empirical validity. For models in which the parameters are estimated using input/output data obtained from dynamic identification experiments assessment of validity involves the following quantitative measures:

a. Examination of whether the parameter estimates actually achieved are sufficiently accurate, for example, for them to lead to useful predictive capability in the model.
b. Examination of the goodness of fit of the model to the data.
c. Testing the statistics of the residual fitting errors to enhance freedom from bias.

After examining the fit of the model, its plausibility is tested in terms of the plausibility of the estimated parameters and of other features of structure, parameters and behaviour. It is then important to consider the extent to which the model is compatible with current physiological knowledge.

If the modelling process is carried out in this fashion, results can be obtained which aid the quantification of effects associated with toxicity. In this manner and by assisting in the design of better dynamic experiments, there is a real prospect of a further reduction in the overall number of animal experiments.

REFERENCES

1. Carson, E.R., Godfrey, K.R. & Reeve, J. (1982a). A review of modelling and the role of dynamic tracer studies in metabolism. In "Quantitative Approaches to Metabolism: the Role of Tracers and Models in Clinical Medicine" (ed. D.G. Cramp), pp. 1-72. Chichester: Wiley.
2. Carson, E.R., Cobelli, C. & Finkelstein, L. (1982b). "Mathematical Modeling of Metabolic and Endocrine Systems" 385 pp. New York: Wiley.
3. DiStefano, J.J. (1980). Design and optimization of tracer experiments in physiology and medicine. Federation Proceedings 39, 84-90.
4. DiStefano, J.J. (1982). Comprehensive dynamics of distribution and metabolism of thyroid hormones in blood and tissue pools using sequentially optimized experiment designs and a priori inequality analyses. In "Proceedings of the 6th IFAC Symposium on Identification and System Parameter Estimation" (ed. G.A. Bekey), pp. 902-907, New York: Pergamon Press.
5. Leaning, M.S., Carson, E.R. & Finkelstein, L. (1983). Model validation. Mathematical Bioscience (in press).

Quantitative Use of Structural Designs

J. C. DEARDEN

INTRODUCTION

Quantitative structure-toxicity studies aim to model a toxic response in terms of molecular descriptors. Ultimately, any biological response to a compound is a function of the electron distribution within that compound, and of the extent to which that distribution can be polarised, e.g. by the approach to a receptor. It is not yet possible, however, to describe biological responses in such fundamental terms, and we must at the moment make do with descriptors that themselves are reflections of electronic behaviour. Dr Tute has indicated that three very important descriptors are lipophilic, electronic and steric terms, although many other descriptors may also be used.

Using such descriptors, it is often possible, *within a*

congeneric series, to quantify the biological response, as in equation (i):

$$\log(1/C) = a.f(A) + b.f(B) + d.f(D) + \ldots \qquad \text{(i)}$$

where C is the concentration (in molar units) of compound required to exert a certain magnitude of response. Inherent in such a relationship is the requirement for all compounds to act in a similar manner at the same receptor site, which is why only compounds within a congeneric series should generally be included in such a correlation. Even within such a series, one often finds that, in LD50 testing, compounds may act at different receptor sites because of the high concentrations used; it is thus notoriously difficult to model LD50 data mathematically. Chronic toxicity testing (which after all is probably more realistic) is more amenable to mathematical description.

The importance of outliers in such descriptions is emphasised, since such compounds may be acting by different mechanisms, and may thus offer clues to greater or lesser toxicity.

THE IMPORTANCE OF EXPERIMENTAL DESIGN

There are a number of important points that must be borne in mind when mathematical modelling is undertaken. First, the resulting equation depends on the descriptors; use the wrong descriptors, or insufficient descriptors, and the resulting equation will be inadequate; i.e. the model is a poor one. Secondly, it is vital to have a good span of parameter space; for example, if all the derivatives tested have substituents of about the same size, one cannot expect the equation to indicate the importance of steric effects. Not only should there be a good range of parameter space, but there should be as even a distribution as possible of values throughout that space.

The foregoing emphasises the necessity for planning a modelling study very carefully, preferably with the help of a statistician. Retrospective QSAR studies are not recommended! There are numerous papers dealing with series design (e.g. 1-3).

SOME OTHER MODELLING TECHNIQUES

In standard multiple regression analysis, exemplified by equation (i), there are restrictions to be observed regarding the ratio of data points to descriptors, and regarding collinearity among descriptors. It is probably true to say that, because of these constraints, such analysis is going out of fashion, and more powerful methods such as principal component analysis (4), discriminant analysis (5), canonical variate analysis (6) and partial least-squares analysis (S. Wold, personal communication) are being more widely used. For example, Rose & Jurs (7), using pattern recognition via discriminant analysis, were able recently to obtain 97% correct classification of a set of 150 nitrosamines as carcinogenic or non-carcinogenic, using 22 molecular descriptors.

A rapidly expanding area of QSAR work is that of molecular graphics, whereby one may postulate receptor characteristics (e.g. by the distance geometry approach of Crippen (8)) or utilise known receptor sites (e.g. from X-ray crystallography of enzymes) to determine the substrate characteristics required for optimal fit. Much work has already been done on dihydrofolate reductase inhibitors in this respect (9).

I anticipate that over the next few years we shall see substantial improvements in the ability of QSAR to predict toxicity, via the above approaches.

I want next to mention two QSAR approaches which utilise more than one biological response. The first is that of Tichý & Trčka (10), who have shown that it is possible to predict toxicity in higher animals from the measurement of some response in lower animals. For example, using a series of alcohols, they have obtained an excellent correlation between LD50 values in mice and inhibition of movement in Tubifex worms. Tichý & Trčka have termed this approach QAAR (quantitative activity-activity relationships).

The second approach has been pioneered by Unger (11), and involves the assessment of multiple responses of animals to single doses of compounds, and then searching for correlations between those responses and some required activity. For example, in screening drugs for neuroleptic activity, Unger assessed 36 behavioural and other responses of mice, and was able to correlate neuroleptic activity well with five of those responses. There is no reason in principle why such an approach should not prove useful for, say, LD50 toxicity studies and thus reduce the number of animals needed for toxicity work.

TIME AS A FACTOR IN MODELLNG STUDIES

Finally, I should like to demonstrate how computer modelling studies of the distribution of xenobiotics in vivo have emphasised the importance of time in the assessment of biological response. Tute (12) has indicated that a QSAR is often parabolic with respect to lipophilicity - that is, biological responses passes through a maximum as lipophilicity increases. This enables one to calculate maximal response in a congeneric series. However, Dearden & Townend (13) have shown that optimal lipophilicity varies markedly with the time interval between dosing and assessment; they also showed that the time to maximal response varied approximately parabolically with lipophilicity, being minimal at intermediate values of lipophilicity. The implication of this for toxicity testing is that quite different answers regarding maximal toxicity within congeneric series may be obtained if different test times are used. Furthermore, if one considers maximal response instead of response at a certain time after dosage, the relationship is not parabolic at all, but becomes asymptotic. Thus a lipophilic compound that may not appear particularly toxic three hours after administration may prove highly toxic if the animal is observed until the toxicant reaches maximal concentration at the appropriate receptor site.

CONCLUSIONS

In summary, mathematical modelling of toxic response often enables one to predict toxicity within a congeneric series, and thus reduces the need for much toxicity testing. Some techniques can enable toxicity predictions to be made on non-congeneric compounds, particularly if information is available regarding the receptor. QSAR may enable much toxicity testing to be transferred to lower orders of animals. Finally, modelling shows that care must be taken with the interpretation of toxicity results in respect of the time interval between dosing and assessment.

REFERENCES

1. Hansch, C. & Unger, S.H. (1973). Strategy in drug design. Cluster analysis as an aid in the selection of substituents. Journal of Medicinal Chemistry 16, 1217-1222.
2. Austel, V. (1983). Design of test series by combined application of 2n factorial schemes and pattern recognition techniques. In "Quantitative Approaches to Drug Design" (ed. J.C. Dearden), pp. 223-229. Amsterdam: Elsevier/North-Holland.
3. Schaper, K-J. (1983). Rational selection of derivatives for QSAR analysis. In "Quantitative Approaches to Drug Design" (ed. J.C. Dearden), pp. 235-236. Amsterdam: Elsevier/North-Holland.
4. Dunn, W.J., Wold, S. & Martin, Y.C. (1978). Structure-activity study of β-adrenergic agents using the SIMCA method of pattern recognition. Journal of Medicinal Chemistry 21, 922-930.
5. Martin, Y.C., Holland, J.B., Jarboe, C.H. & Plotnikoff, N. (1974). Discriminant analysis of the relationship between physical properties and the inhibition of monoamine oxidase by aminotetralins and aminoindans. Journal of Medicinal Chemistry 17, 409-413.

6. Szydlo, R.M., Ford, M.G., Greenwood, R. & Salt, D.W. (1983). The relationship between the physico-chemical properties of substituted benzyl cyclopropane-1-carboxylate esters and their pharmacokinetic, pharmacodynamic and toxicological parameters. In "Quantitative Approaches to Drug Design" (ed. J.C. Dearden), pp. 203-214. Amsterdam: Elsevier/North-Holland.
7. Rose, S.L. & Jurs, P.C. (1982). Computer-assisted studies of structure-activity relationships of N-nitroso compounds using pattern recognition. Journal of Medicinal Chemistry 25, 769-776.
8. Crippen, G.M. (1980). Quantitative structure-activity relationships by distance geometry: systematic analysis of dihydrofolate reductase inhibitors. Journal of Medicinal Chemistry 23, 599-606.
9. Li, R., Hansch, C., Matthews, D., Blaney, J.M., Langridge, R., Delcamp, T.J., Susten, S.S. & Freisheim, J.H. (1982). A comparison by QSAR, crystallography and computer graphics of the inhibition of various dihydrofolate reductases by 5-(benzyl)-2,4-diaminopyrimidines. Quantitative Structure-Activity Relationships 1, 1-7.
10. Tichý, M. & Trčka, V. (1983). Contribution of QSAR analysis to data extrapolation between biological objects. In "Quantitative Approaches to Drug Design" (ed. J.C. Dearden), pp. 33-41. Amsterdam: Elsevier/North-Holland.
11. Unger, S.H. (1980). Consequences of the Hansch paradigm for the pharmaceutical industry. In "Drug Design" (ed. E.J. Ariens), vol. IX, pp. 48-119. New York: Academic Press.
12. Tute, M.S. (1971). Principles and practice of Hansch analysis. Guide to structure-activity correlation for the medicinal chemist. In "Advances in Drug Research" (ed. N.J. Harper & A.B. Simmonds), vol. VI, pp. 1-77. London: Academic Press.
13. Dearden, J.C. & Townend, M. S. (1977). A theoretical approach to structure-activity relationships - some implications for the concept of optimal lipophilicity. In "Herbicides and Fungicides - Factors Affecting their Activity" (ed. N.R. McFarlane), special publn. no. 29, pp. 135-141. London: The Chemical Society.

General Discussion

DAVID MACHIN

Rapporteur

Dr G.M. COHEN addressed a question to Dr Tute, saying that whilst he admired the approach of Hansch and co-workers in trying to optimise the conditions and identify those characteristics which gave a good therapeutic response and separated as far as possible the optimum properties of therapeutic response and the toxic response, he felt that what was happening in the leukaemia study was the optimising of conditions for treating leukaemias in the animal model. But how good was the animal as a model for the human situation? Dr TUTE replied that Dr Cohen had made a very valid point, which applied not only to mathematical models, but to all other types of model, including in vitro models. Modelling the Ames test, for instance, was an example of a particularly bad situation. A certain correlation could be obtained, but this was an artificial system, one removed from man, and in the modelling situation one could not really get away from that. Dr TUTE continued by saying that data from the Home Office Forensic Science Laboratory presented by King & Moffat (1981) illustrated a particular correlation with data in man. They had constructed a somewhat artificial index, but nevertheless an index of fatal toxicity in man. This index is plotted on the vertical scale as lot T, where T is the number of deaths from drug poisoning associated with one million prescriptions for a particular barbiturate. The authors had looked at several groups, i.e. several pharmacological classes, and correlated an index of drug toxicity to man from this particular technique with log P, which is the index turning up frequently in animal studies. There was quite an intriguing linear relationship between log T and log P ($r = 0.992$), showing that the same parameter that turns up in toxicity of barbiturates to mice and in measuring drug blood levels in mice, also turns up in fatal toxicities in man. Thus, there is a relationship, albeit a tenuous one. The way forward is to develop better models.

Mr MACHIN made two closing comments - the first, that a good deal of real data is needed in the building and testing of a mathematical model, and secondly, that any particular model is only likely to be evolutionary, in that as more data, experience and knowledge are accumulated, the model should and could be modified. Thus once a model has been developed it should not be assumed that it will remain in its original form.

Statistical Contributions to Experimental Design

G. F. HEALEY

INTRODUCTION

The importance of statistics in the analysis phase of an experiment is widely acknowledged. However, it is the design of the experiment which largely determines the validity of this analysis. Hence, the contribution of statistical principles at the design phase is also important. This report discusses some of the major design techniques which can be applied to assist the collection of valid and meaningful data. As a result, experiments may not have to be repeated, data may not have to be discarded, and the greatest amount of information may be extracted from the biological material used. There are several excellent texts on experimental design. Three books of considerable historical importance are due to Cochran & Cox (1), Fisher (2) and Cox (3). Many of the principles mentioned in this report are of general use and could be applied to any animal experiments.

REMOVAL OF BIAS

Randomisation

An important principle in experimental design is that the effect of extraneous factors should be controlled. These factors should not be allowed to bias a comparison between treatments. Random-isation ensures, as far as possible, that treatment groups do not differ in some unrecognised factor such as litters or age (4). Hence, all animals have an equal chance of being allocated to any particular treatment group. From a researcher's viewpoint, proper randomisation is a commonsense means of ensuring that allocation bias is kept to a minimum. It does not ensure that the groups are absolutely alike in all relevant aspects. It is somewhat analogous to insurance, in that it is a precaution against disturbances that may or may not occur (1). It also provides the basis of statistical inference which must be related to the purpose of the experiment.

There are many opportunities for systematic bias to creep into animal experiments. Differences between litters, cage heights and positions in the animal house are important examples. Factors which tend to be overlooked include those with a time sequential element in them (5). One example is the day-to-day dosing sequence for a particular group of animals. If a group of animals is to be injected each day, then a different order should be used each day. However, if one had an experiment with, say, four groups of 10, with a different dose-level for each group, randomising all 40 animals each day would be too complicated to carry out. In fact, the randomisation scheme can usually be designed to take account of the study objectives and practical considerations.

Randomisation in animal experiments is no doubt a nuisance. Animals have to be numbered, tables consulted and care taken over allocation (e.g. (6)), but, in comparison with other aspects of design, it is relatively inexpensive in time, effort and cost. Its function is to provide us with valid, unbiased estimates of experimental error variation, treatment means and differences between treatment means (7).

Systematic Operator Bias

One method to remove operator bias is by "blind" operation. This may be useful in at least three stages: the treatment application, the measuring of the response and the data analysis. The idea is that the operator is not told the identity of any particular treatment. At the application stage one would have to ensure that all preparations were indistinguishable and were administered identically. A simple coded labelling system would be needed. "Blind" operation at the measurement stage depends on the type of response. Assays for blood parameters and microbial concentrations in tissues, for example, can often be performed without knowledge of the treatment group. Bias can also occur at the data analysis stage, and it may be beneficial for the statistician to analyse data "blind". This is not always possible, of course, especially when a dose-response is to be investigated.

REDUCTION OF EXPERIMENTAL ERROR

Randomisation assures us of a valid measure of experimental error (7). This experimental error derives from three major sources. First, there is natural variability due to differences between or within the experimental animals. Secondly, there is variation resulting from lack of uniformity in experimental conditions. Thirdly, there is measurement error. Apparent differences between treatment means are measured against various elements of the experimental error. It is important not only to have a valid measure of the error but also to reduce it as far as possible. Two methods of achieving this will be discussed; blocking and the use of concomitant variables.

Blocking

It may be possible before an experiment to identify factors not related to the treatments, but which are almost certain to have an effect on the response. These effects must be allowed for in the experimental design. The simplest method is to use the technique of blocking. Thus, a particular experiment with four treatments might have litters as blocks. If there were five litters with four litter-mates each, one could apply four treatments to each litter, one treatment per animal. The comparisons between treatments could be made free of litter differences. These differences between litters could be removed from the experimental error by analysis of variance. Typical examples of blocking factors in animal experiments are sex, cage tier-level (see (6)), distance from light or ventilation source, body weight and age.

A good example of a situation where blocking might be used to advantage concerns the European Pharmacopoeia pyrogen test in rabbits. Important sources of variation in response appear to be body weight and sex (8). Failure to recognise this may cause high error variation or an imbalance relative to the two factors, resulting in wrong decisions or irreproducibility of results.

Several blocking factors may be used in a single experiment, although in practice the Latin Square, with treatments balanced for two factors, is the most complex of the useful designs. With more factors, allocation of animals to treatments becomes more complicated. If the blocks are sufficiently large (e.g. large litters) it may be possible to arrange that each treatment occurs two or more times within a block. Each block then provides its own "internal replication" which allows treatments to be compared within a block. This would be useful if the blocks were interesting in their own right, e.g. if they were strains or sex (4).

Note that the "levels" of the blocks can be widely different. The same experiment could be performed in several laboratories.

The estimate of any treatment differences is then effectively pooled over the laboratories. This would increase the applicability of the results. It might also be possible to exclude absolute differences in the level of response between laboratories from the experimental error. Another possibility is to use several different inbred strains as blocks. This could be better than using a single outbred strain; the applicability is preserved and the error kept down.

In experiments with blocking there is always the possibility of treatment/block interactions. For example, treatment differences may be large in one litter yet small in another. This can sometimes be overcome by applying transformations to the data, but the interactions may in themselves be interesting if not problematic.

It seems that blocking is not as widely used in animal testing as it is in other applications (9). Certainly, much of the development of these methods was in the field of agriculture. Yet blocking follows naturally from the identification of major sources of variation, as true in animal studies as in field experiments.

Cross-over Designs

A further possibility is to use each single animal as a block and make within-animal comparisons. If two groups of mice are to be given either control or drug, then it may be much more precise to administer them to the same animals sequentially, using a cross-over design. The between-animal variablility is still estimated but, since each treatment occurs in each animal, the individual animals are effectively blocks. The drug-control comparison is done within-animals and does not depend on between-animal variation.

Many types of such design are possible, and reductions in the numbers of animals required may be substantial. The gain will be greatest when there is high variability from animal to animal but low variability within an animal (10). One assumption of such designs is that a particular treatment response is not affected by any previous treatment. An adequate recovery or "wash-out" period between treatments may ensure this. However, residual effects such as high antibody production or increased tolerance may still occur, so these designs need to be used with caution.

A most important factor is whether such experiments are possible within the framework of the Home Office regulations (11). Using the same animal in several phases of an experiment may involve unacceptable suffering, even if it is allowed to fully recover between each stage. Therefore, these designs may not be appropriate for many toxicity studies or those efficacy studies involving prior infection with a pathogen or induction of particular lesions. However, they may be useful for basic pharmacological work or for bioassays where the response measurement involves no significant suffering.

Use of Concomitant Variables

A further method of reducing the error variation is by exploiting the dependence of a response on uncontrolled "concomitant" variables. For example, the frequent dependence of a response on body weight means that doses are usually adjusted according to body weight (mg/kg) before the experiment. This particular proportional adjustment implies a linear relationship, with zero intercept, between response and body weight. However, this may be far too restrictive. It may be better to merely record body weight, administer equal doses and then use analyses of covariance (ANCOVA) to determine the true relationship between response and body weight (10).

In many biological situations the relationship between some response y and a concomitant variable x is of the form y = axb. Such a relationship has been found between basal metabolic rate and body weight, with b = 0.75 (12). A preliminary plot of log y against log x should then show approximate linearity. A slope of 1 would imply y = ax, the proportional adjustment model, whilst a slope of 0 would suggest y = a with no effect of the concomitant variable. If there is clearly some non-zero relationship then an analysis of covariance (with x or log x) would reduce the experimental error and make the study more precise. The extra computational effort is unlikely to be a problem these days, and it is worth pointing out that making adjustments on assumed relationships may cause a loss in precision over non-adjustment if, for example, one made an over-correction for the effect of body weight (10).

To determine the improvement made after a covariate has been used, the "relative efficiency" can be calculated (1,13). A useful study of the effect of covariates on organ weight (with particular reference to beagles) has recently appeared (14).

Other typical covariates are pre-treatment temperature, initial blood glucose level, etc. It is not widely realised that any number of concomitant variables can be used. For example, the researcher could include both body weight and age as covariates. This would be especially recommended at the beginning of a series of assays. If either concomitant factor fails to reduce the error significantly, then after a few assays it may be omitted.

REPLICATION

An experimental unit is the unit of biological material to which one application of treatment is applied. When a treatment appears more than once in an experiment, it is said to be replicated (7). The functions of replication are threefold. First, it allows the estimation of the experimental error with sufficient degrees of freedom (i.e. the effective number of observations). Secondly, it improves the precision of the experiment by reducing the standard error of a treatment mean. Sample size calculations can indicate the numbers required to detect a given treatment difference (e.g. (1)). Thirdly, replication can increase the scope of the inference by appropriate selection of experimental units (7).

Estimation of Experimental Error

The experimental error should be estimated from variation amongst observations on experimental units. Consider the comparison of two treatments, each applied to several animals, where the variable of interest is the frequency of a particular type of cell in the spleen. Each spleen is homogenised, split into three and then assayed. The triplicates only reflect variation in the final part of the assay. This variation will be small compared with the between-animal variation. Such "within-assay" replication may usefully serve as a safeguard against inaccurate measurements, but cannot provide an estimate of error for treatment differences.

The same principle may sometimes apply to the caging of animals. If mice within a treatment group are housed more than one to a cage, their responses may be correlated. This correlation could make the response more similar than if the animals had been caged separately. In this case the cage should become the experimental unit (15) and the replication within a cage would be less important than replication of the cages themselves. When a treatment group consists of several cages each housing more than one animal, then the between-cage and within-cage variation can be estimated separately (10).

It is common in agricultural experiments to take into account the effects of neighbouring plots. Similar effects have been found in animal experiments where cross-infectivity by rhinoviruses may extend for several cages and considerable distances (16). Such effects can reduce the amount of true replication by reducing the independence of the experimental units.

Making large numbers of replicate measurements over time on the same animal may increase the amount of information derived from that animal. The absorption of a chemical over time and the development of a treated lesion over time are two typical examples. There are two problems, however. First, the replication may not be of much use for treatment comparisons, since results at adjacent times will be highly correlated. Secondly, standard summary parameters such as "time-to-peak-response" or "area-under-the-curve" may be highly correlated so that they do not complement each other. The adequate summary of time-curves requires careful thought to maximise the amount of derived information. It may be preferable to increase the number of response variables.

Precision

An experiment should not be over-precise or under-precise, and should therefore have the correct amount of replication. There is little value in performing an experiment if resources do not allow sufficient replication to detect important effects. Conversely, there is no point in using 10 animals per group if 4 would be adequate. In fact, if the result of an animal experiment is so obvious as to not require any statistical analysis, then it is likely that fewer animals could have been used. Much statistical endeavour in the last fifty years has been directed towards inference from small samples.

Scope of Inference

The required scope of inference of an experiment determines the selection of the experimental units. For example, a particular inbred strain of animal may show a treatment effect, but such a result may only have limited applicability. To increase the scope of inference, different strains could be included. The experimental units would be more variable (animals from different strains) and appropriate designs would be needed. Here, replication is over inbred strains rather than, say, within a single outbred strain. The scope of inference is increased and the error variation controlled (17). Treatments are compared within each strain, and how the comparisons vary over the strains can also be seen. The pooling of results over strains may, however, be difficult and is analogous to the problems of pooling data from several experiments (e.g. (13)).

FACTORIAL DESIGN

Two-factor Designs

At the present time, much animal experimentation is carried out with simple experimental designs. A common design is the "completely randomised design" with, say, 10 animals randomly assigned to each of four dosage groups. Subsequent analysis is straightforward. In some situations however, more complex designs can often be used either to increase the precision of the experiment or to obtain more information from the same material.

Increasing the precision of experiments can be achieved by the methods described earlier. To increase the information from the same amount of material one can increase the complexity of the treatment structure. If, for example, three compounds were to be compared in each sex, a 3 x 2 factorial design could be used. There would be six treatment groups, one for each combination of compound and sex. This design, by using every combination of the two factors, allows the average effects of each factor, and their interaction, to be estimated simultaneously. By this approach, the consistency of the difference between the three compounds over the sexes may be tested. If there is no interaction then observations may be pooled over the sexes in making comparisons between compounds (13,18).

A further example of the type of improvement that can be achieved is as follows. Consider the daily administration of an anti-infection drug at a particular dose-level to a certain species of animal. The researcher may want to compare three starting times for dosing, e.g. -1, +1 and +3 days after infection, and three dose regimes, e.g. dosing for one, two or three days. The simplest approach would be to perform two separate completely randomised experiments (each with one factor fixed). With 36 animals available, the two ANOVA (analysis of variance) tables would be:

Source	df
Times	2
Error	15
Total	17

Source	df
Regimes	2
Error	15
Total	17

Instead of two separate experiments of 18 animals, a 3 x 3 factorial design could be used with 4 animals for each of the 9 combinations:

Source	df
Times	2
Regimes	2
Times x Regimes	4
Error	27
Total	35

Hence, with the same number of animals, we have obtained an estimate of error based on more degrees of freedom, and we also have information on the starting times by regimes interaction. Notice that if there was no interaction, then the two factors would be independent. The above experiment could then be considered as a comparison of starting times or as a comparison of regimes, each with 36 observations.

Designs with Several Factors

For screening applications, the complexity of designs with more factors may militate against their use. Sometimes, however, designs with many factors may be worthwhile and, if used, would extract a great amount of information out of relatively little biological material. For example, in growth experiments, a large number of factors might be involved - light, temperature, diet, etc. The one-at-a-time approach, each experiment looking at only one factor, is inefficient. With a factorial design for 4 factors at 2 levels there would be 16 combinations. However, not all combinations need be used. A "fractional factorial design" with only 4 combinations may still allow all major factors to be estimated. Only if there were large "higher-order" interactions (i.e. those involving three or more factors) would there be a problem of interpretation (1).

Allocation in 2 x 2 Designs

Interesting results on the allocation of animals in 2 x 2 factorial experiments designed to study the interaction of two toxic agents have recently been obtained (19). Such experiments will have four groups: untreated control, agent 1, agent 2, and a combination group where both agents are applied at the same time. Given a binary (all-or-none) toxic response variable, it is possible to allocate animals to the four groups so as to maximise the information on the interaction. It is suggested that a greater proportion of animals should be in the combination group than in the control group. Gains of up to 20% in efficiency may be possible. This means that the experiment would need up to 20% fewer animals than the equivalent equi-replicate experiment.

Design Complexity

Despite the apparent complexity of factorial designs, the statistical analysis is quite easy and details are readily found in the literature (e.g. (1)). In general, the labour of statistical analysis for an important experiment would be a small part of the total labour involved and considerations of the complexity should not influence the choice of design (11).

LD50 TESTING

The area of acute toxicity testing has been discussed in detail by Dr V.K. Brown in another section of these Proceedings. The use of LD50 testing will remain widespread for some years to come, partly because of regulatory requirements, partly because alternatives such as computer prediction are not sufficiently developed as yet (20). Some possibilities for improving LD50 estimation will therefore be discussed.

Fixed-dose Testing

For fixed-dose or "classical" testing, the variance of an LD50 estimate is decreased by:

a. improving dose selection;
b. steeper dose-response;
c. reducing systematic variability between dose-levels;
d. increasing the number of animals.

Prior information, such as a small dose-ranging study, should allow the mean of the doses to be fairly close to the LD50. The next stage is to choose a range for the dose-levels. A compromise must be struck to ensure that the range of dose-levels is wide enough to give a good estimate of the dose-response equation, but that the outer doses are not too extreme. This could be achieved by choosing the lowest and highest doses to be around those corresponding to the expected 10% and 90% responses (5).

The dose-response slope depends mainly on the range of tolerance shown by the particular species to the particular compound. Animals of an inbred strain might be expected to respond more similarly to each other than those of an outbred strain. This would result in a steeper slope for the inbred strain and reduced variance of the LD50 estimate. However, the applicability of such a result would have to be considered.

Staircase Testing

One method of ensuring that the majority of animals are tested near the LD50 even without a dose-ranging or pilot study, is by using the "up-and-down" or staircase method of estimation (21). This is a sequential method. Briefly, if the first animal dies the dose is decreased. If the next animal survives the dose is then increased. The tested doses eventually oscillate around the LD50. The test requires a starting dose, a dose step-length (both usually in log terms) and an end-point (the number of trials, N, after and including the first unlike pair of responses). In fact, if a reasonable step-size is chosen, the starting dose is not important (21).

This method has several advantages. The test is "robust" in the sense that estimation does not depend on the choice of dose-response model or tolerance distribution. The calculations are easy and do not require complicated computer programs such as those for probit analysis. Furthermore, few animals are tested at extreme doses.

Using the staircase method it is possible to investigate how the LD50 varies with any factors of interest (for example, by using factorial designs). Each LD50 estimate would be a single observation and analysis of variance could then be applied. With fixed-dose testing such an experiment would be difficult, posing problems of dose selection for each treatment combination. In this context, a useful feature of staircase estimates from short sequences of equal length is that the variance of the estimates is fairly constant whatever the sequence, starting dose or step-length (22).

A disadvantage of the staircase method is that it is not possible to get a direct estimate of variance from a single sequence. A second difficulty associated with this method is that the study may take longer.

Other Aspects

One possible alternative to an LD50 test is, for example, an LD10, the estimation of the dose giving a 10% response. Testing would be carried out at the lower end of the dose-response curve. However, to avoid losing precision on the LD10 estimate, more animals would have to be used. Hence the number of deaths might be reduced but the total "suffering" increased. Furthermore, if terminal sacrifice is carried out, one should reduce the total number of animals used and hence design the experiment for LD50 estimation. Acceptance of tests such as this as replacements for the LD50 would take years to achieve and it may indeed be irrelevant in comparison with more fundamental issues such as interspecies or interlaboratory variations and extrapolation to man (23). The staircase method cannot, of course, be used for other than LD50 estimation.

The opportunity should be taken to pool data whenever appropriate. If several compounds are being tested, application of parallel probit line regression (24) allows an overall slope to be estimated from the pooled data with greatly increased precision over estimates for individual compounds. Computer statistics packages can do such calculations easily (25), but there may be problems of non-linearity and non-parallelism (26).

It is possible that a considerable increase in information in tests with death as an end-point could be achieved by taking into account survival times. In fact, it has been shown recently that an LD50 can be estimated from a plot of survival time versus dose (27). Reductions in animals tested may be possible with this method, although at present several important statistical and design issues remain unsolved. These include the incorporation of survivors into the analysis, and the choice of dose-levels for such a highly non-linear curve.

CARCINOGENICITY

Their complexity of design makes carcinogenicity tests difficult to conduct and interpret correctly without statistical involvement of some depth and sophistication. Major statistical problems in the analysis of these tests include low tumour frequency, the large number of tissue or organ sites, differential survival in treatment groups, the long latent period for most cancers and choice of dose-response models (e.g. 15,28). These problems may occur even in the most well-designed studies.

Recently published guidelines on the design and conduct of carcinogenicity studies reflect a fairly high degree of agreement on such basic factors as size of treatment groups (up to 100 animals), the number of dosage levels (up to 3) and the range of dosage levels (e.g. therapeutic to minimally toxic). Further statistical advice can ensure proper randomisation, and, by adequate range-finding studies, reasonable dose-levels. Computerised data entry and analysis can take much of the burden out of handling the data from a complex study. Three particular aspects will be discussed briefly.

Historical Controls

Incorporation of historical control data into the statistical analysis is possible. There have been recent developments in the statistical theory (29). A test for a dose-related increase in tumour frequency can be carried out using control data pooled over previous experiments. A feature of the test is that very heterogeneous historical data will receive low weight relative to the concurrent control data. Homogeneous data may receive more weight and have a greater impact on the analysis. Clearly, experiments closely similar to the current one are likely to be of most use as a source of such data and preliminary investigation will be needed to identify them.

Reading of Slides

With the large number of slides produced in a study with several hundred animals and up to 40 tissues for each animal, a slight treatment-related bias in the diagnosis could be magnified considerably (15). A statistical ideal might be to perform the microscopic examination in randomised order and "blind", that is, in ignorance of the dose-group. The pathologist would know the sex, tissue-type and <u>all</u> other information on that slide <u>except</u> the dose-level (or treatment identity). The optimum procedure could be a two-stage one. A sample of slides from each group is used (not "blind") to compile a list of important features. The whole set of slides can then be scored "blind" according to this list. If randomisation and "blind" reading prove impractical then, at least, careful standardised recording of information should be carried out.

Context Classification of Tumours

Tumour rates may be difficult to compare when survival differs considerably between different treatment groups. This is because a large proportion of the tumours that may arise do so only in old age, so that animals dying of other causes before old age have had less time to develop cancer. Colworth rats allowed to live for two and a half years have ten times the malignant hepatoma incidence of rats allowed to live only one and a half years (30). However, if tumours are classified as "fatal" or "incidental" then this problem can be overcome (31). Consider the following simple data which compare a toxic non-carcinogen with a control (30):

	Treatment	Control
Animals at risk	100	100
Deaths in 15 months	60	20
Tumours	18	6
FATAL	18/100	6/100
INCIDENTAL	18/60	6/20

The data show that although there were more deaths in the treatment group, the incidental tumour rates are equal, 18/60 and 6/20 (30%). However, if we had known that all tumours at 15 months were fatal, then we could have justifiably concluded that the proportions 18/100 versus 6/100 showed that the treatment was in fact carcinogenic. Thus:

a. For tumours observed in a <u>fatal</u> context in a particular period, tumour rates should be calculated relative to the number of animals at risk at the start of that period.
b. For tumours observed in an <u>incidental</u> context, tumour rates should be calculated relative to the number of animals dying in that period.

It is recognised that the classification of a tumour as "fatal" or "incidental" is not a simple exercise and that data such as those described above may be unlikely to occur in practice, particularly when the dose-levels are well chosen. It has been suggested that, if such a problem is found, then the classification can be carried out retrospectively, though this may be difficult to achieve without bias.

GENOTOXICITY

The relevance of tests for genotoxicity to animal testing lies mainly in the possibility of predicting in vivo genotoxicity, and also in the fact that several tests are themselves in vivo. Spontaneous mutational events are rare, of the order of 1 in 10^6 at any given locus, hence their detection may demand a combination of high dose and large numbers of observations for the relevant end-point. These requirements place a premium on good experimental design and objective assessment of the results using rigorous statistical methods.

Tests should always be repeated and positive controls run concurrently to provide validation data. A range of concentrations not more widely spaced than a factor of five should be used (32). New tests should go through a validation stage. Recent FDA hearings suggested that regulatory authorities will look most favourably on results from established tests of adequate size (33). Other relevant design aspects include adequate numbers of events and cells, randomisation schemes, bias-free conduct of the study and appropriate controls. Three design aspects will be discussed.

Sampling

Randomisation is as important in genotoxicity testing as in any other type of experimentation (34). The principle of random sampling is that all relevant cells in the test system should have an equal chance of being sampled. With sampling from complex organs the cell population must be precisely defined and cell sub-sampling should be carried out over this whole cell population. If the test organ is clearly heterogeneous then some form of proportional sampling or stratified sampling could be considered. Additional problems occur when the cells available may be greatly reduced in treated animals, as in the Micronucleus Test (35).

For quantitative assays, the numbers of cells to be scored can be determined by sample size calculations (e.g. 36,37). The assumption of Poisson occurrence (a distribution of rare events) of genetic events can be incorporated into the equations (34). For sample size calculations, a knowledge of the spontaneous (or vehicle-treated control) occurrence of events is required. This can be taken from historical data and should in fact be known if the test has been adequately validated.

Controls

Appropriate (negative) controls should be used. The toxic effect of mutagens frequently causes differential survival in control and treated groups. This has two major effects. First, if cell death and cell mutation are correlated and there is also differential non-genetic toxicity, then observed mutation rates are difficult to interpret. One would need to be able to distinquish between the two types of death. Secondly, cells surviving non-genetic toxicity presumably have altered population characteristics. This is of some importance in proliferation tests where the end-point is related to colony formation and division rate. Not only may the cells be more vigorous but they will be growing at lower density. Ideally a test should have a control population, such that at every drug dose the two groups of cells defined to be at risk have exactly the same characteristics with respect to vigour, density and number. This problem has been recognised, for example, in the Cell Transformation Test (38) and in the AG-resistance assay in V79 Chinese hamster cells (39).

Standard Errors

A problem with genotoxicity tests is that they may be ad hoc or novel. No statistical methodology will have been developed and, more particularly, it will be difficult to estimate standard errors. It is poor science to quote single figures with no estimate of variance. Either the rejection criteria should be set so that a positive result is a result which could not be explained by experimental variation alone, or the results should be in a form which allows straightforward statistical analysis. In any case, much relies on the end-point being chosen to reflect the response in as direct a way as possible (e.g. Bateman's (40) discussion of the Dominant Lethal Test). Finally, since inter-test variation can be substantial, it may be beneficial to estimate treatment effects over several laboratories or, at least, several different operating conditions.

STRATEGY FOR DRUG SCREENING

A major use of animals in the pharmaceutical industry is in screening for efficacy. Generally, a promising lead compound will be discovered and a number of congenerics will be synthesised, each one differing from the others by, perhaps, only a single chemical group. These congenerics will be screened for biological activity in an assay series comprising in vitro and in vivo assays.

In an early screen, a relatively large number of compounds will be tested. It is unlikely that one will stand out so much as to be statistically significantly better than the second place compound. A more or less continuous range of activities will be found (e.g. 41,42). Compounds showing the highest activity will proceed to the next assay in the series, and may be used as lead compounds in a new cycle of synthesis.

Each assay can have an associated activity criterion. If the result for a particular test compound meets this criterion, then the compound may pass to the next stage. The criterion could be based on statistical significance. For example, all compounds with observed activities significantly greater than the control at the 5% level could be retained. However, for early screens, such a criterion may be too strict and few compounds may pass through to later stages. Because of the many hurdles to be surmounted by a drug during the development process, its overall chance of becoming a marketed product is low. Thus, a reasonably high number of compounds must pass through the earlier screening stages to allow for the unavoidably high drop-out rate and to give a reasonable assurance of an adequate flow of new products to the market place.

A useful indicator of the efficiency of an assay series is the frequency of discovery of truly active compounds. This is related to the probability of discovery and to the average life of a compound. These two factors in turn depend on the distribution of activities in the congeneric series (43) and the chances at each stage of rejecting and accepting compounds with given activities.

Statistical modelling of the assay system may lead to the improvement of the design of the system to reduce the interval between discoveries. Preliminary results (D. Calhoun, personal communication) suggest that in the early in vivo screens it may be beneficial to increase the number of compounds tested, decrease the numbers of animals per group, and increase the range and number of doses. The result will be less information on more structures, but an overall increase in the frequency of discovery (assuming that truly active compounds are entering the system at a steady rate).

The design of each assay and the choice of the activity criterion should therefore be adjusted bearing in mind the relative costs of retaining false-positives and rejecting false-negatives. Decreasing the group sizes in the early assays reduces the chance of obtaining significance at any particular level (e.g. 5%) so that the activity criterion must be relaxed, in a statistical sense, to allow more compounds through. At some stage, however, it becomes too expensive to continue screening many false-positives and the criteria must be tightened up accordingly.

An excellent introduction to this subject has recently appeared in the literature (44). An interesting approach identifies four characteristics of an assay. It is assumed that a compound is either active or inactive, and that the proportion of actives can be estimated from past experience. After testing, a compound will be classified as positive or negative. It is possible to design the assay so as to optimise the following measures (45):

a. "sensitivity" - the ratio of true positives to total actives;
b. "specificity" - the ratio of true negatives to total inactives;
c. "positive accuracy" - the ratio of true to observed positives;
d. "negative accuracy" - the ratio of true to observed negatives.

An advantage of testing more compounds is that it gives the opportunity to average activity evidence over structural classes, or study quantitative structure-activity relationships (QSARs). QSARs can be used to predict the activity of new compounds and thus reduce the chance of in vivo testing on negative compounds (see article by Dr M. Tute, these Proceedings). It can increase the proportion of truly active compounds passing through the system.

In conclusion, it may be said that maximisation of the performance of a series of screening assays requires close collaboration between the biologist, chemist and statistician. It should be noted, however, that screening forms only part of a much larger research and development context (46,47).

SUMMARY AND RECOMMENDATIONS

Summary

Much wastage of animal material could be reduced by improving the experimental design of toxicity and efficacy screening tests. Statistical techniques, such as factorial designs to maximise information from limited material, and analysis of covariance to reduce experimental variation, could be applied more frequently.

The design of an experiment is critical to its ability to show "statistical significance" and to allow proper interpretation of results. Proper interpretation is only possible if the design has allowed for bias from unmeasurable influences. Statistical techniques of randomisation, stratification and, where possible, "blind" operation, allow for systematic bias in the conduct of the study.

Of particular importance in much animal testing is the extrapolation of results to man. In view of the many sources of variability that can affect the interpretation of study results, it is vital that the major sources of variation are identified and accounted for in the experimental design. Such sources may include interlaboratory variation and differences between strains. Experiments should be replicated over these major sources to assist in the interpretation of results relative to man.

Wastage of animals in testing can occur in several ways. First, the statistical parameters may be inefficiently estimated. In LD50 testing, sequential methods or survival time analysis, where appropriate, may be able to produce equally reliable results with fewer animals. Secondly, inadequately designed experiments may give equivocal results and thus have to be repeated. For example, unless all sources of observational bias have been removed, and the context of tumour discovery has been recorded, carcinogenicity studies may produce meaningless results. Thirdly, inappropriate replication can occur. In early preclinical efficacy screening, for example, it may be unnecessary to aim for statistical significance and hence use large numbers of animals per group in individual assays. The role of statistics should be to ensure that the overall testing system has a reasonably high probability of discovering an active compound.

The secret of good experimental design is the close collaboration of the statistician with the researcher. The researcher cannot be expected to pick an experimental layout from a textbook and immediately apply it in the most efficient manner. In consultation with the statistician, however, he can view his experiment more critically and, through careful design, achieve considerable improvement both in the meaning and applicability of his results. He may, as a natural consequence, expand his repertoire of design principles, become more confident with unfamiliar techniques, and generally increase the information he derives from his experimentation.

Recommendations

1. Adequate randomisation should be carried out wherever possible. The effects of bias over time should never be ignored. "Blind" operation should be considered at both the time of treatment application and of response measurement.

2. The technique of blocking and the use of concomitant variables should be more widely used. The resulting reduction of experimental error may allow reduced numbers of animals to be used in subsequent experiments. Cross-over designs may be useful for pharmacological work.

3. The degree of replication should be based on variation between appropriate experimental units. Excessive replication should be avoided by appropriate statistical design and analysis.

4. Factorial designs should be used more frequently. When more than one factor is being investigated, the factorial approach allows the researcher to obtain more information from less material than the single factor approach.

5. LD50 testing may be improved by using sequential methods or survival curves, where appropriate. Reductions in numbers of animals used may result. If traditional methods are necessary, then careful choice of dose-levels and the pooling of data over similar tests may allow fewer animals to be used.

6. The scheme for slide reading should be standardised to remove any treatment related bias that may arise. The context classification of tumours in carcinogenicity experiments is of some importance. Correct interpretation of the results may only be possible if such classification is carried out.

7. It should be recognised that good experimental design is as important in mutagenicity testing as in any other area. Three specific design requirements are; random sampling, adequate controls and estimation of standard errors.

8. In preclinical efficacy testing, highly precise early screens are unnecessary. The involvement of a statistician at the design stage could prevent wastage of biological material whilst maintaining a good chance of discovery.

REFERENCES

1. Cochran, W.G. & Cox, G.M. (1957). "Experimental Designs", 617 pp. New York: Wiley.
2. Fisher, R.A. (1960). "The Design of Experiments", 236 pp. Edinburgh: Oliver & Boyd.
3. Cox, D.R. (1958). "Planning of Experiments", 210 pp. New York: Wiley.
4. Armitage, P. & Remington, R.D. (1970). Experimental design. In "Statistics in Endocrinology" (ed. J.W. McArthur & T. Colton), pp. 3-32. Cambridge, Massachusetts: MIT Press.
5. Finney, D.J. (1952). "Probit Analysis", 318 pp. London: Cambridge University Press.
6. Mantel, N. (1980). Assessing laboratory evidence for neoplastic activity. Biometrics 36, 381-400.
7. Steel, R.G.D. & Torrie, J.H. (1960). "Principles and Procedures of Statistics", 481 pp. New York: McGraw-Hill.
8. El-Khalik, A.F.A. & Benoliel, D.M. (1982). Effects of weight and sex of rabbits on the results of the testing of chorionic gonadotrophin injection according to the European Pharmacopoeia. Journal of Pharmacy and Pharmacology 34, 209.
9. Chanter, D.O. (1982). Protocols for routine toxicity studies, a statistician's view. Archives of Toxicology suppl. 5, 40-44.
10. Finney, D.J. (1971). "Statistical Method in Biological Assay", 668 pp. London: Griffin.
11. Home Office. (1981). Report of the Advisory Committee on

Animal Experiments, 40 pp. London: HMSO.
12. Martin, R.C. (1981). Relative brain size and basal metabolic rate in terrestrial vertebrates. Nature, London 293, 57-60.
13. John, J.A. & Quenouille, M.H. (1977). "Experiments: Design and Analysis", 296 pp. London: Griffin.
14. Shirley, E.A.C. (1982). The use of background data in the analysis of covariance. Statistics in Medicine 1, 281-292.
15. Society of Toxicology. (1981). Re-examination of the ED01 study. Fundamental and Applied Toxicology 1, 26-128.
16. Squires, S. & Belyavin, G. (1976). Free contact infection in ferret groups. In "Chemotherapy and Control of Influenza" (ed. J.S. Oxford & J.D. Williams), pp. 35-42. New York: Academic Press.
17. Festing, M.F.W. (1975). A case for using inbred strains of laboratory animals in evaluating the safety of drugs. Food and Cosmetic Toxicology 13, 369-375.
18. Armitage, P. (1971). "Statistical Methods in Medical Research", 504 pp. Oxford: Blackwell.
19. Wahrendorf, J., Zentgraf, R. & Brown, C.C. (1981). Optimal designs for the analysis of interactive effects of two carcinogens or other toxicants. Biometrics 37, 45-54.
20. Rekker, R.F. (1980). LD50 values: are they about to become predictable? Trends in Pharmaceutical Sciences 1, 383-384.
21. Dixon, W.J. (1970). Quantal response variable experimentation: the up-and-down method. In "Statistics in Endocrinology" (ed. J.W. McArthur & T. Colton), pp. 251-268. Cambridge, Massachusetts: MIT Press.
22. Dixon, W.J. (1980). Efficient analysis of experimental observations. Annual Reviews of Pharmacology and Toxicology 20, 441-462.
23. Finney, D.J. (1980). Review of "Report on LD50 Test". Biometrics 36, 361.
24. Yeh, C. (1981). Use of bioassay in drug development: dose-response relationships. In "Statistics in the Pharmaceutical Industry" (ed. C.R. Buncher & J. Tsay), pp. 43-74. New York: Marcel Dekker.
25. Chanter, D.O. & Heywood, R. (1982). The LD50 test: some considerations of precision. Toxicology Letters 10, 303-307.
26. Cornfield, J. (1970). Invalidity in bioassays. In "Statistics in Endocrinology" (ed. J.W. McArthur & T. Colton), pp. 145-162. Cambridge, Massachusetts: MIT Press.
27. Molinengo, L. (1979). The curve doses versus survival time in the evaluation of acute toxicity. Journal of Pharmacy and Pharmacology 31, 343-344.
28. Crump, K.S. (1979). Dose-response problems in carcinogenesis. Biometrics 35, 157-168.
29. Tarone, R.E. (1982). The use of historical control information in testing for a trend in proportions. Biometrics 38, 215-220.

30. IARC. (1980). Long-term and short-term screening assays for carcinogens: a critical appraisal (annex). IARC Monographs, suppl. 2, 311-426. Lyon: International Agency for Research on Cancer.
31. Peto, R. (1974). Guidelines on the analysis of tumour rates and death rates in experimental animals. British Journal of Cancer 29, 101-105.
32. Anon. (1981). Grahame-Smith's recommendations in MAL 4. Scrip 648, 3-4.
33. FDA. (1980). Report on cyclamates. Federal Register 45, 61474-61530.
34. Ehrenberg, L. (1977). Aspects of statistical inference in testing for genetic toxicity. In "Handbook of Mutagenicity Test Procedures" (ed. B.J. Kilbey, M. Legator, W. Nichols & C. Remel), pp. 419-460. Amsterdam: Elsevier/North-Holland.
35. Schmid, W. (1977). The micronucleus test. In "Handbook of Mutagenicity Test Procedures" (ed. B.J. Kilbey, M. Legator, W. Nichols & C. Remel), pp. 235-242. Amsterdam: Elsevier/North-Holland.
36. Aleong, J. & Bartlett, D.E. (1979). Improved graphs for calculating sample sizes when comparing two independent binomial distributions. Biometrics 35, 875-881.
37. Katz, A.J. (1978). Design and analysis of experiments on mutagenicity. I. Minimal sample sizes. Mutation Research 50, 301-307.
38. Styles, J.A. (1977). A method for detecting carcinogenic organic chemicals using mammalian cells in culture. British Journal of Cancer 36, 558-563.
39. Arlett, C.F. (1977). Mutagenicity testing with V79 Chinese hamster cells. In "Handbook of Mutagenicity Test Procedures" (ed. B.J. Kilbey, M. Legator, W. Nichols & C. Remel), pp. 175-192. Amsterdam: Elsevier/North-Holland.
40. Bateman, A.J. (1977). The dominant lethal assay in the male mouse. In "Handbook of Mutagenicity Test Procedures" (ed. B.J. Kilbey, M. Legator, W. Nichols & C. Remel), pp. 325-334. Amsterdam: Elsevier/North-Holland.
41. Boyd, J.C., Millership, J.S. & Woolfson, A.D. (1982). A comparison of log p and molecular connectivity in the structure-activity analysis of some antimicrobial agents. Journal of Pharmacy and Pharmacology 34, 158-161.
42. Martin, Y.C. (1978). "Quantitative Drug Design" 425 pp. New York: Marcel Dekker.
43. Davies, O.L. (1958). The design of screening tests in the pharmaceutical industry. Bulletin of the Institute of International Statistics 36, 1-16.
44. Redman, C.E. (1981). Screening compounds for clinically active drugs. In "Statistics in the Pharmaceutical Industry" (ed. C.R. Buncher & J. Tsay), pp. 19-42. New York: Marcel Dekker.
45. Dunnett, C.W. (1972). The never-ending search for new and

better drugs. In "Statistics: Guide to the Unknown" (ed. J. Tanur), pp. 23-33. San Francisco: Holden-Day.
46. Davies, O.L. (1963). The design of screening tests. Technometrics 5, 481-489.
47. Dunnett, C.W. (1961). The statistical theory of drug screening. In "Quantitative Methods in Pharmacology" (ed. H. Dejonge), pp. 212-231. Amsterdam: Elsevier/North-Holland.

Statistics and the Objectives of FRAME

D. O. CHANTER

INTRODUCTION

The role of statistics in toxicology is usually regarded by toxicologists as being concerned with the analysis of data. By some it is even thought of as a necessary evil, a kind of ritual which has to be undertaken to satisfy regulatory authorities or journal editors that the proper inferences have been drawn, but which is in fact quite unnecessary because really the toxicologist is perfectly capable of interpreting his own data without assistance from the statistician. Salsburg makes a similar point in a paper which is well worth reading (1).

In reality though, statistics is concerned with much more than just the analysis of data; it is concerned with the whole process referred to as "the scientific method". There are basically two ways of obtaining new knowledge: one is by the observation of nature as it is, i.e. without interfering with it, and the other is by experiment, i.e. by interfering with nature in a controlled way. Statistics, in its broadest sense, is concerned with both these processes, but for our present purposes I shall confine my attention to the second.

Experimentation is the process of obtaining information from experimental material. Statistics is the study of how to do this efficiently, that is, how to use experimental resources in such a way that the maximum amount of information is obtained, whilst ensuring that this information is both precise and accurate. This process has two main components, design and analysis. Most discussions of statistics in toxicology centre around the latter, and we are indebted to Graham Healey for presenting a paper which concentrates on design and which sets out several principles which can be used to improve the efficiency of toxicological experimentation.

REDUCING NUMBERS OF ANIMALS USED IN EXPERIMENTS

It is unfortunate that some statisticians have given toxicologists the impression that, if consulted about the design of an experiment, they will always ask for more animals to be used. This view is so widespread that some toxicologists believe it is only worth using statistical methods to analyse data when large numbers of animals have been used; when only small numbers are involved they see statistical methods as too prone to lead to misleading conclusions. In fact, proper statistical thinking becomes more important, rather than less, as the number of animals used becomes smaller. With large numbers, underlying trends should be clear (except with parameters such as tumour incidence, which needs to be disentangled from mortality effects), but with small numbers such trends are not so easily seen, and it is important to have a proper objective method of making inferences.

When I am consulted about the design of a toxicology study, I very rarely recommend any increase in the number of animals to be used. Instead, I approach the problem as one of using the resources which the toxicologist has allocated in such a way as to obtain as much precision as possible. Since the designs (and analyses) favoured by toxicologists are often very inefficient, there is considerable scope for reducing animal numbers and offsetting the resulting reduction in precision by using more efficient methods of design and analysis. A necessary prerequisite for this, however, is freedom to treat guideline protocols as guidelines rather than as requirements.

ALTERNATIVES

Statistics also has an important role to play in the development of alternative test systems. For example, if a test system is based on a cell culture, there is a temptation to argue that because a very large number of cells can be used in a single test, random variability is no longer important and statistical analysis unnecessary. This might be true if all the cells were independent of one another, but they are not. The number of independent experimental units in such a test is often very small; the independent units are often the culture flasks or the containers in which exposure to the test substance takes place. Often there are very few of these, and in the statistical sense such experiments are analogous to animal experiments with only one or two animals at each dose-level.

STATISTICS AND THE OBJECTIVES OF TOXICOLOGY

Many toxicological experiments are carried out in which observations are made on one species in the hope that the conclusions reached will be applicable to some other species (often man). If data are available for both species for a variety of toxicants, it is possible to correlate the results for the two species to see whether the extrapolation process is justified. Often such data are not available, and non-statistical justification of the extrapolation is required. This can be provided only when there is a sound scientific understanding of the biological processes involved, and when this is available the non-statistical justification supersedes the statistical one. However, with our current state of knowledge, there is still room for uncertainty about the validity of extrapolating from a particular animal toxicity study to man when a new substance is being tested. This uncertainty is sometimes taken as a justification for not bothering to apply proper statistical principles of design and analysis when carrying out the animal experiment. Such arguments, of course, are ethically untenable. If an experiment is irrelevant to the question asked, then there is no point in doing the experiment. If the experiment is relevant (however slightly), then if that experiment uses animals there is an ethical requirement for it to be carried out to the highest possible scientific standards. It is for the toxicologist to decide which experiments are sufficiently relevant to be worth doing and which are not. Once that issue has been decided, any statistical techniques which are known to be capable of improving the efficiency of experimentation should be used.

USING STATISTICAL IDEAS IN TOXICOLOGY

I have tried to show that the proper use of statistical thinking in toxicology provides one of the means by which the objectives of FRAME might be achieved (particularly the reduction of animal numbers in the kinds of study at present in use). In my view, it is unfortunate that the statistical ideas which are available for this purpose have been included in this report as a separate paper, comprehensive though that paper is. These ideas are of no help unless they are actually used, and in my view they would be more likely to be used had they been incorporated into individual working party reports, wherever relevant. There are not many statisticians specialising in applications in toxicology; it is important that their contribution be used as effectively as possible.

REFERENCE

1. Salsburg, D.S. (1981). Statistics and toxicology: an overview. In "Scientific Considerations in Monitoring and Evaluating Toxicological Research" (ed. E.J. Gralla), pp. 123-136. Washington: Hemisphere.

Design and Analysis of Carcinogenicity Studies

P. N. LEE

The important part the statistician has to play in animal experiments has been emphasised by a number of speakers. It is vital to ensure that experiments wasteful of animals are not conducted and that the maximum valid information is obtained from the available data. I would like to make a few comments on the question of design and analysis of carcinogenicity experiments, an area of particular interest to me.

Mr Healey has recommended the reading of slides "blind" and in a randomised order, to avoid two dangers - first, that the knowledge of the treatment might effect the classification of a lesion and, second, that systematic bias might occur over time. One should be aware, however, that "blind" reading, while fine in principle, not only leads to a small increased chance of animals being wrongly identified in the unscrambling, but is also without point when on occasion the pathologists can identify the treatment from the slide, e.g. when a high dose of a food colouring causes abnormal pigmentation of some tissues. Furthermore, though diagnostic drift is certainly a very real problem indeed, especially for grading certain non-neoplastic lesions such as those related to senescence, it should be realised that, provided the pathologist is aware of the problem, strict randomisation is not actually necessary to deal with it.

More important than strict blindness and randomisation of the order of slide reading, in my view, is that the pathologist should have a systematic approach to the recording of information that bears in mind the problems of statistical analysis. In the worst method of recording, the non-quantitative pathologist dictates a report in which he follows no standard procedure. He may describe the same lesion in a variety of different ways. He may record only the most severe or interesting lesions present. He may fail to indicate clearly and in a standard way the size, severity, multiplicity, and other characteristics of a lesion. Faced with this, the statistician trying to obtain a valid comparison of the incidence of a particular lesion in the different groups has the following problems:

a. The sheer labour of finding the occurrences of that lesion described in different ways among a mass of text.
b. The doubt whether failure to mention a lesion implies: it was there, but something more interesting came up, so it was over-looked or the section was so inadequate that one could not tell whether or not it was there.
c. The difficulty of dealing with a lesion mentioned as present/not present in some animals, but graded in others.

A far better procedure is for the pathologist to decide, for all those conditions that are likely to be worth statistical analysis, to record information in a standard way. Dr Francis Roe and I have been involved in the development of a computer program which allows the pathologist, having defined a set of conditions, to enter simple numerical values indicating presence/absence, grade, size, etc. The computer will then not only produce the full text of the histopathological report, but also the appropriate statistical tables and analyses. Such a system not only produces more valid data, but it is also quicker for the pathologist to use, and cuts down enormously the delay between completion of slide reading and the analysis of the results.

Let us turn now to the question of analysis. Particular attention has been given in recent years to the importance of classification of tumours as either "fatal" (causing or contributing to the death of an animal) or "incidental" (observed only because the animal dies of another cause). The FRAME Toxicity Committee's Preliminary Report suggests this classification should be done routinely for each tumour that occurs, but my experience suggests that in fact this exercise is often without point. As most statisticians working in this field know, the basis for this suggestion comes from an analysis by Peto _et al._ (1) of the pituitary tumour data from the large BIBRA nitrosamine experiment. This showed that if all tumours were classified as incidental there appeared to be a reducing effect of treatment, whereas if all tumours were classed as fatal there appeared to be an enhancing effect. When, however, a separate judgement was made for each tumour treatment, this was (correctly) found to be without effect. The impression has grown from this that such separate judgements are necessary for each tumour that occurs before statistical analysis can be attempted, and this has caused some concern, as it is, in some cases, a difficult and subjective procedure. In fact, beautiful as this analysis was, in some ways it has taken the eyes of statisticians off the ball, because, though it is quite common that adjustment for differential between group survival under either extreme assumption (all tumours fatal or all tumours incidental) can come up with different conclusions from an incorrect, simple analysis ignoring survival, it is in fact quite rare that the answers using either extreme assumption actually do differ materially. Only when these answers differ and there is real doubt as to how the great majority should be classified on general principles is it worth going through the classification procedure for individual tumours.

Three other general principles are worth mentioning in the analysis of carcinogenicity study data:

1. Use of the full information from an experiment carried out at a number of dose-levels by calculating the significance of the trend statistic (1). This method can be much more sensitive at picking up the true difference than the commonly used procedure of comparing each treatment group individually with the controls.

2. Use of any available information on the size and severity of the lesions in the analysis. It is clearly wasteful for the pathologist to record such data if the statistician is going to treat analysis simply as a comparison of proportions of animals having the lesion.

3. Taking into account relevant non-neoplastic information in the interpretation of the neoplastic data. It is a mistake to assume that, just because cancer is the end-point, attention should be given only to tumour incidence. I have analysed a study in which mammary gland tumour incidence was raised in the treated animals, but the statistical significance was marginal, so the conclusion from these data alone was equivocal. However, there was a strikingly clear dose-related trend in mammary gland hyperplasia which gave considerable strength to the view that the raised tumour incidence was not a chance finding.

REFERENCE

1. Peto, R., Pike, M.C., Day, N.E., Gray, R.G., Lee, P.N., Parish, S., Peto, J., Richards, S. & Wahrendorf, J. (1980). Guidelines for simple, sensitive significance tests for carcinogenic effects in long-term animal experiments. In "Long-term and Short-term Screening Tests for Carcinogens: a Critical Approach", IARC Monographs on the Evaluation of Carcinogenic Risk to Humans, suppl. 2, pp. 311-426. Lyon: IARC.

General Discussion

DAVID MACHIN

Rapporteur

Dr L. BERRYMAN said that Mr Healey was talking about randomisation as a way of eliminating bias and one of the points he had raised was that, in a three-hour dosing procedure, groups of animals should be dosed randomly. He disagreed with that point because, in a three-hour dosing procedure with a six-hour variation in daily dosing time, a group of animals might be dosed only 20 hours after the last dose on one occasion, but after 27 hours on another occasion. This could effect the plasma level of a test compound with long half-life, with a subsequent effect on the pharmacology.

Professor A. GOLDBERG asked whether a generalisation could be made by either looking at a fixed number of animals or doing a repeat study using lower numbers of animals. In other words, could more information be obtained from two experiments with three animals each as compared to one experiment with six animals.

Mr HEALEY replied briefly, and later in writing, as follows:

In replying to Dr Berryman: "If you recognise that variation within the day is a problem, block accordingly, recognising that factor. It is also a question of designing the experiment to remove the effects of the factor. If it is necessary to preserve the 24 hour interval between successive dosing, then the design should incorporate this as far as possible. Randomising within a day and having a fixed-interval between doses are to some extent confounded, but by having an interval of greater than 24 hours (e.g. 27 hours) some interesting designs are possible. The reply to Professor Goldberg depends on what between-experiment variation one has, and the intended applicability of the result. If the result is likely to vary when the experiment is done under different conditions, then you could certainly argue that increasing the number of experiments increases your scope of inference. Thus, the average effect pooled over your several experiments will be a better estimate of the so-called "true" effect. If there isn't much between-experiment variation, on the whole it is better to do a single large experiment than several small experiments. This is a general principle."

Mr MACHIN said "Perhaps I could just make one comment from the chair before we close, and that is, that much of what has been said by Mr Healey in this session is not new; that is, in the statistical sense it is not new. In particular, the advantages of blocking were first described by Fisher some 50 years ago. So what has been said may not be new but nevertheless has certainly taken, or is taking, a long time to percolate through to all aspects of experimental work. This is particularly important, as has already been stressed, with respect to the work of FRAME, in that efficient designs imply the use of fewer animals."

Reproductive Toxicity

C. L. BERRY

INTRODUCTION

It is not possible to predict the effects of chemicals on the reproductive process from their structure alone, although certain potentially dangerous compounds may be identified in this way. In considering the range of processes that are involved in the production of male and female gametes, their coming together in fertilisation, implantation and subsequent development, this is perhaps not surprising.

To consider the post-implantation embryo alone, it will be evident that the temporally-regulated transcription and translation of genetic messages which underlies the complex interplay of cell proliferation, cell death, differentiation, and migration which collectively constitutes the process of development may be interrupted at many stages and in many ways. Each interruption may produce a cascade effect, or its effects may be rapidly negated by the processes of repair which are active in the embryo and fetus. A major problem in attempting to predict the likely effects of chemicals on the developing conceptus is the evaluation of the effects of the metabolic role of the mother and of the placenta in the handling of a chemical.

The complexity of these processes is indicated by the frequency with which they go wrong. More than 70% of all human conceptions fail to result in an established pregnancy, and there is ample evidence to suggest that the vast majority of those embryos and fetuses eliminated are abnormal. Similar findings may apply to other species; early embryonic and fetal wastage is well documented in rodents. In man, this process, which is effective in preventing abnormal births, greatly complicates epidemiological attempts to identify human teratogens; if minor changes in fertility or abortion rates occur, they would be very difficult to identify. Teratogens which do not produce significant early embryonic mortality will be most readily identified by this type of study.

There is considerable lack of awareness amongst those who consider the effects of chemicals on development of the presently available data on human reproductive wastage. Acquisition of new data in this field would be of major importance in estimating putative risks from chemicals and for determining priorities in the use of animals.

The number of human conceptions is unknown. Although 2.5-3% of deliveries have a major malformation present at birth, numerous studies have shown a higher rate in early pregnancy - more than 90% of anomalies as diverse as cebocephaly, Turner's syndrome and neural tube defects are aborted (see (1) for bibliography). In spontaneous first trimester abortions, around 60% exhibit chromosomal aberrations, mostly trisomies, monosomy or triploidy (2). This spontaneous wastage of early conceptuses is documented not only by the clinical observations of a 15-20% abortion rate, but also by recent studies demonstrating massive embryonic loss after implantation. Using specific B-HCG assays for early pregnancy as a method of demonstrating the occurrence of implantation (the hormone is only produced when the trophoblast grows into the uterine wall), it has recently been shown that even in a group of women who might be expected to have good reproductive performances (adequate social background, aged in their mid-twenties), almost 50% of implanted embryos fail to continue to develop to term (3). More recent data on *in vitro* human fertilisation support these observations and calculations (4).

With this background, we have looked critically at current practice in teratology testing, identified problems, and considered alternatives. We wish to emphasise that our view is that whole animal tests are still necessary in safety evaluation, but that the number of animals used might be reduced. It is also important to note that some of the agents tested are made for the benefit of animals.

CURRENT TESTING

Most countries require that a new chemical is tested with regard to effects on maturation of the gonads, mating, gestation, parturition, lactation and, in some instances, through to the development and maturation of the filial generation, before marketing is permitted. For drugs, there are three basic components to such testing:

a. A fertility/general reproductive study is required, in which one species (usually the rat) is dosed prior to and through mating and early gestation, and perhaps through to weaning of reared offspring. For drugs intended for long-term use (e.g. anti-hypertensives, anti-rheumatics, etc.), it may be recommended that offspring be reared untreated and kept to maturity in order to examine them for possible adverse effects on later development.
b. Teratology studies in two species (usually the rat and the rabbit) are recommended. The test material is administered to pregnant females during organogenesis, and the animals are killed just prior to parturition to determine resorption rates and to obtain fetuses for examination.
c. A perinatal and postnatal study in at least one species, usually the rat, is required by most countries for drugs and comprises the administration of the test compound to pregnant females during late gestation and throughout lactation. In some countries it is recommended that a proportion of offspring are reared to maturity. In all parts of these tests, administration is via the route(s) of clinical use and three doses are used, the highest of which should produce some toxic effect in the mother, or be the largest practical or tolerated dosage.

For non-pharmaceuticals, test systems are less ordered, although for more established types of chemical, such as pesticides or food additives, the main emphasis is on performance of a multigeneration study; often, teratology studies in at least one species are also required, either within, or separate from, the multigeneration study.

Unfortunately, designs vary not only between countries, but also within countries where different agencies are responsible for different types of chemical. Additionally, in some countries changes in design occur at not infrequent intervals and are continuing to occur. In such circumstances, duplication of experimentation tends to occur.

PRACTICAL CONSIDERATIONS

Factors affecting the developing conceptus (embryotoxicity, teratogenicity) inevitably form the central focus in any discussion of reproductive toxicity. It is convenient, therefore, to use the same basis for discussing practical aspects, since many will also apply to other aspects of reproduction.

Species

In our view, factors other than scientific ones are sometimes involved in the choice of species in these studies. Clearly, companies investigating antibiotics may not use animals where essential gut flora is disturbed by them. The regulatory requirements of countries like Japan and France that dislike the use of two rodent species in teratology studies might be disputed scientifically; this assumption of unsuitability is not rational.

The suitability or otherwise of a test species is governed by a multitude of factors, ranging from cost and availability through ease of handling, housing and lifespan to similarity to man in respect of developmental processes and pharmacokinetics. Too often, however, the choice is based on a limited and unbalanced set of factors; for example, sub-human primates are often suggested because in terms of phylogeny and pharmacokinetics they are more similar to man than other species. This works well when the objective is to confirm a positive response to a potent material, such as that to thalidomide, but can be completely misleading in assessing whether or not an unknown material presents some hazard, particularly if the metabolism of the test compound differs between man and primate. Even if there is metabolic similarity to man, primates would be inadequate for detecting moderate to low levels of activity or providing assurance of lack of activity. The reason for this is that cost and availability preclude use of the large numbers that would be required for detection of low frequency phenomena such as malformations, a problem exaggerated by the fact that, being monotocous (like man), there is a tendency to conserve resources by aborting or terminating abnormal pregnancies. In other words, to be effective for detection of low level, but nevertheless important, effects, one would need to use numbers of sub-human primates in the same order as those required for epidemiological surveys in humans, i.e. thousands.

It may be expected that if alternative species are used, companies will naturally exploit species they normally keep for other work; the background data they may possess is of obvious value.

Dosages and Dose-levels

This is a difficult matter, involving careful balance of dosage with intervals between dosages, the number of animals in each group, and a value judgement about the type of effect most likely to occur. Errors are most often made because of a failure to use evidence from other studies effectively in choosing dose levels. This requires good co-operation between general and reproductive toxicologists. However, we consider that the usual requirement is for one negative control and three test groups, with that at the highest dosage preferably providing evidence of minimal adult toxicity. This requirement is sometimes taken to extremes. Alternatively, the use of a single "limit" dose (equivalent to a high dosage) for materials of low toxicity is an effective screening procedure. Also, it is rarely, if ever, necessary to use more than three dosages or to span ridiculous ranges (e.g. 5 to 5000 mg/kg) in a single study.

Number of Animals

The number of animals used is often decided empirically rather than scientifically. Compounds should not be rejected at the regulatory level because 18 instead of an intended 20 rodents in a group are pregnant; it should be remembered that to make any increase in the value of a study the size of a group must usually be increased from around 10 to 20 or 15 to 30. If a low frequency phenomenon is to be evaluated, hundreds (or even thousands) of litters per group would be used. Large studies are difficult to control, not least because of chronological dispersion, and thus may lose their value.

We believe that a major difficulty which results in the use of more animals than necessary is the non-heterogeneity of the requirements of regulatory agencies, both in written form and in the stances adopted in interpretation.

Route of Administration

There are sometimes difficulties in this area, particularly with non-pharmaceuticals. Pharmacokinetic data may reduce the necessity to examine a large number of routes. Inhalation studies with face-only exposure are difficult and unpleasant for the animals. We believe that the less stressful whole-body exposure should be accepted more readily and would reduce the number of confounding variables, particularly when stress itself may be teratogenic in rodents.

Timing and Duration of Treatment

For embryotoxicity/teratology studies with pharmaceuticals, there is perhaps less dispute about requirements than in most areas. In general, divergence from the standard requirements will be accepted if rational scientific argument and supportive data are provided. Examples would include dosing depot preparations at intervals of 3 or 4 days, or performance of two studies with short complementary dosing periods, instead of a single study with the standard dosing period, for materials showing marked enzyme induction or marked cumulative toxicity.

Maternal Observation

Awareness of maternal responses to the test compound derived both from reproductive studies and associated non-reproductive studies is essential for proper interpretation. Daily observation, regular weighing, which should be weekly in quiescent periods of a study (e.g. pre-mating) and more frequent in rapidly changing phases (e.g. gestation and lactation) should be routine; macroscopic examination of maternal tissues at termination, supported by preservation of tissues for histopathological examination (if necessary), is also advisable. Collection of such data may reduce the need for further studies.

Fetal Examinations

The methodology in this field is well established and described, but many studies have to be repeated due to inadequate examination of the fetuses or to poor interpretation and presentation of results. We believe that some regulatory authorities are also poor at assessing this type of data.

SCREENING TESTS

It is essential to have a clear view of what is expected of a screening test. The major requirement is for a test that will detect unwanted effects of relatively unknown compounds with a high degree of sensitivity and good fidelity. Screening tests cannot establish mechanisms of malformation, a desirable but academic study. For reasons discussed earlier, screening will involve the use of intact mammals, especially where the safety of man and domestic animals is concerned. An exception to this may be the target requiring protection.

Knowledge of mechanisms may permit the use of a valuable compound shown to be hazardous in animals - the mechanism may not operate in man. It is at this stage that we believe that there is a greater scope for the use of *in vitro* or non-mammalian systems.

It is apparent that for humans there is a generally falling rate of malformations and a lack of evidence of any new powerful teratogens (i.e. similar to thalidomide), despite the operation of many congenital malformation registries and increasing facility for the detection of adverse effects; this supports the concept that selective embryotoxicity is a rare phenomenon. In contrast, screening tests performed to date indicate a slightly greater potential hazard to other aspects of reproduction, which, whilst they may be less marked, may be more detrimental in the long run.

STRATEGY

Given the above basis, a strategy intended to make the most effective use of current requirements can be initiated.

The first priority in this plan would be to harmonise international requirements, thereby reducing unnecessary duplication of studies or exaggerated dimensions within studies. This applies particularly to general reproductive and multi-generation studies. Secondly, a more flexible approach should be adopted, rather than the slavish following of regulations or the adoption of arbitary compartmentalisation of studies. In respect of the latter, performances of a dominant lethal assay, because it comes under the heading of "mutagenicity" and is additional to examination of male fertility, which comes under the heading of "reproductive toxicology", more often than not represents an unnecessary waste of resources.

Usually, it will be most practical to initiate reproductive toxicology testing with the embryotoxicity (teratogenicity) tests in rats or mice. There is usually information available, from pharmacological screening, acute toxicity and, sometimes, in vivo cytogenetic studies, to enable there to be a reasonable chance of selecting appropriate dosages. The study can thus be initiated at, or shortly after, the subacute preliminary toxicity study, the advantage being not only the chance of earlier detection of reproductive hazard, but also the chance of earlier detection of general toxicity: the latter arises because the stress of pregnancy often creates a sensitivity that allows responses to occur more rapidly.

Particularly for non-pharmaceuticals, the process can be extended with care to the performance of a combination subacute/short reproduction study to provide a single, rather than a dual, stepping stone to the more critical chronic toxicity and reproductive studies.

Provided that the test material is not abandoned at this stage, the next most common step would be initiation of the preliminary and main investigations of embryotoxicity in a second species. In a number of situations a useful alternative would be initiation of the perinatal and postnatal study, as parturition, early neonatal survival and early lactation form the second stressful watershed in the reproductive process.

INTERPRETATION OF THE RESULTS OF STUDIES

Here there are major difficulties, usually relating to incidence of malformations, anomalies or variants. These difficulties are compounded by what appears to be widespread ignorance of the frequencies of minor malformations/variations, the relevance of growth retardation to teratogenesis, and the background of reproductive wastage. What is the significance of one rarely seen major defect in the high dose group, when none are seen in any other group, including controls? Similarly, what is the significance of a marked increase in a commonly occurring variant seen only at a dose-level associated with marked maternal toxicity? These questions are often answered intuitively in the absence of a scientific basis for the assessment of teratogenic risk. We do not have dose-response relationships for human teratogens in a variety of species - there are not enough compounds known to be teratogenic to give us a reasonable base of this kind. The ratio of teratogenic dose to pharmacological levels, toxic levels or death is only a crude approximation to this, and the exceptions to compounds fitting in an apparent framework would be the danger. In general, the closer the teratogenic dose to toxicological effects, the safer the compound is for the human conceptus.

ALTERNATIVE TEST METHODS

Suggestions for alternative methodology have included _in vitro_ methods such as cell, tissue, organ, limb or whole embryo culture, and _in vivo_ systems using chick embryos, bacteria, hydra, planaria, echinoderms, fish, and other non-mammalian systems. Attention has been focussed almost entirely on the developing conceptus (teratogenicity), although in some respects there would appear to be more opportunity for alternatives in other aspects of reproduction.

Many investigators currently employing mammals would be among those most interested in suitable alternative systems, the likelihood of reduced costs of experimentation providing a strong motivating force.

To date, attempts to introduce alternative non-mammalian methods into reproductive toxicology have been ineffective, largely due to:

a. the failure of proponents to become conversant with the necessity, scope and reasons for current studies;
b. lack of understanding by supporters of a particular method that, whilst it may be a success in a specific closed situation, over-extrapolation of this success to the broader, more complex field of safety evaluation is inappropriate without adequate validation;
c. poor understanding of the processes that lead to malformation; the implications of their natural occurrence as low frequency phenomena, allied to the limitation of chemically-induced malformations to a narrow range of dosages, are not fully appreciated. Documented and established evidence that materials capable of inducing malformations do not necessarily constitute an appreciable hazard to the species in question or to other

species is often ignored, as is the fact that some materials with "teratogenic potential" are essential to life, e.g. cortisone, selenium, vitamin A.

It becomes apparent in assessing the results of many studies that simple detection of a potential to cause adverse effects, especially malformations, is insufficient. It needs to be followed by or allied with the capacity to evaluate degrees of risk. Unfortunately, proponents of alternative systems set sensitivity as their primary goal, forgetting that increased sensitivity is usually attained at the expense of fidelity. Consequently, over-enthusiastic persuance of the goal of sensitivity may well generate apprehension, which in turn may increase the need to do more mammalian tests to provide the fidelity that will allow evaluation of hazards. The integrated process of mammalian reproduction, involving internal fertilisation, the development of the conceptus in the protected environment provided by the dynamic combination of embryonic membranes, placenta and dam, and neonatal care and nourishment of offspring, is unique to the animal kingdom. In vitro or non-mammalian systems may be able to mimic parts of the process, but not all, and certainly will not mimic the entire integrated system.

In the final analysis, therefore, it is impossible to envisage a situation where the use of intact mammalian systems can be avoided entirely. Consequently, development of alternative non-mammalian systems with a view to supporting, integrating with, and increasing the efficiency of mammalian systems, rather than replacing them entirely, would appear to provide the greatest opportunity to reduce the numbers of mammals used in reproductive toxicology.

PERINATAL AND POSTNATAL TOXICITY STUDIES

Although there are disagreements in this area, we do not think that perinatal and postnatal studies are necessary for all compounds, since in many instances their aims will be covered by fertility and general reproductive studies. The decision not to require these tests would greatly reduce the number of animals used in reproductivity tests. However, used properly, these tests, if done before the general reproduction study, may help in designing this and multigeneration studies. To consider specific points, as before:

1. Choice of species. The rat is used almost invariably.

2. Dose-levels. No additional comments.

3. Number of animals. No additional comments.

4. Route. Cross-fostering experiments may be useful.

5. Timing and duration of treatment. It is important that some flexibility in design is used to alleviate problems such as transient maternal neglect. Treatment usually starts from day 15-17 and ceases at weaning (variously defined as 21 or 25 days).

6. Maternal examinations. The same considerations apply as in teratology studies.

7. Pup examinations. We believe these to be important, and if the test is to be done, they represent its centre point. There should be proper counts, examinations and weighing at birth, 4,8,12 and 21 days postpartum.

FERTILITY AND GENERAL REPRODUCTIVE PERFORMANCE STUDY

Many of the general comments made above also apply here:

1. Species. The rat is normally used, but the mouse is an acceptable alternative.

2. Dosages, dose-levels. These should be set for the most susceptible sex, since in safety evaluation we are concerned with establishing the lowest dose causing an adverse effect.

3. Number of animals. We believe there are major problems here, as a result of heterogeneous regulatory requirements, "unwritten rules" and, the poor design of many studies.

4. Route. Usually constrained by problems of practicability.

5. Timing and duration of administration. There are major differences in requirements of regulatory authorities which greatly complicate experimental design. We believe it is the responsibility of both industry and a co-ordinating body (OECD, for example) to agree protocols and resolve difficulties. To illustrate one simple point, it is possible to avoid repetition of a study by continuing the dosing of males after mating and until litter values have been determined. Where results are equivocal, males can be re-mated to a second batch of females, instead of the whole study having to be started again.

6. Maternal behaviour. There would be advantages in better observation of maternal behaviour if compounds are considered to affect reproduction by altering coital frequency, etc.

7. Fetal examination. In general, this is not necessary, unless undertaken in order to amplify the teratology study.

8. Behavioural studies. In our opinion, these are problematic and seldom reproduced exactly between laboratories. Gross differences are rare, but other, probably significant changes, are virtually impossible to assess. Academic studies have been carried out with highly potent compounds which have resulted in the induction of these procedures into the context of safety evaluation by those not sufficiently familiar with the scope, aims and philosophy of this area.

REFERENCES

1. Berry, C.L. (1981). Congenital malformation. In "Paediatric Pathology" (ed. C.L. Berry), pp. 1-31. Heidelberg: Springer-Verlag.
2. Boue, J., Boue, A. & Lazar, P. (1975). Retrospective and prospective epidemiological studies of 1500 karyotyped spontaneous human abortions. Teratology 12, 1-26.
3. Craft, I., McLeod, F., Green, S., Djahanbakhach, O., Bernard, A. & Twigg, H. (1982). Human pregnancy following oocyte and sperm transfer to the uterus. Lancet i, 1031-1034.
4. Miller, J.F., Williamson, E., Glue, J., Gordon, Y.B., Grudzinskas, J.G. & Sykes, A. (1980). Fetal loss after implantation. A prospective study. Lancet ii, 554-556.

In Vitro Reproductive Toxicity Studies

KEITH SNELL

IN VITRO TERATOGENICITY TESTS

It is clear that in the area of reproductive or developmental toxicology it would be impossible to devise a single alternative test system to supplant the use of live animals in toxicity testing. The reproductive toxicity study seeks to evaluate the possible toxic impact of an agent on germ cell maturation, fertility, embryogenesis, fetal development, parturition, neonatal development, reproductive capacity and efficiency, and maturation. For much of the ontogenic period, more than a single organism or biological compartment is under scrutiny. For example, during gestation the maternal-placental-fetal developmental unit is being exposed to the agent, and during lactation it is the maternal-mammary-infant developmental unit. These units are characterised by heavily interdependent biological compartments functioning together as an integral whole. The individual components each have their own unique susceptibilities in terms of target sites of toxicity, and superimposed on this are the interactive processes co-ordinating the functions of the components. In addition, the unit as a whole introduces considerable complexity in terms of pharmacokinetic inter-relationships.

Nevertheless, certain defined aspects of development are amenable to investigation using in vitro procedures based on cell or organ culture techniques. The area that has received the most attention in this respect has been teratogenesis and its evaluation using whole embryos, isolated embryonic tissue or embryonic cells in culture (see (1-4), for reviews). Of course, such techniques are themselves dependent on the use of live animals as a source of material, but on a much reduced scale compared with toxicity studies in vivo. Rather little use has been made of established cell lines, which are propagated entirely in vitro. This is perhaps understandable in view of the loss of differentiated functions associated with many cell lines. However, a number of them are capable of undergoing differentiation, such as embryonal teratocarcinoma and 3T3-L1 pre-adipocyte cells, and their evaluation for teratogenicity investigations should be promoted.

Undoubtedly, the major value of in vitro methods is in the delineation of teratogenicity mechanisms in order to develop meaningful theoretical concepts on which to base testing procedures. The entirely empirical basis of current developmental toxicity evaluation is a reflection of the paucity of knowledge concerning pathogenetic mechanisms in teratogenesis. Indeed, it could be argued that legislative guidelines are woefully inadequate in this respect, in that they are explicitly designed to optimise the identification of the final manifestations of toxicity of known teratogens (such as thalidomide), rather than to detect mechanistic correlates earlier in the pathogenetic sequence that might serve as more general indicators of teratogenic potential. In particular, the preoccupation with anatomical malformations as end-point indicators of developmental toxicity is of dubious scientific validity and is an impediment to innovative progress in this area. The ease with which visible morphological abnormalities in experimental animals can be anthropomorphised implies a fidelity in the extrapolation to human hazard which is illusory and which tends to over-inflate their value as indicators of developmental toxicity. Thus, anatomical malformations are only one of a number of other significant final manifestations of developmental toxicity, which also include growth retardation and a variety of metabolic and functional defects. They are certainly not a guide to the nature of any human defect, since not only are particular malformations notoriously species-specific, but even within the same species the type of malformation is entirely dependent on the gestational age at the time of exposure to the teratogen. Furthermore, the appearance of an anatomical defect is such a late event in the pathogenetic sequence that there is a much greater possibility for the intervention of developmental repair and adaptive mechanisms, which themselves may be age-specific and species-specific, that could reverse or mitigate toxicity. The operation of repair processes is partly the explanation for the extreme rarity of observable malformations, which in itself is a drawback of this particular end-point indicator, requiring as it does very large numbers of animals in order to detect a statistically-significant increase in incidence after exposure to a teratogen. Taken together, these various considerations suggest that the use of more mechanistic correlates adaptable to *in vitro* measurement might prove a useful alternative in certain circumstances to the standard *in vivo* procedures. Along the lines of *in vitro* testing for mutagenicity/carcinogenicity potential, such methods would be particularly valuable in rapid prescreening tests for evaluating relative teratogenic potentials of a series of chemical compounds. Of course, as with *in vitro* carcinogenicity tests, hazard assessment has also to take account of other important factors, particularly in relation to pharmacokinetics. In addition, as pointed out by Brown in this discussion and elsewhere (2,5), it is essential to make a quantitative comparison of dose-response relationships for adult toxicity and embryo/feto-toxicity.

Mechanistically, mammalian development is based on a sequence of cytodifferentiation and morphogenetic events. With respect to cytodifferentiation, this is characterised by the cellular elaboration of new enzymes and other protein determinants of function. Interference with their elaboration constitutes a sensitive and quantifiable indicator system for the identification of developmental defects and is a more mechanistic correlate of developmental aberration. Some studies have been carried out using the elaboration of developmental phase-specific proteins *in vitro* (3) and enzymes *in vivo* (6,7). With respect to cell morphogenesis, this is known to be critically dependent on cell surface properties and functions, and an *in vitro* system for its evaluation based on cell adhesion to a lectin-coated substratum has been described by Braun *et al.* (8,9) and used for teratogenicity measurement. A comprehensive approach to *in vitro* teratogenicity testing based on a combination of cytodifferentiation and cellular morphogenetic assays will play an increasing role in the future, akin to the developments in carcinogenicity testing, and investment in this area should be a priority.

FUNCTIONAL POSTNATAL DEVELOPMENTAL TOXICITY

The susceptibility of the developing organism to toxic insult is not confined to prenatal life, since much development and functional differentiation, even in man, continues after birth, particularly in the central nervous sytem. Even when the critical primary teratogenic interaction does take place before birth, the defect or disturbance may be functional rather than structural, and may remain cryptic or latent until these functions or other interactive processes become operational at a later maturational stage, even in postnatal life, Metabolic teratogenesis (7) and psychoteratogenesis (10) are terms which describe the perinatal and postnatal development of two types of functional disorder after early gestational exposure of the developing conceptus to a toxic agent (e.g. low dose methyl mercury exposure). Again, because of the guidelines relating to teratogenicity studies require animals to be killed just prior to parturition for morphological examination, precluding their assessment for postnatal functional disorders. On the other hand, the perinatal and postnatal study, which does allow for functional toxicity testing, recommends dosing over the final third of gestation and lactation, thus omitting the period of organogenesis and precluding the assessment of cryptic functional teratogenesis. Regulations governing this latter study, however, do recommend dosing throughout lactation. Given the propensity of certain lipophilic chemicals (such as halogenated hydrocarbon insecticides) to concentrate in breast milk, postnatal translactational exposure is a significant route for the developing infant, and at a period when integrative functional development is at its greatest. Although data are not plentiful, it appears that the dose-response curves for functional disturbances lie to the left of those relating to embryotoxicity and structural malformations. Taking these considerations together, it seems likely that functional developmental abnormalities constitute the most serious hazardous effect of toxic agents to which developing organisms may be exposed.

To avoid prohibitive expense, evaluation of functional disturbances should be at the earliest possible developmental stage and should ideally be quantifiable, in order to investigate dose-response relationships and to establish threshold levels. These criteria are satisfied by the use of developmental phase-specific enzyme clusters (developmental enzyme pathology), as proposed by Andrew & Lytz (11) and Snell (7). In rodent liver, the acquisition of new enzymes during development occurs in a series of distinct steps - at the late fetal, neonatal and weanling stages - and enzymes showing marked developmental increases at any of these phases are designated as belonging to that cognate enzyme cluster (Fig. 1). If it is accepted that there is an underlying biochemical basis for physiological dysfunction, then lesions at the biochemical level will precede other manifestations of pathophysiology, and developmental enzyme pathology will serve as a reliable and sensitive indicator system for functional developmental toxicity. The measurement of organ-specific developmental enzyme profiles allows for the functional evaluation of a number of target organs. However, in practice, the dependence of developmental enzyme accumulations in the liver on the very precise co-ordinated response of neural and endocrine networks means that hepatic developmental enzyme profiles will serve as more-general indicators of the impairment of body functions, including those governed by the central nervous system.

Other methods for the evaluation of functional developmental toxicity have been described, and these include: observations of morphological characteristics (physical appearance, posture), growth (body-weight and organ-weight gain) and maturational events (ear and eye opening, incisor eruption, acquisition of fur); measurements of behavioural characteristics such as specific reflexes (righting reflex, corneal reflex, swimming reflex), activity parameters (open-field tests), neuromuscular co-ordination (locomotion tests), learning ability (maze tests, conditioning response tests) and sensory capacities (vibrissal and visual placing); measurements of reproductive capacities and of immunological competence. Many of these alternative methods are difficult to quantify and involve subjective evaluations. All of them operate at later and more remote stages of the pathogenetic sequence than enzymic correlates. Moreover, many of the methods require complex experimentation and are very demanding in terms of financial expense and personnel time. The rapidity and ease of enzymic determinations, together with accurate and reproducible quantitation, make them attractive indicator systems for assessing functional toxicity. In addition, for direct-acting agents, it would be possible to measure organ-specific development enzyme changes in tissue or cell culture systems <u>in vitro</u>.

At the present time, it is vitally important to initiate validation studies in order to correlate the application of developmental enzyme pathology with the other indicator systems used for evaluating functional developmental toxicity. In particular, it is necessary to establish the relative sensitivity of the biochemical approach as well as its predictivity in relation to functional abnormalities. The benefits to be derived from this simple and rapid approach to toxicity evaluation are analagous to the contributions of clinical chemistry in the present day diagnosis of human disease.

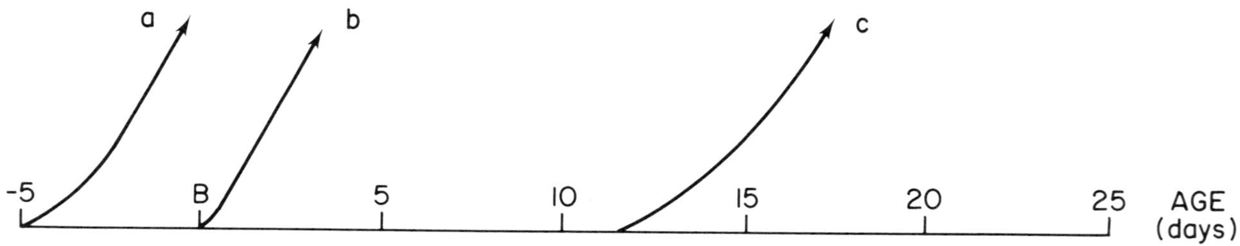

(a) glycogen
glucose 6-phosphatase
glycogen synthetase
glycogen phosphorylase
NADPH-cytochrome *c* dehydrogenase

(b) PEP carboxykinase
serine aminotransferase
glyoxylate aminotransferase
fructokinase
palmityl CoA synthetase
glycerol kinase
glucose 6-phosphatase
alanine aminotransferase

(c) glucokinase
alanine aminotransferase
tryptophan dioxygenase
NADP-malate dehydrogenase
ATP-citrate lyase
xanthine oxidase

Figure 1 Enzyme Clusters During Neonatal Development of Rat Liver. (a) Fetal cluster; (b) neonatal cluster; (c) weanling cluster. Enzymes appearing in more than one cluster show a biphasic developmental accumulation. B: birth.

REFERENCES

1. Beck, F. (1982). Model systems in teratology. In "Developmental Toxicology" (ed. K. Snell), pp. 11-29. London: Croom Helm.
2. Brown, N.A. & Fabro, S.E. (1982). The in vitro approach to teratogenicity testing. In "Developmental Toxicology" (ed. K. Snell), pp. 31-57. London: Croom Helm.
3. Clayton, R.M. & Zehir, A. (1982). The use of cell culture methods for exploring teratogenic susceptibility. In "Developmental Toxicology" (ed. K. Snell), pp. 59-92. London: Croom Helm.
4. Kochlar, D.M. (1981). Embryo explants and organ cultures in screening of chemicals for teratogenic effects. In "Developmental Toxicology" (ed. C.A. Kimmel & J. Buelke-Sam), pp. 303-319. New York: Raven Press.
5. Fabro, S., Shull, G. & Brown, N.A. (1982). The relative teratogenic index and teratogenic potency: proposed component of developmental toxicity risk assessment. Teratogenesis, Mutagenesis and Carcinogenesis 2, 61-76.
6. Kwasigroch, T.E. & Neubert, D. (1978). A simple method to test chondrogenic and myogenic tissues for differential effects of drugs. In "Role of Pharmacokinetics in Prenatal and Perinatal Toxicology" (ed. D. Neubert, H.J. Merker, H. Nam & J. Langman), pp. 621-630. Stuttgart: Georg Thieme.
7. Snell, K. (1982). Developmental enzyme pathology. In "Developmental Toxicology" (ed. K. Snell), pp. 299-339. London: Croom Helm.
8. Braun, A.G., Emerson, D.J. & Nichinson, B.B. (1979). Teratogenic drugs inhibit tumour cell attachment to lectin-coated surfaces. Nature, London 282, 507-509.
9. Braun, A.G., Buckner, C.A., Emerson, D.J. & Nichinson, B.B. (1982). Quantitative correspondence between the in vivo and in vitro activity of teratogenic agents. Proceedings of the National Academy of Sciences, USA 79, 2056-2060.
10. Vorhees, C.V. & Butcher, R.E. (1982). Behavioural teratogenicity. In "Developmental Toxicology" (ed. K. Snell), pp. 247-298. London: Croom Helm.
11. Andrew, F.D. & Lytz, P.S. (1981). Biochemical disturbances associated with developmental toxicity. In "Developmental Toxicology" (ed. C.A. Kimmel & J. Buelke-Sam), pp. 145-165. New York: Raven Press.

Problems in Current Reproductive Toxicity Testing

N. A. BROWN

TYPES OF REPRODUCTIVE FAILURE AND THE DIVISION OF RESOURCES

The vast majority of research efforts in reproductive toxicology, particularly those which might increase our understanding of mechanisms and of extrapolation to man, are concerned with structural birth defects. There appears to be little rationale for this emphasis, either from animal or human data. Some will argue that a malformed child is a greater cause for concern than cases of infertility or spontaneous abortion, particularly in an increasingly overpopulated world. Others will say that the impact of a loss of pregnancy or an inability to conceive is not to be dismissed lightly. Leaving aside such arguments, it seems safe to say that we do not know which aspects of the human reproductive cycle are most sensitive to environmental insult and, therefore, whether we are using our resources appropriately in this area.

Available human data suggest that single chemical agents are rarely the cause of birth defects and that other stages of reproduction may be more liable to disruption. However, current information is far from complete. It is important that there should be careful collection and analysis of epidemiological data on geographical, occupational and migrant variations in infertility, spontaneous abortion rates, retarded growth, impared mental function and other manifestations of human reproductive failure. Although these are difficult tasks to perform, the information generated may identify unexpected sources of risk or perhaps interacting factors, and should provide a rational basis for deciding where our precious animal resources should best be utilised.

INTERPRETATION OF CURRENT "TERATOGENICITY" TESTS

In the area of mandatory screening for reproductive toxicants there is also undue emphasis on structural birth defects, compounded by unsophisticated interpretation of test results. It is a common misconception that the aim of teratogenicity tests should be to detect teratogens. This is incorrect on two counts. First, tests should be designed to evaluate all possible manifestations of embryotoxicity, not just major structural abnormalities. Variations in fetal weights or the incidences of minor variants or resorptions may be just as important as gross malformations and are frequently more-sensitive indicators. Secondly, it is likely that there is no chemical which is non-teratogenic or, more correctly, non-embryotoxic. Karnofsky first argued that all agents are teratogenic, provided a sufficiently high dose can be administered to a susceptible strain or species. It is a law which is difficult to disprove. Thus, it is not good practice to label chemicals as either "teratogens" or "non-teratogens", nor to speak of tests to detect teratogens; all chemicals have teratogenic potential.

However, the vast majority of chemicals are able to disrupt development only at doses which are also toxic to the adult organism. Very few agents are selectively toxic to developmental processes. Such agents might be termed as having a high teratogenic hazard. Teratogenic hazard is the ratio of teratogenic doses to adult toxic doses and is the parameter of primary importance in teratogenicity testing. It may be of no interest that a compound has extreme teratogenic potency, say 1ng/kg, if dams are killed at 1.5ng/kg. However, a chemical which induces embryotoxicity at doses which are an order of magnitude lower than those which cause any toxicity in the adult may be a significant reproductive hazard to man and may be regulated on that basis. At least the initial aim of any teratogenicity test *in vivo* or *in vitro* should be to detect agents with high teratogenic hazard. Estimation of the magnitude of the hazard, the teratogenic potency (absolute dosages which cause defects) and the spectrum of defects are the secondary aims. Any proposed teratogenicity test, either *in vivo* or *in vitro*, which does not enable some estimate of teratogenic hazard to be made is likely to be a waste of valuable resources.

Teratogenic hazard can be expressed by any one of several indices. We have proposed a "Relative Teratogenic Index" (RTI), calculated from the ratio LD01/td05 and have discussed its merits and likely alternatives (1). Carefully performed traditional teratogenicity tests do estimate teratogenic hazard, although it is rarely expressed numerically or even discussed as an entity. A good study will always carefully monitor maternal response to the administered agent, and this data can provide the numerator in a hazard ratio. The denominator should be the lowest dose which influences embryo/fetal development, whatever the manifestation.

An example of the use of the concept of teratogenic hazard is provided by our studies of various anticonvulsant drugs, particularly sodium valproate (Epilim, Depakene). From standard testing in the whole mouse (1), the RTI for valproate is relatively high at 4.1 which is the same order of magnitude as the "active" human teratogen, trimethadione (4.0, ref. 1,2) and considerably higher than that of phenytoin (1.6, ref. 3), which is considered a weak human teratogen. The major malformation induced by valproate was exencephaly. Parallel experiments *in vitro*, using cultured post-implantation embryos from mice and rats (4), showed that valproate directly inhibited neural tube closure, with a minimum effective concentration of 0.6mM (about 90µg/ml). Thus, teratogenicity was due to the parent compund, not a rodent-specific metabolite, and effective concentrations are of the same order of magnitude as human serum concentrations (40-100µg/ml, ref. 5). These data prompted us to search for data on human exposure to valproate in early pregnancy (6), and very recently, several examples of neural tube defects in the offspring of mothers taking valproate have been reported (7-9). This example shows how careful interpretation of data from standard animal testing, integrated with information from *in vitro* techniques, can enable a better estimate of human risk.

SOME LIMITATIONS OF *IN VITRO* TESTS

The potential and the limitations of *in vitro* screening systems (as distinct from *in vitro* systems in general) for reproductive toxicity are fairly easy to define, but perhaps not widely appreciated. It is clear that there is no foreseeable alternative to the whole animal for a complete reproductive toxicity study. It is unlikely that *in vitro* tests will ever be developed that could detect chemicals which might affect parturition or lactation, or those which might induce impotence. However, there are areas where *in vitro* screens should be of use, and several of these are poorly studied by toxicologists. As examples, several aspects of spermatogenesis, oogenesis and fertilisation are amenable to study *in vitro*, but have rarely been utilised in toxicology. In fact, virtually all *in vitro* screens in reproductive toxicology have had the limited aim of "detecting" teratogens. There has been a tendency for experimental embryologists to propose each of their model systems as *in vitro* screens, with too little thought of the practical requirements of a screening system. Of all the proposed screens, none have been fully validated, but several show promise, including those using frog embryos (10), mouse limb bud mesenchyme (11,12), and tumour cell attachment (13). Although others may be modified, only one test system has been specifically designed to estimate teratogenic hazard: the hydra-based system (14), and this must currently be considered the *in vitro* screen of choice.

FINAL COMMENTS

As a final note, all of these tests in reproductive toxicology provide information on toxic potential, potency or hazard, under defined circumstances. Risk to man depends upon actual exposure conditions. To extrapolate to man in the area of reproductive toxicology, as in all other areas of toxicology, it is necessary to evaluate or estimate the physiological disposition of the agent in man. Embryo/fetal or gonadal exposure levels, time periods, and the nature of metabolites or reactive intermediates determine a toxic effect. From the test system and from man, such information must be collected, if risk and safely evaluation are to be more than an intelligent guesses.

REFERENCES

1. Fabro, S., Shull, G. & Brown, N.A. (1982). The relative teratogenic index and teratogenic potency: proposed components of developmental toxicity risk assessment. Teratogenesis, Carcinogenesis and Mutagenesis 2, 61-76.
2. Brown, N.A., Shull, G. & Fabro, S. (1979). Assessment of the teratogenic potential of trimethadione in the CD-1 mouse, Toxicology & Applied Pharmacology 51, 49-71.
3. Brown, N.A., Shull, G., Kao, J., Goulding, E.H. & Fabro, S. (1982). Teratogenicity and lethality of hydantoin derivatives in the mouse: Structure-toxicity relationships. Toxicology & Applied Pharmacology 64, 271-288.
4. Kao, J., Brown, N.A., Schmidt, B., Goulding, E.H. & Fabro, S. (1981). Teratogenicity of valproic acid: in vivo and in vitro investigations. Teratogenesis, Carcinogenesis and Mutagenesis 1, 376 382.
5. Medical Letter (1979). Drugs for Epilcpsy 21, 25.
6. Brown, N.A., Kao, J. & Fabro, S. (1980). Teratogenic potential of valproic acid. Lancet i, 660-661.
7. Robert, E. & Guibaud, P. (1982). Maternal valproic acid and congenital neural tube defects. Lancet ii, 937.
8. Bjerkedal, T., Czeizel, A., Goujard, J., Kallen, B., Mastroiacova, P., Nevin, N., Oakley, G. & Robert, E. (1982). Valproic acid and spina bifida. Lancet ii, 1096.
9. Editorial. (1982). Valproate and malformations. Lancet ii, 1313-1314.
10. Dumont, J.N., Schultz, T.N. & Newman, S.M. (1982). A frog embryo teratogenesis assay: Xenopus (FETAX) - a model for teratogen screening. Teratology 25, 37A.
11. Hassell, J.R. & Horigan, E.A. (1982). Chondrogenesis: a model development system for measuring teratogenic potential of compounds. Teratogenesis, Carcinogenesis and Mutagenesis 2, 325-332.
12. Flint, O.P. (1982). An in vitro assay for teratogens using

embryonic cells exposed to compounds in utero or directly in culture. Teratology 25, 40A.
13. Braun, A.G., Emerson, D.J. & Nichinson, B.B. (1979). Teratogenic drugs inhibit tumour cell attachment to lectin-coated surfaces. Nature, London 282, 507-509.
14. Johnson, E.M. (1980). A subvertebrate system for rapid determination of potential teratogenic hazards. Journal of Environmental Pathology and Toxicology 4, 153-156.

Alternative Methods

A. K. PALMER

Generally, mention of reproductive toxicology provokes an immediate assumption that this means teratology, i.e. the induction of malformations. Proposals for non-mammalian or *in vitro* test methods to all intents and purposes have been promulgated in this direction. Because of this, the FRAME document has also had to be channelled towards this emphasis. However, frightening the induction of malformation may be, objectively, in the broader spectrum of mammalian reproduction it is perhaps the most unlikely adverse event that may occur. Moreover, if it does occur it may have far less long-term consequences than other adverse effects, e.g. female or male sterility.

In its broader aspects, mammalian reproduction is unique in the animal kingdom, particularly in respect of the co-ordination and integration of the processes of maturation, copulation, fertilisation, development of the embryo and fetus in a protective maternal envelope, parturition and lactation. Those actively involved in safety evaluation, especially at initial screening stages, perform studies to cover all these aspects. By and large, proponents of alternative systems have paid insufficient attention to the broader aspects of reproductive toxicity testing and have failed to understand the importance of its integrated nature.

Most non-mammalian exercises have been confined to specific restricted aspects and specific cases, and have been followed by faulty extrapolation from the specific to the general. Perhaps this is because it is difficult to envisage non-mammalian systems that could be used to explore effects on behavioural aspects of mating and nursing or effects on the process of parturition. Even in the area that has been explored to the greatest extent, namely, effects on embryonic development, proponents of _in vitro_ systems - some of which may necessitate use of mammals as source material - have tended to overlook the importance of the extensive defence mechanism provided by the maternal organism and, in later stages, by the placenta. Thus, it is pointless to apply materials directly to a developing embryo or proliferating tissue until one is certain that the same material reaches the embryo in the same quantity.

There is also a lack of awareness of some basic principles of toxicology, namely, that "all substances are poisonous, only the dose determines that a substance does not poison" (Paracelsus). In other words, toxicity and its counterpart, safety, are relative. Even more prevalent is lack of awareness of the different approach required for initial screening of materials of unknown potential and for toxicological or teratological investigation of materials with known potential. Thus, use of a system that merely indicates a potential hazard without providing means by which it can be established, whether or not this can be transposed to a real life situation, is likely to do more harm than good.

In pressing the claims for alternative methodology, proponents have emphasised aspects of economy and sensitivity, but have neglected the equally, if not more important, aspects of fidelity. Already, whole animal tests have provided us with problems in this area, since many materials have been shown to induce malformations in animals whilst relatively few have been shown to represent a teratogenic hazard to man. Increasing this sensitivity with _in vitro_ systems may only add to the existing dilemma and the consequent alarm that may be raised could well lead to increased use of mammals to put the results of the _in vitro_ tests in perspective.

That there is a wide discrepancy between the number of agents shown to be "teratogenic" in animals but affording no proven risk to man, indicates that it would be naive to asume that teratogenic potential is always synonymous with lack of safety; the reverse also applies.

Particularly for drugs and pesticides, which are intended to interfere with biological processes, it should be obvious that there will always be a balance between adverse and beneficial consequences according to dosage and conditions of usage. Tests of such materials, therefore, must place especial emphasis on perspective, with a view to establishing not just whether an agent will affect the developing embryo, but whether the effect is likely to occur under conditions of usage.

For relatively well defined agents with a relatively well defined usage, the investment placed into development of a specific agent or group of agents is such that they would neither be abandoned nor considered safe on the basis of results obtained in systems lacking fidelity: therefore, in vitro "screening" tests would merely represent an additional expense in most cases.

By continuing to neglect the broader aspects of mammalian reproduction and the basic principles of toxicology, and by continuing to press the claims of alternate methodology for screening, proponents of alternate systems may actually frustrate the cause for reduced usage of intact mammals.

First, they are diverting attention away from usage of alternative systems in second and fundamental investigations, both of which in the long-term could lead to greater understanding of toxicological processes, and therefore more efficient testing procedures.

Secondly, they are introducing more confusing factors in an existing confused situation and, thereby, may divert attention away from improving interpretation of, and extrapolation from, mammalian studies. In turn, this could delay attempts to harmonise national and international regulations.

If there is a place for using alternate methodology in a screening role, it is within poorly-defined areas for which, as yet, toxicity testing programmes are non-existent or in their infancy. In such areas as environmental pollution with a complex mixture of agents of natural, agricultural or industrial origin, use of mammals to test the importance of every agent or intermediate that may be present in marked, moderate or minute quantities, would be untenable. The most logical approach would be to consult with conservationists (e.g. NCC) to see if there had been an impact on ecosystems. According to the information provided, alternate test systems, such as those using hydra, or fish breeding, could be devised to identify the components of the mix likely to afford the greatest hazard.

At this stage, sufficient information may be generated to allow action to be taken to remove the source of pollution, not because it may be harmful for humans or other mammals, but because we wish to preserve the environment. However, if action cannot be taken at this point, the alternate methodology can be used to select priorities for investigations in higher systems, including mammals.

For similar sources of mixed pollution, i.e. in the work place, the more likely sequence would be use of human surveillance and, perhaps, mammalian studies to provide information on potential hazards of the overall mix of agents present or of the most predominant types present. Concurrently, or afterwards, alternate methods could be used to check the potential of the many minor components.

Finally, it must be stated that the most immediately productive and effective way to reduce the usage of intact mammals in testing for reproductive toxicity would be to harmonise testing requirements. Too often, studies are repeated or are of excessive dimensions because of an inconsequential difference between regulatory authorities. Indeed, the differences may be so slight that all that would be required for harmonisation would be reaffirmation that the suggested procedures are "guidelines" not mandatory requirements.

Responsibility for achieving this objective lies not just with the agencies, but with the scientific community as a whole. The key would be to look at screening tests as an applied science not as a nuisance to which we must pay token homage, nor as a medium to advertise an individual skill or technique in a specific narrow situation.

REFERENCES

1. Palmer, A.K. (1977), Incidence of sporadic malformations, anomalies and variations in random bred laboratory animals. In "Methods in Prenatal Toxicology" (ed. D. Neubert, H.J. Merker & T.E. Kwasigroch), pp. 52-71. Stuttgart: Georg Thieme.
2. Palmer, A.K. (1978). The design of subprimate animal studies. In "Handbook of Teratology" (ed. J.G. Wilson & F.C. Fraser), vol. IV, pp. 215-253. New York: Plenum Publishing Corporation.
3. Palmer, A.K. (1976). Assessment of current test procedures. Environmental Health Perspectives 18, 97-104.
4. Palmer, A.K. (1981). Regulatory requirements for reproductive toxicology: theory and practice. In "Developmental Toxicology" (ed. C.A. Kimmel & J. Buelke-Sam), pp. 259-287. New York: Raven Press.
5. Palmer, A.K. (1982). Use of mammalian models in teratology. Proceedings of Conference Mondiale "Prevention des Anomalies Congenitales Physiques et Mentales" New York: Alan Liss (in press).

Hazards of Development

RUTH CLAYTON

It is evident that the effects of environmental hazards to the normal development and continuing normal function of an individual are distributed over the entire life-cycle, and developmental toxicology might be considered to embrace that part of it stretching from the production of normal gametes at one extreme to the end of the weaning period at the other. In an environment increasingly loaded with potentially hazardous substances, and in the face of restrictions on the time available, how might the cost effectiveness of different possible patterns of the allocation of resources be assessed?

The answer must surely be in operational terms. If there is to be inequality of research effort should not the bias be weighted by the social consequences of disturbances of different parts of the life-cycle, as well as the changing biological susceptibilities of the organism?

On this basis, we might be forced to conclude that, tragic although infertility is to any particular couple, heart rending although it is to lose a child during gestation or shortly after delivery, by far the most devastating social and psychological consequences follow the birth of a live child with gross mental or physical handicaps. The cost to society of medical or custodial care, the cost to family stability and inter-personal relations, the effects on the self-image of the growing child are all considerable (families with a severely handicapped child are known to break up more often than families with normal children). It might even be added here that long-term demographic and economic trends point to requirements of population control which are at variance with the wish to increase human fertility by studies on the effects of toxic agencies on gametogenesis, fertilisation and implantation. The premise in the outline that follows is therefore that an area of major concern is the identification of agencies which may affect the development or subsequent function of individuals exposed *in utero* or shortly after birth.

The major problems of testing for substances which may be teratogenic to man include the questions of the overall reliability of animal or *in vitro* tests, which encompasses questions of species differences in placental structure and pharmacogenetics, and the relationship between developmental processes and cell properties *in vitro*, and such specific questions as the methods of assessment of effect, including the assessment of genetic variations in response within a species. These questions have been discussed *in extenso* elsewhere (1,2).

Although all the earlier work on teratogenesis involved assessments of disturbances of organogenesis and the development of morphological defects, there is increasing evidence that the susceptibility of the developing brain to certain agencies may lead to permanent changes recognised by effects on postnatal learning and behaviour (3). Behavioural teratogens are at present assessed when the offspring are old enough for tests of performance. Testing for behavioural teratogens is therefore clearly a lengthy procedure, and we have begun to investigate the effects of behavioural teratogens on brain or retina cells in cell culture; preliminary data is presented elsewhere (4).

A subject specifically discussed at this Meeting, namely, the Draize test, fails to touch certain specific questions, one of which is the possibility of differences in the response of juvenile corneas to agencies at levels different from those affecting the adult; another is the possibility that substances at non-irritant levels may penetrate the cornea and exert low-level effects on ocular tissues, which may affect vision, either in the short-term or long-term, with the added possibility of different levels of susceptibility between adults and juvenile tissues (4). I will touch briefly here on one problem; the effect of surfactants on the juvenile eye.

Surfactants are used as additives to topical ophthalmic solutions, in part because the uptake of drugs into the eye is facilitated (5), and in part as bacteriostatic agents. Similarly, surfactants are used in contact lens solutions, and also in the form of shampoos or soaps, which may enter the eye inadvertently. We have undertaken a preliminary investigation using a ^{3}H-labelled anionic detergent, at levels which are wholly non-irritant (Clayton, Green, Zehir & Wilson, in preparation). Our findings may be summarised as follows:

a. Surfactant penetrates the cornea, and is found in all ocular tissues. This uptake is much greater in juvenile than in adult eyes (Fig. 1).
b. The rate of release is much slower than that found for drugs such as pilocarpine (6).
c. After repeated applications, which still produced no visible irritant effect, the level of label in ocular tissues had increased, and label was also detected in plasma, brain, liver, kidney, spleen and heart (Fig. 2).
d. Repeated application in juvenile animals brought the calculated level in some ocular tissues close to levels found to affect axonal outgrowth of neural retina cells in cell culture.

The requirement for Draize tests of every new formulation of substances already known to be highly irritant (such as alkalis) has been strongly and justifiably criticised. I would add another caveat: that there may be potential hazards to the growing eye which the Draize test is incompetent to reveal. It is possible that, once the kinetics and distribution of a substance in the eye (following external administration) has been assessed in juvenile as well as adult tissues, *in vitro* methods might prove a helpful adjunct to further assessment.

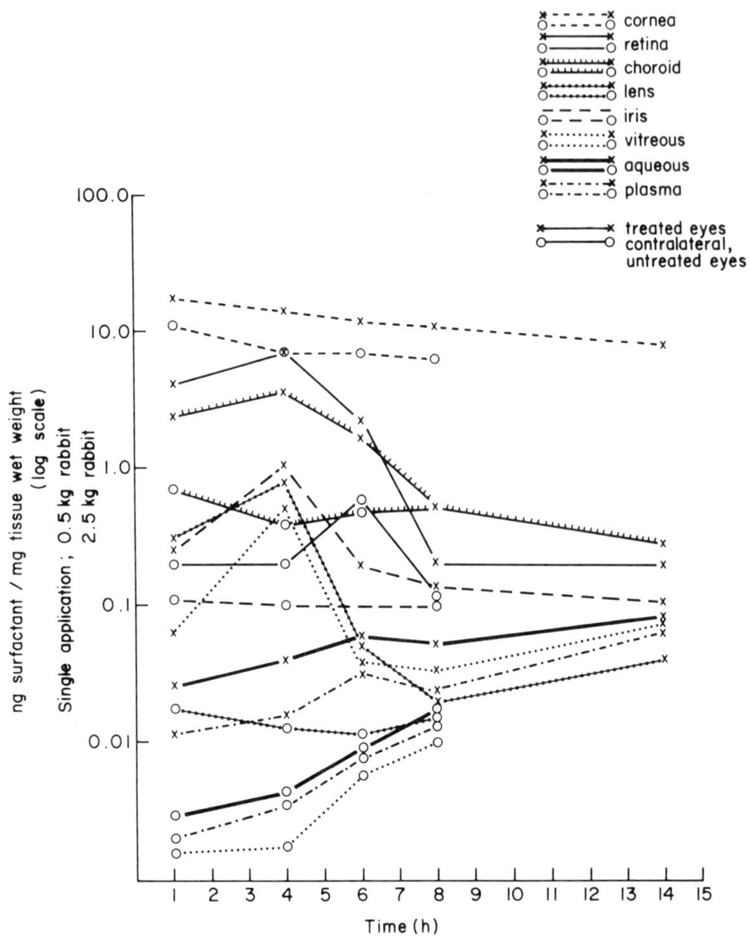

Figure 1 A comparison of the rates of uptake and release from ocular tissues of anionic surfactant applied to the corneas of rabbits of 2.5kg and 0.5kg body weights respectively (modified from Clayton, Green, Zehir & Wilson, submitted for publication).

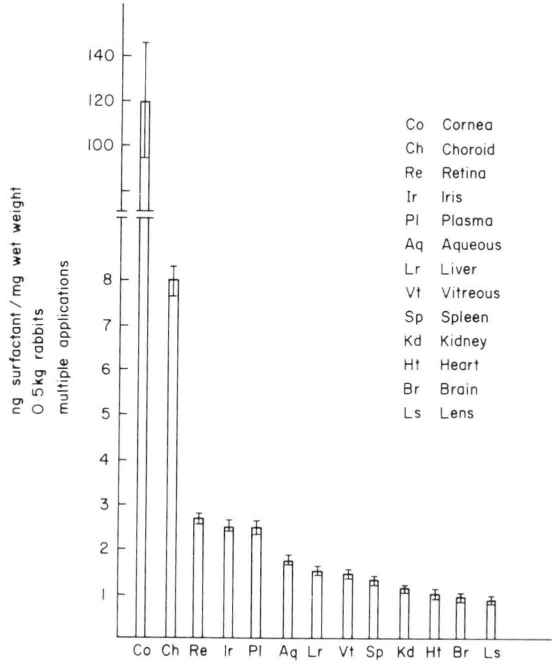

Figure 2 Levels in some tissues of 1kg rabbits after multiple applications, exposed as ng surfactant per mg tissue wet weight (modified from Clayton, Green, Zehir & Wilson, submitted for publication).

ACKNOWLEDGEMENTS

We are grateful to the Humane Research Trust, Medical Research Council and Health and Safety Executive for their support of various aspects of our work.

REFERENCES

1. Clayton, R.M. (1980). An in vitro system for teratogenicity testing. In "The Use of Alternatives in Drug Research" (ed. A.N. Rowan & C.J. Stratman), pp. 153-173. London: Macmillan.
2. Clayton, R.M. & Zehir, A. (1982). The use of cell culture methods for exploring teratogenic susceptibility. In "Developmental Toxicology" (ed. K. Snell), pp. 59-92. London: Croom Helm.
3. Voorhees, C.U. & Butcher, R.E. (1982). Behavioural terato-

genicity. In "Developmental Toxicology" (ed. K. Snell), pp. 247-298. London: Croom Helm.
4. Clayton, R.M., Zehir, A. & Sedowofia, K. (1983). Testing for delayed effects on development and differentiation: some open questions. In "Alternative Methods in Scientific Research" (ed. P. Turner). London: Macmillan (in press).
5. Marsh, R.J. & Maurice, D.M. (1971). The influence of non-ionic detergents and other surfactants on human corneal permeability. Experimental Eye Research 11, 43-48.
6. Mishima, S. (1981). Clinical pharmacogenetics of the eye. Investigative Ophthalmology 21, 504-541.

General Discussion

A. N. WORDEN

Rapporteur

Dr Olga UVAROV asked Dr Palmer how he thought it would be possible to achieve harmonisation of regulations in view of the many obstacles that existed, and whether he could envisage a test that would satisfy all the different regulatory authorities. Dr PALMER replied that he thought that scientists had to get their own house in order first and sit down honestly to work out what could be done with each test - what could be done now, and what might be done in the future. He was not against in vitro systems, but felt that they could be used much more effectively than at present, though not by regarding them as competitive with existing tests. He felt that in vitro investigations should feed off existing problems and should be used to help solve those problems by recycling back, so that we could achieve better testing procedures all round. He had, in fact, already written up a comprehensive test which he felt could replace all existing variations now required for reproductive studies and which therefore utilised excessive numbers of animals. He felt that the OECD and the EPA were beginning to come round to consideration of an all-embracing test, although, unfortunately, they had left in minor aberrations which would cause problems because of the slavish way in which people tended to follow guidelines.

Professor POSWILLO commented that the philosophy that seemed to be emerging was that we should be looking for simple tests for non-teratogenicity rather than for teratogenicity.

Professor BERRY said that the clinical significance of malformation had not been discounted, but that if one took malformation as an end-point, this would significantly underestimate reproductive toxicology. It was comforting that most of the variables that could be measured in man appeared to be on the decrease. Thus, paediatric tumours had decreased by the order of 12% over the last 15 years, to judge from crude mortality statistics. Malformation rates were falling significantly, even allowing for the advent of the remarkable effects of vitamin supplementation, as indicated by current preventative studies. In this particular sense, therefore, things were apparently getting better. However, he added that we did not appear to be assessing changes in fertility, but he took Dr Clayton's point that perhaps a minor decrease in fertility would not be a disaster for many countries; nonetheless, it was still a toxic effect that should be detected.

Neurotoxicity

A.J. DEWAR

INTRODUCTION

The purpose of neurotoxicity testing is to determine whether the chemical under investigation causes any deviations from the "normal" functioning and structure of the nervous system, i.e. to determine whether the chemical has the inherent ability to cause adverse neurobiological effects. Whether such effects, once identified, constitute a hazard depends on other criteria, notably the conditions and extent of possible exposure. Thus, an ability to alter mood may be regarded as a desirable property in a chemical designed to be administered under controlled conditions as a drug for the management of an affective disorder, but would be regarded as a potential hazard in a chemical designed for use as a food additive or a household insecticide.

The object of this report is to survey some of the methods currently available for evaluating the neurotoxicity of compounds and, in particular, to explore the possibilities for using in vitro methodology. As a prelude to this survey, some of the more important features of neurotoxicity will be discussed. An appreciation of these features is essential in order to understand some of the formidable difficulties confronting a toxicologist wishing to devise a strategy for evaluating the neurotoxicity of a compound.

Range of Neurotoxic Phenomena

It is a truism that the nervous system is the most complex organ of all in terms of both structure and function, and it is hardly surprising that this complexity of the nervous system is reflected in the very wide diversity of toxic actions that can be exerted upon it. Many neurotoxins can differentially affect specific regions of the central or peripheral nervous system, specific cell types (e.g. neurones, astrocytes, oligodendroglia/Schwann cells, microglia), blood vessels, or specific functions within cells.

The diversity of neurotoxic phenomena is illustrated in Table I. This summarises some of the symptomatology that has been reported in humans exposed to neurotoxic chemicals. Further illustration is provided by consideration of the types of chemical which can be regarded as "neurotoxins". These include industrial chemicals and solvents such as acrylamide and n-hexane; metals such as lead, aluminium, mercury and tin; pesticides such as DDT and the pyrethroids; psychoactive drugs such as neuroleptics, anti-convulsants, anaesthetics, anti-depressants, sedatives, hallucinogens and stimulants; anti-microbials such as the nitrofurans and hexachlorophene; chemotherapeutic agents such as vincristine, misonidazole and dapsone; and neurotoxins of biological origin such as snake venoms, tetrodotoxin, diphtheria toxin and curare.

Classification of Neurotoxicity

On reviewing the many types of neurotoxic reaction to chemicals it is possible to draw a crude distinction between acute neurotoxic effects and chronic neurotoxic effects. Acute neurotoxic effects are generally due to functional changes in the nervous system, not necessarily involving structural damage or degeneration of the cellular elements. They are often reversible, may occur after a single large dose, and are often due to "pharmacological" actions on nerve cell membranes or synaptic transmission. In contrast, most chronic neurotoxic effects involving structural changes with degeneration of the cellular elements are not readily reversible, and may require repeated doses. These effects may be due to metabolic lesions in the neurones and their axons or in the supporting cells such as Schwann cells and glia, or to interference with the cerebral vasculature.

It must be emphasised that, as with many other over-simple generalisations, there are exceptions. It is sometimes possible, for example, to obtain chronic neurotoxic effects following a single dose of a chemical (e.g. some organophosphates can produce a delayed peripheral neuropathy after a single dose (1)). Furthermore, it is also possible to identify chronic neurotoxic effects that are attributable to functional rather than structural or degenerative changes - the tardive dyskinesia (due to dopamine receptor hypersensitivity) that can result from prolonged phenothiazine therapy being a good example (2).

A further complication is that many compounds can exert both

1. Motor disorders e.g. weakness and inco-ordination of limbs, paralysis, fatigue, slurred speech, rigidity, tremor, convulsions.

2. Sensory disorders e.g. parasthesiae in limb extremities, spontaneous pain, auditory deficits, tinnitus, visual deficits.

3. Disturbances of autonomic function e.g. impaired sexual function, impotence, postural hypotension, lacrimation, excessive salivation, sweating, incontinence, altered heart rate, vomiting, gastrointestinal troubles.

4. Increase in the state of excitability of the central nervous system e.g. hyperactivity, nervousness, agitation, irritability, hallucination, euphoria, mania, seizures.

5. Decrease in the state of excitability of the central nervous system e.g. narcosis, lethargy, apathy, depression, repetitive stereotyped behaviour, coma.

6. Impairment of short-term or long-term memory, disorientation, confusion.

7. Sleep disorders.

8. Psychiatric disturbances e.g. psychosis.

9. Impaired temperature regulation - hypothermia or hyperthermia.

10. Alterations in appetite, weight gain or weight loss.

Table I Types of Symptomatology Associated with Neurotoxicity in Humans

acute and chronic neurotoxicity, at different dose-levels and by independent mechanisms. For example, n-hexane produces a pharmacological and reversible central nervous system narcosis in rodents if administered at 30,000 ppm for 10 minutes, but if administered at far lower concentrations (400-600 ppm) for more prolonged periods (several weeks), it will produce degeneration in peripheral nerves (3).

Chronic neurotoxic effects on the mature nervous system are commonly classified on the basis of the primary site of tissue damage. Four main types of chemically-induced structural damage can be identified: neuropathy, axonopathy, myelinopathy and neurovasculopathy (4,5), and these can be subdivided further when it is possible to define the target site more precisely. Thus, axonopathies can be subdivided into distal axonopathies, where the primary site of damage is the distal portion of the axon, and proximal axonopathies, where it is the proximal axon that is primarily affected. A classification based on that of Spencer & Schaumburg (4) is summarised in Table II. The primary structural changes outlined in this table are frequently followed by secondary and tertiary changes. Thus, the toxic effects of methyl mercury on the neurones of the dorsal root ganglion lead to axonal degeneration and secondary loss of myelin in the sensory fibres of the sciatic nerve (6). Similarly, the primary axonal degeneration seen in distal axonopathies is followed by a secondary loss of myelin.

One of the most common reactions of the nervous system to chronic exposure to neurotoxic chemicals is the development of peripheral neuropathy. By far the most common type of chemically-induced peripheral neuropathy is distal axonopathy (7). The other types of peripheral neuropathy (see Table II) are relatively rare.

Classification of acute neurotoxic effects of a pharmacological nature is generally made on the basis of mode of action or, when this is not possible, on the basis of symptomatology. With the relatively sparse knowledge of the mechanistic aspects of a wide variety of neurotoxic phenomena that exists at present, classification on the basis of mechanism is frequently difficult.

Mechanisms of Neurotoxicity

It is not possible within the space available to discuss mechanisms of neurotoxicity in any detail, since neurotoxicity may be brought about by a large variety of different physiological, pharmacological and biochemical mechanisms. For example, toxins can selectively interfere with basic metabolic processes such as energy metabolism, lipid metabolism and RNA and protein synthesis, with biochemical reactions responsible for the maintenance of myelin, with axonal transport, with nerve membrane permeability, and with the conduction of action

TYPE	PRIMARY SITE OF ATTACK	SUBDIVISION	EXAMPLES
Neuronopathy	Neuronal cell bodies	Cytoplasm	Methyl mercury, Aluminium
		Nucleus	Adriamycin (doxorubicin)
		Postsynaptic membrane	Glutamate
Axonopathy	Axons	Proximal axon	β-Iminodipropionitrile
		Distal axon	Acrylamide, Carbon disulphide, Tri-o-cresyl phosphate n-Hexane
Myelinopathy	Myelinating cells	Schwann cells (PNS)	Diptheria toxin
		Oligodendrocytes (CNS)	Cuprizone
		Myelin sheath	Triethyltin, Hexachlorophene, Acetyl ethyl tetramethyl tetralin
Neurovasculopathy	Neural vasculature		Cadmium, Lead

Table II

A Summary of the Main Types of Chemically-induced Structural Damage in the Mature Nervous System

potentials or with synaptic transmission.

As a result of the explosive increase in the knowledge of the biochemistry and pharmacology of the central nervous system within the last two decades, it is now possible to identify many metabolic changes that, when they occur, are likely to be associated either with neurotoxicity (if produced by an exogenous chemical) or with disease (if produced endogenously). Tables III and IV list some abnormalities believed to be associated with acute or chronic neurotoxicity. These lists are by no means exhaustive and are given merely to illustrate the range of potential mechanisms of neurotoxicity.

To assume from the lists in Tables III and IV that our knowledge of mechanisms of neurotoxicity is at an advanced stage, however, would be erroneous. Although it is true that a great deal is known of potential mechanisms of neurotoxicity, our knowledge of the precise modes of action of many existing neurotoxins is still extremely sparse. This is particularly true of the neurotoxins that produce structural damage such as peripheral neuropathy or encephalopathy. Furthermore, although our understanding of the biochemistry and physiology of the nervous system has grown dramatically in recent years, in absolute terms our state of knowledge remains rudimentary relative to the complexity of the systems being studied. The biochemical and physiological bases of many important neurobiological functions are still far from being completely understood - mood, sleep and memory being good examples. There may also be systems and functions that remain to be discovered and these too may be targets for neurotoxins.

Neurotoxicity and the Developing Nervous System

The previous sections have been primarily concerned with toxic effects on the functioning mature nervous system. However, the immature and developing nervous system has particular vulnerabilities to toxic insult and there has been a growing interest in neonatal and perinatal neurotoxicology.

The development of the nervous system proceeds in a series of interphased stages, commencing with the embryological events and ending with maturity. These stages may be summarised as: organogenesis and neuronal multiplication; a maturation period (known as the "growth spurt") during which there is axonal growth, dendritic arborisation, synaptogenesis and myelination; and a period of generalised growth in size. The onset of these various events occurs at different times (in relation to birth) in different species. In man, the growth spurt (the time of the greatest rate of increase in the net weight of the whole brain) commences before birth and extends for a period of up to two years after birth. Man is thus termed a perinatal brain developer. In contrast, the growth spurt of the Rhesus monkey is predominantly prenatal, that of the guinea-pig is exclusively prenatal, and that of the rat is postnatal.

ABNORMALITY	EXAMPLES
Adverse effects on nerve membranes, e.g. effects on ionic permeablility, effects on active transport systems.	Tetrodotoxin, saxitoxin (blockage of Na^+ channel) 4-Aminopyridine (blockage of K^+ current) DDT, pyrethroids (changes in Na^+ channel)
Adverse effects on neurotransmission, e.g.	
(1) effects on synthesis, release, re-uptake or breakdown of neurotransmitters and putative neurotransmitters such as acetylcholine, noradrenaline, dopamine, serotonin, and amino-butyric acid, glycine, glutamate, taurine, substance P and other peptides.	Botulinum toxin (blockage of acetylcholine release), Organophosphates (inhibition of cholinesterase), Tetanospasmin (blockage of glycine release), Tricyclic antidepressants (blockage of presynaptic amine re-uptake mechanisms).
(2) effects on receptor binding	Bungarotoxin (binding to acetylcholine receptors)
(3) effects on receptor sensitivity	Phenothiazines (long term blockage of dopamine receptors leading to dopamine receptor supersensitivity)*
(4) effects on neurotransmitter-stimulated adenyl cyclase, activation of protein kinase and membrane protein phosphorylation.	Lead (inhibitor of adenyl cyclase), caffeine (inhibitor of phosphodiesterase).
Adverse effects on energy metabolism e.g. depression of respiration, uncoupling of oxidative phosphorylation, inhibition of cytochrome oxidase, interference with oxygen supply to brain.	Barbiturates, halothane (depression of respiration) 2,4-dinitrophenol (DNP) (uncoupler of oxidative phosphorylation), Cyanide (inhibition of cytochrome oxidase), carbon monoxide (interference with oxygen-carrying capacity of haemoglobin).

* a chronic neurotoxic effect but of a functional rather than a structural nature.

Table III Some Abnormalities Potentially Associated with Acute Neurotoxicity

ABNORMALITIES	SYSTEMS, ENZYMES OR COFACTORS INVOLVED	EXAMPLES	
		TOXIC CONDITIONS	DISEASE STATES
Disorders of DNA metabolism	DNA synthesis (developing brain)	Methylazoxymethanol, 5-Azacytidine	
Disorders of lipid and lipoprotein metabolism	Cholesterol biosynthesis (developing brain)	Triparanol	
	Enzymes responsible for lipid catabolism (neuronal lysosomal enzymes)	Chloroquine, chlorphentermine, amiodaron, perhexiline maleate	Many "storage diseases" such as mucolipidoses, sphingolipidoses, e.g. Tay-Sachs's disease, Gaucher's disease, Niemann Pick disease
	Lipid peroxidation Deposition of ceroid lipopigment	Acetyl ethyl tetramethyl (AETT) tetralin	Batten's disease, Ceroid lipofuscinosis
Disorders of axoplasmic transport	Microtubules	Vincristine	
	Neurofilaments	Hexacarbons	
Disorders of neurovasculature - increased vascular permeability, oedema	Vascular endothelial cells	Cadmium	
	Capillaries in the developing brain	Lead	
Edoneurial oedema	Inhibiton of membrane ATPase	Ouabain	
	Myelin sheath	Triethyltin, hexachlorophane	
Excessive stimulation of excitatory synapses leading ultimately to cell death	Excitatory receptors on dendrosomal surfaces	"Excitotoxins" such as glutamate, aspartate, Kainic acid	? Huntington's disease

Table IV

Some Abnormalities Believed to Cause Structural Damage in the Nervous System

ABNORMALITIES	SYSTEMS, ENZYMES OR COFACTORS INVOLVED	EXAMPLES	
		TOXIC CONDITIONS	DISEASE STATES
Disorders of energy metabolism	Thiamine	Nitrofurans	Thiamine deficiency, Beri Beri
	Lipoate	Arsenic	
	Pantothenic acid		Pantothenic acid deficiency (swine)
	Nicotinamide		Pellagra, Harnup'S disease
	Enzymes of glycolysis or Krebs cycle	Methyl n-butyl ketone, carbon disulphide, acrylamide, 2',5'-hexamedione	
	Electron transport chain and oxidative phosphorylation	Thallium	Riboflavin deficiency
	Interference with blood supply of glucose and oxygen.	Carbon monoxide, bismuth	Hypoxia
Disorders of amino acid metabolism	Enzymes of the Krebs-Henseleit cycle and other enzymes involved in amino acid metabolism	NH_4^+ excess	Hyperammonaemia hyperglycinemia
	Pyridoxal phosphate	Isoniazid	Porphyria, pyridoxine deficiency
Disorders of RNA and protein metabolism	RNA synthesis	Actinomycin D, anthracycline antibiotics	
	Protein synthesis (in neuron)	Methyl mercury	Minimata disease
	Protein synthesis (in Schwann cell)	Diphtheria toxin	
	Immune mechanisms	Antitetanus serum, gold, organic arsenic	Hereditary sensory neuropathy, neuropathies associated with disorders of the reticuloendothelial system

Table IV (cont.)

Largely as a result of studies on the effects of malnutrition, hormonal imbalances and inborn errors of metabolism, it is apparent that the period of fastest developmental change is a period of heightened vulnerability. In the human this "vulnerable period" extends to two years after birth (8). In humans, malnutrition during the first two postnatal years, but not later, can result in irreversible intellectual deficit and a smaller brain weight. Glial multiplication and myelination is affected, and neuronal connectivity is reduced by interference with dendritic arborisation and synaptogenesis. The brain areas that develop more rapidly than others after birth (notably the cerebellum) are often especially vulnerable. Hormonal imbalances arising during the vulnerable period can result in permanent damage, whereas in the adult, mental changes produced by endocrine dysfunction are generally reversible (9). Similarly, many of the inborn errors of metabolism produce their most deleterious effects during this period. Both phenylketonuria and leucinosis can result in severe mental retardation, but this can be avoided if, during the early postnatal period, the abnormally high concentrations of phenylalanine and leucine are reduced and low concentrations are maintained by dietary restriction. High concentrations of phenylalanine have relatively little effect on the higher mental function in adults (10).

Many materials that are not overtly neurotoxic to the mature nervous system are neurotoxic to the developing nervous system. One of the most studied of such chemicals is methylazoxymethanol (MAM), a material that has no apparent neurological effect on adult rats, but if administered to pregnant rats produces microcephaly in the offspring. Similar effects can be produced by 5-azacytidine and ethylnitrosourea (11). Neonatal administration of MAM interferes with cellular proliferation and differentiation in the cerebellum (12). MAM is believed to interfere with DNA synthesis (Table IV), so it is not surprising that this material is neurotoxic only during the period when cellular proliferation is occurring in the central nervous system. In a similar way, inhibitors of cholesterol biosynthesis, such as triparanol, exert their maximum neurotoxicity during the period of active myelination (13).

Some neurotoxic substances can affect both the mature and immature nervous systems, but in different ways. The best known examples are the heavy metals and, in particular, lead. Lead intoxication in children can produce encephalopathy, whereas in adults a more common neurological manifestation of lead intoxication is peripheral neuropathy (14).

Species Differences

As in other branches of toxicology, the problems of choosing an appropriate animal model is a major difficulty. In most cases, neurotoxicity testing is performed to obtain some measure of the potential of doing harm to the human nervous system. However, there are many examples where species differ markedly in their response to neurotoxic chemicals, and this makes the extrapolation of animal data to man a risky procedure. Mainly for reasons of expediency and economics, a large proportion of neurotoxicity testing is conducted using rodent species, but it is possible to cite many examples where rodent species have been found to be relatively resistant compared with other species and man; for example, to the delayed neuropathy produced by some organophosphates (where the hen is the most sensitive species (15)), and to the retino-toxicity of the aminodiphenoxyalkanes (where cats, monkeys and man are the most sensitive species (16)).

NEUROTOXICITY TESTING METHODS

Introduction

It should be apparent from the foregoing discussion that it is impossible to envisage a simple test of universal validity for neurotoxicity screening. Neurotoxicity testing of a novel compound ideally requires both acute and chronic exposure to the toxicant, the study of sufficient species to ensure that the most appropriate animal model is being used, and exposure of neonates as well as adults. Furthermore, no one category of experimental technique is capable of detecting all the different types of toxic response that could potentially be encountered and therefore a multi-disciplinary approach is essential. Probably more than in any other branch of toxicology, the use of stereotyped predetermined tests is inappropriate. The testing of the neurotoxicity of a novel compound demands a structured scientific investigation tailored to the type of neurotoxic effect under review.

That this is the case is illustrated by the fact that in the testing guidelines issued by regulatory authorities very few "neurotoxicity tests" per se are specified, other than those pertaining to the testing of organophosphates and carbamates for "delayed neurotoxicity" (peripheral neuropathy) (17-19). Nevertheless, it is tacitly assumed that many neurotoxic phenomena will initially manifest themselves either in the course of acute toxicity testing (i.e. during LD50 determinations) or during the longer term animal tests such as thirteen-week feeding studies. However, although this is doubtless true in some cases, it cannot be assumed that all neurotoxic phenomena will be detected in the course of routine acute and chronic tests in rodents. As we have seen, marked species differences do occur; furthermore, there are some types of neurotoxicity occurring in man that are difficult to detect in the course of animal tests. Effects such as loss of drive, sleep disorders, memory impairment and alterations of mood come into this category. The prediction of idiosyncratic responses of individuals to neurotoxins is another problem.

Before surveying the range of neurotoxicity testing methods currently available, it is useful to draw a distinction between what may be termed first-order, second-order and third-order tests (Fig. 1). At one extreme a novel compound of hitherto unknown properties may be being tested and at the other the compound under investigation may be a member of a class of related compounds whose neurotoxic properties and mode of action are known. Clearly, the testing strategy and the methods used would differ considerably in the two cases.

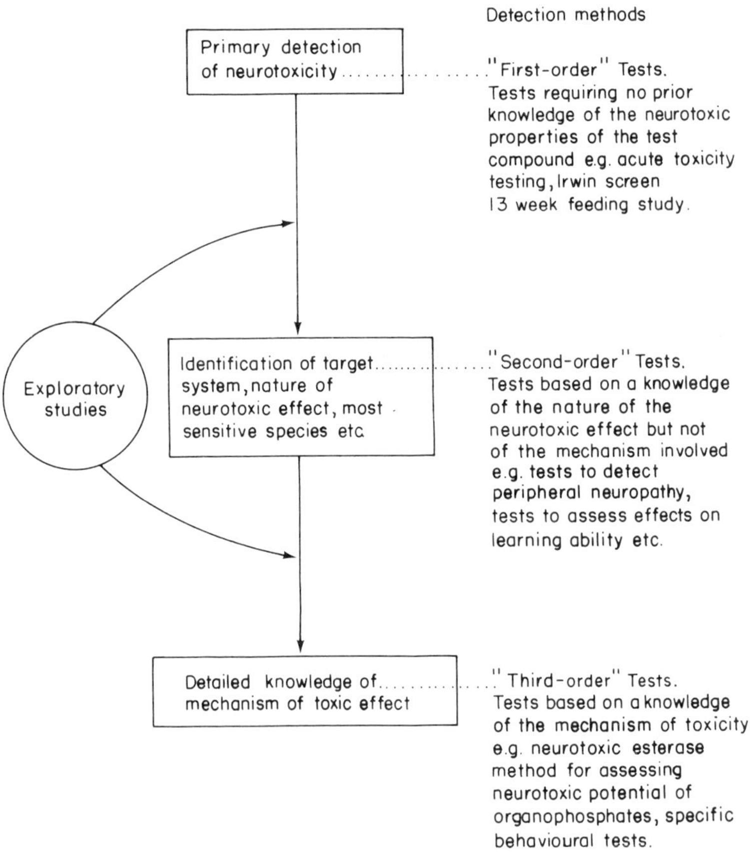

Figure 1 Orders of Neurotoxicity Testing

The use of *in vitro* tests for the detection of neurotoxicity is, and will be, essentially limited to the second-order and third-order type of test. Valid *in vitro* methods for the detection of toxicity require either:

a. detailed knowledge of the mechanism (biochemical, structural or electrophysiological) of the toxic effect under consideration or;
b. a good structural model of the target system incorporating all the factors that could influence toxicity.

Since there is no single "mechanism of neurotoxicity", but a multiplicity of potential mechanisms, it follows that there is no *in vitro* biochemical or electrophysiological screening test capable of detecting all types of neurotoxic phenomena - nor is it probable that one could be developed in the future. Similarly, it is impossible to conceive of an *in vitro* model system that could even approach the complexity of even a simple animal nervous system. Even if it was possible to develop a model with all the requisite cell types, having an ability to integrate sensory input and motor output and having the equivalent of a blood/brain barrier and a metabolic transformation system, the problem of detecting behavioural disturbance, mood change, memory defects and other functional disturbances would remain and one would still have to fall back on animal tests. Thus, it is impossible to envisage an all-embracing *in vitro* screening test for neurotoxicity using a structural model. Nevertheless, it is possible to envisage *in vitro* methods for detecting specific types of neurotoxicity and these will be described under the appropriate headings in the survey of available testing methods that follows.

Clinical Observation and Functional/Behavioural Tests

Behaviour is the outward expression of the net interaction between the sensory, motor arousal and integrative components of the central and peripheral nervous systems (20). Consequently, behavioural disturbances following the administration of a toxicant are valuable indicators of neurotoxicity. It follows that careful observation of the appearance and behaviour of dosed animals is one of the most important methods for the initial detection of neurotoxicity. In order to ensure that observations are as objective as possible and to quantify the results, specific aspects of behaviour can be scored for their presence or absence and, if possible, their degree. A commonly used procedure for doing this is that published by Irwin (21). Irwin's screening procedure requires no equipment other than a pair of forceps and a needle and depends on detailed observation and scoring of forty clinical signs indicative of change in awareness, mood, motor activity, CNS excitation, posture, motor inco-ordination, muscle tone, reflexes and autonomic functions. If it is suspected on the basis of these observations that abnormalities are present, they can be defined further by the use of additional behavioural and functional tests.

Techniques for assessing behavioural deficits range in complexity from simple screening tests used merely to indicate the presence or absence of neurotoxicity (i.e. first-order tests) to more complex techniques designed to investigate certain types of neurotoxicological phenomena in more detail once they have been identified. The screening methods are designed to be used in the routine examination of large numbers of different compounds and do not involve, as a rule, extensive pre-training of the animal. They are relatively inexpensive, albeit labour intensive. The more sophisticated methods can involve pre-training of the animals and the use of specialised (and often automated) equipment. These tests tend to be more objective and sensitive than screening tests, but are less amenable to use on a large scale. Some specialised tests combine behavioural techniques with surgical and pharmacological manipulations.

In the space of a review, the primary aim of which is to point to viable alternatives to animal testing, it is clearly impossible to do justice to the range of behavioural methods currently available. This would demand a lengthy review in itself. Examples of the range of tests suitable for screening are given in Table V, and tests of a more specialised nature are given in Table VI. For further practical details of these methods the interested reader is referred to the original references (also listed in the tables) and to a recent review by Tilson & Mitchell (59). A manner in which these disparate tests can be structured into a testing strategy for assessing the behavioural effects of a compound is described by Tilson & Cabe (60).

Behavioural methods are of considerable importance in the detection and investigation of neurotoxicity, and it may be said that this category of testing method has the greatest general applicability of any neurotoxicity testing method. Behavioural tests can yield information that is not readily obtainable by any other means and, consequently, for some types of neurotoxicity - particularly of the functional type - it is difficult to see them being replaced effectively by any *in vitro* alternative. However, the effective use of behavioural methods in the context of routine acute and chronic toxicity testing could contribute to the reduction in the number of experimental animals required for neurotoxicity testing by:

a. increasing the quantity and quality of information regarding neurotoxicity gained from each animal used in routine acute and chronic testing;

FUNCTION	TEST	REFERENCE
General	Structured clinical observation (e.g. Irwin screen).	Irwin, 1964 (21)
Motor:		
Spontaneous activity	Activity in activity monitor Open field test, Exploratory behaviour	Tilson & Cabe, 1979 (22) Finger, 1972 (23), Delini Stula *et al.*, 1979 (24)
Impairment of motor co-ordination	Inclined plane test Rotarod test, Electrorod test	Graham *et al.*, 1957 (25) Kaplan & Murphy, 1972 (26)
	Narrowing bridge test	Dewar, 1980 (27)
Muscular weakness	Forelimb grip Hindlimb extensor	Boissier & Simon, 1960 (28) Cabe & Tilson, 1978 (29) Tilson *et al.*, 1980 (30)
Fatigability	Swimming endurance	Bhagat & Wheeler, 1973 (31)
Sensory:		
General responsiveness	Startle response e.g. to puff of air	Tilson & Cabe, 1979 (22)
Visual	Optokinetic drum Evaluation of ocular reflexes: light reflex, menace reflex and corneal reflex Localisation and orientation Visual cliff test	Wallman, 1975 (32) Conquer *et al.*, 1979 (33) Marshall, 1975 (34) Sloane *et al.*, 1978 (35)
Olfactory	Orientation in response to odour	Marshall, 1975 (34)
Auditory	Startle response Measurement of threshold sound intensity for Preyer's reflex	Barlow *et al.*, 1978 (36) Baird & Carter, 1979 (37)
Somatosensory/pain/ temperature sensitivity	Tail flick test, hot plate test, Minnesota Thermal Disks	Jansen *et al.*, 1963 (38)
Orientation in space	Negative geotaxis	Fox, 1965 (39)
Physiological behaviour/ Thermoregulation	Measurement of core body, temperature, measurement of ingestion of food and water.	Simonds & Uretsky 1970 (40) Peters *et al.*, 1979 (41)
Learning and memory	One way avoidance task	Clark, 1966 (42)

Table V Examples of Functional and Behavioural Tests Suitable for Screening

FUNCTION	TEST	REFERENCE
Motor		
Fine motor control	Operant response force (conditioning of rats to press a lever attached to a force transducer with a designated force for a given period of time)	Falk, 1970 (43)
Sensory		
Sensory deficits	Maze discriminating tests using sensory cues, e.g. T-maze test using visual discrimination	Zenick *et al.*, 1978 (44)
Visual, auditory, olfactory	Psychophysical studies - operant responding	Chiba & Ando, 1976 (45)
Somatosensory	Vibration sensitivity assessment	Maurissen & Weiss, 1980 (46)
Gustatory	Taste discrimination (using quinine)	Kodama *et al.*, 1978 (47)
Learning memory	Two-way avoidance	Sobotka *et al.*, 1975 (48)
	Discriminative Y-maze	Vorhees, 1974 (49)
	Multiple T water maze	Vorhees, *et al.*,
Affective - emotional		
CNS excitability	Electrical self-stimulation of the brain	Annau, 1978 (51) Ornstein, 1979 (52)
Dissociation from environment	Conditioned avoidance response	Corsico, 1979 (53)
Physiological/ Thermoregulation	Study of circadian rhythms	Stephan & Nunez, 1977 (54)
Specific tests for:		
Monoamine oxidase inhibitory activity	Potentiation of head twitches by 5 hydroxy-	Corne *et al.*, 1963 (55)
	Reserpine reversal	Chessin *et al.*, 1957 (56)
Induction of anaesthesia	Potentiation of 2-methoxy-4-allylphenoxy acetic acid diethylamide-induced anaesthesia	Corsico, 1979 (53)
Extrapyramidal effects (e.g. side-effects of neuroleptics)	Catalepsy test	Burki, 1979 (2)
	Test for dopamine receptor hypersensitivity using apomorphine-induced stereotyped behaviour	Worms & Lloyd, 1979, (57)
Drug dependence liability	Single dose suppression test (Primates)	Swain, 1979 (58)

Table VI Examples of Second-order and Third-order Behavioural Tests

b. enabling specific neurotoxicity tests to be designed on the basis of better preliminary information, thus helping to reduce unnecessary repetition of experiments.

The use of behavioural tests in routine toxicity testing has obvious advantages and has already been advocated and implemented in some quarters. The rat toxicity screen developed at ICI by Fowler and his colleagues (61) serves to replace conventional acute LD50 determinations with a more comprehensive preliminary evaluation of pharmacological and toxicological properties, including neurotoxicity. Brimblecombe (62) has suggested behavioural tests suitable for incorporation into acute and chronic tests. The potential usefulness of behavioural tests to investigate developmental neurotoxicity in the offspring of animals used in teratology studies is also well realised.

Of course, the extent to which behavioural methods can be used in routine testing is limited by the overall objectives of the routine tests. Thus, techniques that induce appreciable stress or involve surgical or pharmacological intervention are clearly unsuitable under most circumstances, because they could significantly influence the outcome of the experiment as a whole. Furthermore, there is the problem that some behavioural testing procedures can be incompatible with the overall experimental design. This is particularly true in the case of techniques involving training procedures before dosing commences. Ideally, behavioural tests used in routine toxicity should be simple, non-invasive and involve the minimum of interference with the animal. However, it is dangerous to over-generalise. The essential factor is that protocols be designed with sufficient flexibility to permit the toxicologist to adopt whatever tests he considers appropriate in the context of his investigation. Unfortunately, in the current climate of rigidly defined tests and Good Laboratory Practice regulations, this flexibility is often difficult to achieve in practice. However, there are some encouraging signs that the arguments in favour of a more flexible approach to toxicity testing are becoming more widely appreciated (e.g. (63)).

Electrophysiological Methods

Electrophysiological techniques, such as electroencephalography, and electroneuronography, have been used extensively in human clinical studies for both the detection and the diagnosis of a wide range of neurological diseases. They have also been used in the context of epidemiological investigations, clinical studies of neurotoxic disorders, and as an aid for monitoring neuromuscular functions in workers exposed to a variety of potentially neurotoxic chemicals (64-69).

Many of the electrophysiological methods developed for use in human clinical investigations have been modified so that they can be employed in neurotoxicological investigations in experimental animals. However, it may be said that in spite of the theoretical availability of such methods they have not been adopted on a large scale for use in routine neurotoxicity testing. The problem is that much of the necessary equipment is expensive, and many of the procedures are complex and require specialised expertise. Furthermore, some of the simple electrophysiological techniques (such as measurement of the maximal motor nerve conduction velocity [MCV]) that are relatively accessible to the non-specialist tend to be rather insensitive and therefore of limited value as screening procedures. The MCV is capable of detecting damage to the largest and most heavily myelinated motor fibres, but if these fibres are not affected the MCV hardly changes. Early damage produced by many axonal toxins would go undetected by MCV measurements, and even when, as in the case of acrylamide neuropathy, the largest diameter fibres are affected, the MCV still decreases by only approximately 20% - even in relatively severe cases (70). Only in cases where there is primary damage to the myelin sheath does the MCV drop dramatically (71).

Nevertheless, electrophysiological methods, in the right hands, are potentially of great value in neurotoxicological investigations. However, for most electrophysiological techniques to be chosen and applied effectively, some preliminary knowledge of the neurotoxic effect under investigation is required, i.e. those techniques are essentially second-order or third-order tests. The sensitivity of the tests is being enhanced by the progressive improvement in electronic instrumentation, so that now even biopotentials in the microvolt range can be recorded. Furthermore, the power of such measurements is considerably enhanced by developments of digital computing techniques which assist in the analysis of the data.

As in the case of behavioural methods, space does not permit a detailed review of all the electrophysiological techniques potentially available, but the main techniques are summarised in Table VII. Electrophysiological techniques, like behavioural testing, have the advantage in that repeated measurements can be made on the same animal over a period of time, and they thus provide a means of monitoring the onset and duration of neurotoxic effects. Ideally, one would like to see an increase in the use of electrophysiological methods in the context of routine chronic toxicological studies. However, although this would serve to increase the quality of neurotoxicological information provided by such studies, it must be admitted that the practical problems would be great. As yet, only MCV measurements have been used to any significant degree in routine toxicological studies to monitor peripheral nerve functions (e.g. (79)). However, as stated above, this measure is of limited effectiveness. Measurement of sensory nerve action potentials is likely to be of far greater value.

TEST	FUNCTION TESTED	COMMENTS	REFERENCES
Maximum motor nerve conduction velocity (MCV)	Function of large diameter motor fibres in peripheral nerve.	Relatively widely used as an indication of peripheral nerve damage but relatively insensitive.	Fullerton, 1966 (72) Fullerton & Barnes, 1966 (70)
Partial antidromic block - conduction velocity of slower fibres (CVSF)	Function of slower (smaller diameter) motor fibres in peripheral nerve.	At present not used to any significant extent in neurotoxicology.	Sepaläinen & Hernberg, 1972 (67)
Sensory nerve conduction (SNV)	Function of sensory fibres in peripheral nerve.	At present relatively underutilised in neurotoxicology. Technique is more difficult than MCV measurement but potentially more useful.	Le Quesne, 1978 (64,65) de Jesus *et al.*, 1978 (73)
Electromyography (EMG)	Neuromuscular function.	Extensively used in clinical studies but as yet not widely used in animal studies.	Gougold & Eberstein, 1977 (69) Mendell *et al.*, 1974 (74)
Stimulus strength duration testing (S-D curves)	Detects denervation of muscles (innervated and denervated muscles differ in their thresholds to excitation).	Little used in neurotoxicology at present.	Johnson, 1980 (75)
Electroencephalography (EEG)	Spontaneous electrical activity of the brain.	Particularly useful for study of effects of sleep.	Takeuchi & Hisanaga, 1977 (76)
Electroretinography (ERG)	Retinal function, susceptibility of rods and cones to toxic effects.	Feasible to include ERG measurements in chronic studies in dogs.	Liverani & Schaeppi, 1979 (77)
Sensory evoked potentials, average evoked potentials (AEP)	Function of different sensory modalities. The AEP indicates the neural activity of the brain involved in processing sensory input.	Techniques are available for use in rodents.	Niemeyer, 1979 (78)

Table VII Electrophysiological Methods in Neurotoxicity Testing

A recent review of electrophysiological methods in neurotoxicity testing (75) made no reference to *in vitro* methods. Most methods of the type outlined in Table VII rely on the use of experimental animals, and it is difficult to envisage an alternative to animals in most of these cases. However, there are indications that for some purposes electrophysiological investigations could be performed *in vitro*. Niemeyer (78) has described the use of the isolated perfused cat eye as a tool in neurobiological research. Homeostatic perfusion of the feline eye with a serum-enriched, oxygenated tissue culture medium gave a preparation that was electrically responsive to physiological stimuli. The mechanical stability of this preparation, due to the lack of cardiovascular pulsations and respiratory movements, permits not only the recording of the ERG, but also intracellular recordings from single neurones. This preparation allows the effects of chemicals on retinal functions to be followed electrophysiologically at the multi-neuronal or single cell level for periods of up to 10 hours. However, its potential for detecting neurotoxicity of the more chronic structural type (i.e. chemically-induced retinopathy), as opposed to toxicity of the functional or pharmacological type, does not appear to have been considered.

Electrophysiological methods have been extensively used in the study of mechanisms of neurotoxicity - particularly neurotoxicity of a pharmacological nature. The techniques involved are far more complex than those outlined in Table VII, since they often involve such procedures as intracellular recordings from specific neuronal types or a measuring effect on ionic permeability in nerve membranes. Techniques of this type yield information not readily obtainable by other methods. For instance, permeability changes in nerve membranes are too rapid to be detected by routine chemical or radioisotope methods, but can be followed by the use of such techniques as the voltage clamp.

Electrophysiological methods utilising nerves from arthropods, molluscs such as squid, and from some lower vertebrates such as the frog and *Xenopus*, have been used to test potential neurotoxins for effects on nerve membrane permeability, and for studying their mechanism of toxic action in detail. Examples of compounds that have been studied in this way are DDT, the pyrethroid insecticides, and neurotoxins of biological origin, such as tetrodotoxin and saxitoxin (80-83). Such methods are essentially third-order methods since they depend on an indication of the putative mechanism of neurotoxicity. They have the advantage that they can often be performed *in vitro* using preparations from non-vertebrate species. The problem is the usual one of whether the results obtained are directly applicable to higher mammals or man. For example, pyrethroids, which are very active on arthropod nerve fibres, have virtually no blocking action on peripheral nerves of the rat and the frog

(82). This problem has, to some extent, been alleviated by advances in tissue culture techniques which allow, in some cases, electrophysiological studies to be performed on mammalian nervous tissue in culture. Jacques et al. (84) demonstrated that intracellular recordings of mouse neuroblastoma cells in culture offer an effective way of investigating the effects of chemicals on ionic channels in nerve membranes, and have used this method in conjunction with $^{22}Na^+$ uptake measurement in the study of the neurotoxicity of pyrethroids.

Neuropathological Methods

Fundamental to an understanding of the effects of a neurotoxic chemical on the nervous system is pathological examination of animals exposed to that chemical. Such examinations will help confirm whether the neurotoxicity is of a pharmacological or structural nature and, if the latter, will determine the localisation of that damage within the central or peripheral nervous system. Examination of animals at different periods after exposure to the chemical will help determine the primary target of the neurotoxicant, the cell type, and the cellular component involved. It will also assist in determining the rate of progress of the damage and the rate (or likelihood) of repair.

The examination of such an intricate structure as the nervous system is an enormous task and to perform the type of detailed morphological analysis that is ideally required for the elucidation of the effect of a new neurotoxic chemical, entailing as it does the use of many specialised fixation and staining methods and quantitative techniques (e.g. (7)), is virtually impossible in the context of routine toxicity testing. Here, simple (and inexpensive) screening methods are generally used, and it is only if a presumptive abnormality is detected that more-specialised methods are employed (85). The problem with this type of approach, however, is that the conventional methods of tissue analysis using light microscopic examination of formaldehyde-fixed and paraffin-embedded autopsy material are often insufficiently sensitive to detect the subtle changes that can occur. Indeed, Dayan (85) estimated that, using these relatively simple techniques, any change involving a loss of less than 20-30% of cells or fibres would be unlikely to be detected. This lack of sensitivity is primarily due to poor structural resolution resulting from fixation technique.

These conventional methods, although effective for the detection of many of the pathological phenomena of interest to toxicologists, such as tumours and necrotic lesions, are of relatively limited value in neurotoxicology, except in cases where changes are sufficiently gross (e.g. in neurotoxic disorders of brain development in neonates). Unfortunately, in many toxicology laboratories the requirement to examine large numbers of different tissue samples from large numbers of animals from rigidly defined chronic toxicity tests has meant that in many cases no other type of approach is considered feasible. There is, therefore, from a neurological viewpoint, considerable scope for improving the quality of information gained from animals in chronic tests.

The last 20-30 years has seen the development of many improved methods for the preparation and examination of nervous tissue and these have been widely used in a research context. Resolution has been enhanced considerably by the use of buffered-glutaraldehyde fixation (either by immersion or, preferably, by whole body perfusion), post-fixation in osmium tetroxide, and the use of thin plastic sections (86-88). Some of these techniques initially arose from the demands of electron microscopy, but have proved of immense value in light microscopy. Increased resolution has permitted quantitative analysis of such features as the relative distribution of nerve fibre diameters. Quantitation has, in turn, been facilitated by the evolution of appropriate computing techniques to assist in the collection and evaluation of data. Another powerful diagnostic aid that can be used quantitatively is the technique of nerve fibre teasing (89). This allows the examination of individual nerve fibres in three dimensions and is particularly useful for detecting abnormalities in the axon and myelin sheath of peripheral nerves.

Spencer et al. (88) have described how some of these more modern techniques can be employed in routine neurotoxicity testing, and have suggested an examination procedure that could serve as a screen for the main types of chronic neurotoxicity. By sampling six crucial areas of the peripheral nervous system and eight in the central nervous system (e.g. the tibial nerve of the knee and the medulla oblongata), they consider that it should be possible to detect and distinguish between distal axonopathies, neuronopathies and myelinopathies, even in their early stages. This procedure thus attempts to reconcile the need to use more sophisticated and sensitive preparation techniques with the practical need to reduce the areas of the nervous system examined to a minimum.

In addition to techniques of general applicability (i.e. suitable as first-order tests), there have also been many developments in the use of more-specialised techniques, such as electron microscopy and histochemistry. Electron microscopy is of considerable value in investigating a known lesion in depth, but is totally unsuitable as a routine screening technique. The same is essentially true of histochemistry. One of its potential uses in neurotoxicology is in investigating the effects of neurotoxicants on neuronal structures containing biogenic amines. Functional and structural changes in these neuronal systems can be detected and quantified by the use of flourescence histochemistry and microfluorimetry (90).

There is little likelihood of the disappearance of pathological examination of animals exposed to neurotoxicants as an essential requirement of neurotoxicity testing. However, the numbers of animals required could be minimised and the quality of information maximised if the fullest use could be made of contemporary improved methodology. In a neurotoxicological investigation, it is infinitely preferable to examine the nervous system of a relatively small number of animals in a scientifically rigorous and investigative manner using the most sensitive and appropriate methods than to cursorily examine a small number of pre-chosen areas from a large number of animals using techniques that are acknowledged to be of limited sensitivity.

Biochemical Methods

Biochemical approaches to the detection or prediction of neurotoxicity fall into three main categories: methods based on the use of neurochemical correlates of neuropathological change, methods based on a knowledge of the biochemical basis of the neurotoxicity under investigation, and methods based on a knowledge of biochemical changes likely to produce, or be associated with, neurotoxicity. In essence, methods in the first category offer alternatives and, in some cases, improved methods of obtaining neurotoxicological information from experimental animals. The advantages of such methods are in terms of speed, relatively low cost, objectivity, quantitation and a reduction in sampling error (a particular problem of neuropathological methods). Methods in the last two categories offer a potential means of replacing the use of experimental animals by *in vitro* tests, but, as yet, relatively few such methods exist and those that do are often performed *in vivo/in vitro* (i.e. using tissue from dosed animals).

Neurochemical Correlates of Neuropathological Change

Central nervous system. In recent years the search for the neurochemical basis of certain important neurological diseases, such as multiple sclerosis and Alzheimer's disease, has led to an awareness of the usefulness of certain biochemical markers for detecting neuropathological changes, and there have been claims that appropriate neurochemical measurements can detect some pathological changes within the CNS prior to the appearance of unequivocal histopathological alterations (e.g. (91)). Some of the chemo-anatomical indices of potential use in studies of chemically-induced CNS degeneration are shown in Table VIII.

The manner in which these indices are utilised can be varied, depending on the nature of the degenerative change being investigated. When gross changes are being looked for, measurements on homogenates of either whole brain or such areas as the

BIOCHEMICAL MARKER	INDEX OF:
DNA	Cellularity
RNA/DNA, protein/DNA	Relative number of neurones
β-Galactosidase	Degeneration of neuronal perikarya
β-Glucuronidase	Glial cell proliferation
Carbonic anhydrase) S-100 protein)	Glial cells
14-3-2 protein	Neurones
2':3'-cyclic nucleotide) 3'-phosphohydrolase (CNP)) Cerebrosides, sulphatides) Cholesterol)	Myelin
Gangliosides	Synaptic membranes
Dopamine	Dopaminergic neurones
Dopamine β-hydroxylase) Noradrenaline)	Noradrenergic neurones
Tryptophan hydroxylase) 5-Hydroxytryptamine)	5-Hydroxytryptamine neurones
Glutamic acid decarboxylase) γ-Amino butyric acid)	γ-Amino butyric acid neurones
Choline acetyl transferase) Acetylcholine) Acetylcholinesterase)	Cholinergic neurones

Table VIII Chemo-anatomical Indices of Potential Use in Studies of Chemically-induced CNS Degeneration

cerebral cortex or cerebellum may be adequate.

β-Glucuronidase is a very sensitive indicator of cellular reaction to degeneration, provided that a feature of the degeneration is microglial and astrocytic hypertrophy. Whole brain β-glucuronidase activity has been reported to increase by as much as 500-1000% in anoxia-induced degeneration (92) and by several hundred per cent in the encephalopathy produced by such neurotoxins as cuprizone (93).

A decrease in brain β-galactosidase appears to accompany the extensive neuronal loss produced by such agents as Semliki Forest virus (95), and decreases of cerebellar β-galactosidase have been shown to parallel the loss of Purkinje cells in acrylamide-dosed rats (187). A decrease in cerebellar β-galactosidase has also been reported in rats dosed with misonidazole (94).

The results of work related to senile dementia, Huntingdon's Chorea and Parkinson's disease (reviewed by Bowen & Davison (95)) have shown that measurements of the activities of the various neurotransmitter-related enzymes (such as choline acetyl transferase, glutamic acid decarboxylase and aromatic acid decarboxylase) could be of value in detecting differences in the vulnerability of different neuronal systems to toxic agents. For example, the effects of such substances as 6-hydroxydopamine that destroy catecholamine-containing neurones can be readily detected by measuring whole brain noradrenaline or dopamine levels (96).

In addition to offering a rapid method of detecting gross changes and providing a convenient way of investigating the vulnerability of different neuronal systems, chemo-anatomical indices can be used to complement detailed neuropathology and to assist in quantitation. This can be done whether at a relatively gross level or at a more detailed level. A method for combining histological examination and microchemical analysis of serial frozen sections of histologically complex regions of the CNS has been described by Hess & Pope (91), but as yet this type of approach does not appear to have been used to any significant extent in neurotoxicity testing.

Developing nervous system. A potentially very useful application of chemo-anatomical indices is in the detection of neurotoxic effects during brain development - indeed a significant proportion of our current knowledge of the sequence of developmental events was obtained by the use of such indices (for a review, see (97)). Furthermore, biochemical markers have been widely used in detecting, defining and quantifying deleterious effects of factors such as undernutrition and hormone deficiences during the "growth spurt" (98-100). It is possible to envisage a strategy for using a combination of DNA, RNA, protein, 2',3'-cyclic nucleotide 3'-phosphohydrolase (CNP), acetylcholinesterase and ganglioside measurements to evaluate the effects of neurotoxic chemicals on the major stages of brain development.

At present, behavioural methods are most often employed for evaluating the toxic effects on brain development, but there are indications that the usefulness of biochemical methods is beginning to be appreciated. Chanda et al. (101) used DNA, RNA, and protein measurements to examine the effects of the alkylating agent methylazoxymethanol on the developing rat cerebellum, and Dudley et al. (102) used a similar approach to study the effects of exposure to halothane on brain development. CNP has been used in studies of the toxic effects of triethyl lead on myelination in the developing rat forebrain (103,104) and measurements of a variety of neurotransmitters and their associated enzymes have been made in studies of the effects of methyl mercury on brain development. However, although the use of these markers offers many advantages in terms of speed and relative cheapness, it is essential that one remains critically aware of their limitations. Although 2',3'-cyclic AMP phosphohydrolase is generally accepted as a reasonable marker for myelin (105), problems have been identified with its use as a myelin marker during brain development. The specific activity of the enzymes in purified myelin has been shown to change with age and undernutrition (106) and in studies of the effect of triethyl tin on myelination it was found that the decreases in forebrain CNP did not correlate well with the loss of isolatable myelin (107).

Peripheral nervous system. If a peripheral nerve is cut or crushed, the part of the nerve distal to the point of section undergoes a type of axonal degeneration known as Wallerian degeneration (108). The biochemical correlates of Wallerian degeneration have been intensively studied, and changes in virtually all the major constituents and associated enzyme systems have been reported (for a summary of the literature with references, see (109)). Since the bulk of chemically-induced neuropathies are either of the primary axonal type or feature secondary axonal degeneration, the idea of using some of the more dramatic correlates of Wallerian degeneration as the basis of a simple biochemical test for chemically-induced peripheral neuropathy has been explored.

For reasons that have been outlined elsewhere (27), attention has been focussed on the two lysomal enzymes, β-glucuronidase and β-galactosidase - enzymes that can be readily measured using simple colorimetry or fluorimetry and that increase by up to 2000-3000% and 1500% respectively, in nerves undergoing Wallerian degeneration (110,111).

Validation studies using compounds of proven neurotoxicity (e.g. acrylamide and methyl mercury) indicated that such compounds elicit substantial increases in the activities of both these enzymes in peripheral nerves of dosed animals, and that the magnitude of these increases was related to the dose of compound administered and to the degree of functional impairment produced (26,109). Furthermore, the distribution of the enzyme increases along the nerve was consistent with the known distribution of the nerve damage. Compounds known not to produce peripheral neuropathy (e.g. dimethyl sulphoxide) had no effect on peripheral β-glucuronidase and β-galactosidase even if administered in near-lethal doses.

Measurement of peripheral nerve β-glucuronidase and β-galactosidase (commonly used in conjunction with clinical observation and functional testing) has been used with success for screening a variety of pesticides, industrial chemicals and drugs for their capacity to induce peripheral neuropathy in a number of species (112). It has also been used effectively in conjunction with behavioural and pathological methods for evaluating the effectiveness of treatment against methyl mercury poisoning (113). The technique has proved a sensitive and useful one, capable of detecting sub-clinical nerve damage barely visible by conventional paraffin histology, e.g. the very sparse axonal degeneration produced by near-lethal doses of some pyrethroid insecticides and the relatively minor distal axonopathy produced by the radiosensitising drug, misonidazole (94). In addition to its sensitivity, the method has the advantage of technical simplicity, objectivity, and rapidity (80-100 nerve samples can be processed comfortably in a day by two people). The data generated are quantitative, can be subjected to statistical analysis, and are suitable for the construction of dose-response graphs and the determination of "no-effect" levels.

A variation on this biochemical method for detecting peripheral nerve damage has been the use of a cytochemical assay for measuring the lysosomal enzymes. This was developed by Clarke et al. (114) for studying the neurotoxicity of misonidazole. Both the cytochemical and the biochemical methods for measuring peripheral nerve β-glucuronidase have been used successfully for screening a series of nitroimidazole radiation sensitisers for neurotoxicity (115,116). The two methods gave mutually consistent results.

Retina. The retina is very rich in DNA owing to the large numbers of nuclei present in the photoreceptor cell layer. Consequently, measurement of retinal DNA offers a very simple and rapid method of obtaining an indication of chemically-induced retinal degeneration, and such measurements could easily be incorporated into routine chronic toxicity testing. Loss of retinal DNA closely accompanies degeneration and loss of photoreceptors and is extremely easy to measure using a simple colorimetric method (117). This method has been used successfully in the study of the long-term effects of drugs and light deprivation on retinal degeneration in rats (118,119).

Tests for Specific Neurotoxins Based on a Knowledge of Their Mechanism of Action

Although it is possible to envisage a number of short-term biochemical tests for detecting specific acute neurotoxic effects (e.g. cholinesterase measurements for organophosphate-induced acute neurotoxicity), the development of equivalent tests for structural neurotoxicity is considerably more problematic and, at present, only one such method exists. This is the so-called neurotoxic esterase method for predicting the delayed neurotoxicity of organophosphates (120).

Organophosphates are examples of a class of compounds that can exert two types of neurotoxicity. Their acute neurotoxicity arises as a result of inhibition of acetylcholinesterase (AChE) by phosphorylation of the active site (for review, see (121)). Some organophosphates can also produce a distal axonopathy (delayed neurotoxicity). Organophosphates that cause delayed neurotoxicity phosphorylate a characteristic nervous tissue protein and inhibit its activity as an esterase (122). This protein has been termed "neurotoxic esterase" (NTE) and is widely distributed in the nervous system. Subcellular fractionation studies in hen brain have revealed it to be bound firmly to small membranes which may be of synaptosomal origin (123). The delayed neurotoxic effect of organophosphates does not occur because of this loss of esterase activity (since phosphates can also inhibit NTE, but are not neurotoxic), but depends on the chemistry of the inhibited enzyme (1,124). After the neurotoxic esterase has been inhibited by neurotoxic organophosphates, it undergoes a process known as "ageing", which leaves a charged acidic group attached to the membrane-bound esterase (125). How this alteration of the protein subsequently leads to axonal degeneration is, as yet, unknown. However, the knowledge that organophosphates that produce delayed neurotoxicity inhibit neurotoxic esterase has been used as the basis of a test for measuring the neurotoxic potential of these compounds (123). This test has an extensive bibliography and for a succinct summary of the "state of the art" the reader is referred to Johnson (126).

In essence, this method involves assaying <u>in vitro</u> the NTE activity of brain or spinal cord from hens (the most sensitive species) that have been dosed with the organophosphate under investigation 24 or 48 hours previously. Since hen brain contains at least four other esterases in addition to NTE, NTE is assayed by a differential assay in which two samples are pre-incubated with paraoxon plus mipafox. Paraoxon is an inhibitor of all esterases, including NTE. The rate of hydrolysis of the substrate phenylvalerate is determined under both conditions and the difference represents the NTE activity. By comparing this activity with that of control hens, it is possible to calculate the extent to which NTE has been inhibited by the organophosphate. Extensive studies *in vivo* and *in vitro* have demonstrated that an NTE inhibition of 70-80% is required to precipitate delayed neurotoxicity. Less inhibition, even for prolonged periods, does not result in neuropathy (127).

Although the above method *in vivo/in vitro* is the one most commonly employed, the NTE method can be used wholly *in vitro*, the organophosphates being added to the assay medium. Lotti & Johnson (128) demonstrated that the inhibitory power (I50) of organophosphates against hen brain NTE *in vitro* correlates well with their ability to produce a neuropathy *in vivo*. Since the I50 of organophosphates against AChE *in vitro* correlates with their acute toxicity *in vivo*, the ratio I50 AChE/I50 NTE provides a good index of the hazard of delayed neurotoxicity. Thus, a ratio of greater than 1 is found with organophosphates capable of producing a neuropathy after being administered in doses less than the LD50, but a ratio of less than 0.025 is found (with one exception) in organophosphates that do not produce neuropathy. Ratios of less than 1, but greater than 0.025 are characteristic of organophosphates that can produce neuropathy if given in doses in excess of the LD50. However, in these cases the birds would have to be protected against the acute neurotoxicity with atropine and oximes.

An exciting feature of this technique is that it permits the direct prediction of neurotoxicity in man. Lotti & Johnson (128,129) have been able to map the distribution of NTE in the human nervous system and have studied the sensitivity of NTE and related esterases from biopsy and autopsy samples of human central and peripheral nervous systems. Using *post-mortem* brain tissue *in vitro* they determined the ratios I50 AChE/I50 NTE for a series of organophosphates and were able to compare the results directly with comparable *in vitro* data from hen tissue. In general, the ranking of the neurotoxicities of the compounds was similar in both man and the hen, but for some compounds the ratio for human enzymes was higher, and for some lower, than the corresponding hen ratio. A further ratio representing human enzymes I50 ratio/hen enzymes I50 ratio gives a direct indication of the relative neurotoxic potential of a compound in man and the hen.

Because of its ultimate potential for making realistic predictions of neurotoxicity to man, this type of mechanism-based biochemical test offers enormous practical benefits, and has the potential to substantially reduce, if not totally eliminate, the need for live animal experimentation. It is more objective and sensitive than conventional testing procedures, is cheaper and requires far less of the test material - an important factor when one is dealing with a new development compound that may be in short supply. Furthermore, even if it is performed *in vivo/in vitro*, the hens are sacrificed before they suffer any of the clinical signs of neuropathy.

For these reasons, it is to be hoped that the neurotoxic

esterase method could largely replace the so-called hen "demyelination assay", particularly during the early stages of development of new organophosphorus compounds. The conventional demyelination assay involves dosing hens, waiting until they show gross functional impairment, and then examining formalin-fixed, paraffin-embedded sections of spinal cord. This assay, although widely used and commonly requested by regulatory authorities, has been heavily criticised both scientifically and technically for its lack of sensitivity (e.g. (88)). Another problem with this assay is that in the minds of many non-specialists it is often regarded as the neurotoxicity test and therefore suitable for the testing of a wide range of pesticides. It is not. The hen happens to be the most sensitive species for organophosphate neurotoxicity, but not for many other chemically-induced neuropathies.

Although the neurotoxic esterase test is the only short-term biochemical method that exists for structural neurotoxicity, biochemical methods have been used for screening neuroleptic drugs for their ability to induce chronic extrapyramidal side-effects. There is evidence to suggest that the antipsychotic action of neuroleptics is mainly due to blocking of dopamine (DA) receptors in the limbic system, whereas the Parkinsonoid side-effects are due to blocking of DA receptors in the striatum (130). Effects on DA turnover in the striatum, anterior limbic complex and limbic cortex can be measured and a low ratio of striatal/limbic activity can be taken as predictive of a low incidence of extrapyramidal side-effects (131). A method of assessing neurotransmitter/receptor interaction is to measure neurotransmitter-stimulated adenylate cyclase activity - hence a method for predicting antipsychotic activity is to measure the inhibition of DA-stimulated adenylate cyclase activity (132).

Tests Based on a Knowledge of Biochemical Properties Associated with Neurotoxicity

As discussed in earlier sections of this review, there are many biochemical properties associated with the different forms of neurotoxicity, and for this reason there is no realistic prospect of a simple all-embracing biochemical test being developed for neurotoxicity screening purposes. Any future biochemical screening approach would have to involve a whole battery of tests. Although nothing appears to have been published regarding the development of such a comprehensive and integrated screening battery, there are some indications of interest in developing more-limited testing strategies based on the investigation of biochemical processes of particular importance to the nervous system.

Energy metabolism. The nervous system has a very high metabolic rate and in humans accounts for approximately 10% of the total energy expenditure of the body at rest. The oxygen consumption of the brain is nearly 25% of the total oxygen consumption, although the brain accounts for only approximately 2% of the body weight (133). This huge energy expenditure is required to maintain the integrity of a very complex structure and for the performance of many endergonic functions, synthetic processes and active transport systems. The brain, in contrast to other organs, is uniquely dependent on glucose for its energy metabolism, and any disturbance of glucose metabolism will be expected to have far reaching consequences on brain function.

In recent years methods have been developed for measuring glucose utilisation in different regions of the brain, using radioactively labelled 2-deoxyglucose (134,135). This permits an analysis of the functional activity of brain regions in response to either functional stimuli or chemicals (136,137). The relevance of this approach to neurotoxicity screening is currently being evaluated. Potentially, it could not only assist in the detection of neurotoxicity, but could also throw light on mechanisms of action.

Further interest in energy metabolism has been aroused in relation to peripheral neuropathy. There is evidence that the most common type of toxic neuropathy, distal axonopathy, is caused in part by an interference with enzymes and their co-factors concerned with energy metabolism in the axon (138,139). It has been suggested (140) that an inability of the neuronal system to supply new enzymes or co-factors to compensate for the inhibitor leads to degeneration at points further from the source of supply, i.e. the distal portion of the nerve. Another hypothesis is that the neurofilaments in the axon could be a target site for toxic action (141,142).

The metabolic basis of toxic distal axonopathies is still a matter of active debate and is far more complex than indicated by the oversimplified summary given in the previous paragraph (see (143)). However, the fact that there is sufficient information available to warrant the generation of even preliminary hypotheses is encouraging. Whether these hypotheses will ultimately lead to a viable biochemical test for predicting the ability to produce distal axonopathy remains to be seen, but the possibility has already been discussed in the literature (144). However, as Cavanagh (145) has pointed out, it is conceivable that certain types of chronic neurotoxicity could be due to relatively minor metabolic defects that may be difficult to detect within the short timescale of most test tube biochemical methods.

Neurotransmission. Chemical neurotransmission is a unique feature of the nervous system and is of considerable significance as a potential target for neurotoxins. Consequently, there is a huge literature on the effects of toxicants on various aspects of neurotransmission (for a survey, see (146)).

The study of effects on neurotransmission generally plays an important part in the evaluation of new drugs and it is probable that the study of neurotransmitter effects will play an increasingly important part in the toxicological evaluation of other xenobiotics (17).

Although there are many reports of effects of toxicants on neurotransmission, most have concentrated on cholinergic and monoaminergic systems. The effects of such putative neurotransmitters as glycine, serotonin (5-HT), gamma-aminobutyric acid (GABA), substance P, glutamate, and taurine have been relatively neglected. Furthermore, many past studies concentrated simply on levels of neurotransmitter rather than on the dynamics of synaptic function.

The neurochemical literature is full of elegant and sensitive methods for assessing neurotransmitter levels, synthesis, release, re-uptake and breakdown. Many techniques are available for studying the dynamic aspects of transmitter metabolism release _in vitro_ using isolated nerve terminals (e.g. (147)), but, apart from a few examples (e.g. (148)), there has been little published on the use of these neurochemical methods for neurotoxicity testing. However, these techniques have been used for studying the effects of specific toxicants such as organic and inorganic lead and mercury (149), and p-chloroamphetamine (150).

More recently, there has been growing interest in the binding of neurotransmitters to their receptors and the associated stimulation of adenylate cyclase which leads in turn to activation of protein kinases and phosphorylation of membrane proteins. In a recent detailed paper, Bondy (151) has advocated the use of neurotransmitter binding interactions in screening for neurotoxicity. Binding studies can be performed either by the screening of receptor sites within dosed animals using radio-labelled ligands (e.g. ^{3}H-spiroperidol for dopamine receptors) or by measurements of the direct effect of toxicants on receptor-ligand binding _in vitro_. Bondy's suggestion does not only relate to neurotoxicity of a purely pharmacological nature. He considers that the modulation of receptors may be an inescapable concomitant of neurotoxicity in general. Bondy has carried out some work on acrylamide and heavy metals in his system, and the initial results appear encouraging. However, this approach to neurotoxicity testing is very much in its infancy and further validation work is required before its general applicability and practicality can be assessed.

Comments on Biochemical Tests for Neurotoxicity Based on Mechanism

Biochemical methods based on a knowledge of mechanism have considerable power in that they ultimately allow direct prediction of neurotoxicity to man. Furthermore, they have the potential to be performed wholly *in vitro*. Because of their obvious scientific and humanitarian advantages it is clearly desirable that, wherever possible, further methods based on mechanism be developed.

The difficulties involved, however, must not be underestimated, particularly in the field of structural neurotoxicity. The neurotoxic esterase method was the outcome of over forty years of basic research on the nature and mechanism of organophosphate neurotoxicity and, in spite of considerable efforts, equivalent methods do not yet exist for any other classes of neurotoxins. Furthermore, although methods geared to the mechanism of specific classes of neurotoxins are of considerable power, they are of somewhat limited applicability. Consequently, the research effort involved in their generation may be thought justified only in support of families of compounds of sufficient economic importance. It is also necessary to appreciate that the development and validation of such methods will necessitate some animal experimentation, although this can be kept to a minimum by the use of appropriate tissue culture methods or by the use of such *in vitro* biochemical techniques as brain slices, isolated neurones, glia or synaptosomes.

In spite of their many advantages, biochemical tests conducted totally *in vitro* do have some drawbacks. *In vitro* techniques in which the toxicant is added to the biochemical assay system allow direct interactions at the molecular level to be studied in a controlled environment. However, they eliminate such critical factors to *in vivo* toxicity as absorption, penetration of the blood/brain barrier, excretion, and secondary and indirect effects. Consequently, from a toxicological point of view, it is necessary that at some stage tests are performed *in vivo/in vitro* using tissue from dosed animals. Thus, even if it proves possible to develop a range of mechanism-based biochemical tests for neurotoxicity, the need for experimental animals, although considerably reduced, would not be completely eliminated.

Tissue Culture

Tissue culture is defined as the study of organs, tissues or cells maintained or grown *in vitro* for more than 24 hours and can be classified into three types: organ culture (the maintenance of an organ *in vitro*), tissue culture (the maintenance of tissue fragments or "explants" in culture), and cell culture (the growth of single cells that have been disassociated from their tissue of origin) (152). Nervous tissue was amongst the earliest tissues to be cultured. A technique for maintaining frog spinal cord *in vitro* was described as early as 1907. However, despite this early start, techniques for the culture of materials of nervous origin are only now approaching the state of development where they could be said to be routine, and maintenance of such cultures still demands specialised expertise.

The success of cell culture techniques in the field of mutagenicity and carcinogenicity testing has led to interest in the possible use of appropriate culture techniques in neurotoxicity testing. If this could be done successfully the need for animals in neurotoxicity testing could be reduced substantially. However, there are many difficulties involved. Tests for carcinogenicity involve looking for genetic mutations and disturbances in the control of cellular growth and proliferation. They can therefore employ relatively simple single cell cultures and the effects being looked for are clearly defined. In contrast, in neurotoxicity testing one needs to study differentiated cell systems whose principal component, the neurone, has lost the ability to divide. The problems involved in obtaining controllable and predictable nervous tissue culture, are legion and techniques are time-consuming and expensive. Apart from the scientific problem, it is probable that the widespread use of tissue culture techniques in neurotoxicity testing could be constrained by economic factors.

All three types of tissue culture have been used in the study of neurotoxic chemicals. Indicators of specific toxic effects on motor and sensory neurones have been obtained by studying ciliary ganglia and root ganglia ("organ cultures") respectively (e.g. (153)). The mouse neuroblastoma C-1300 and rat glioma C-6 cell lines have been used for a variety of neurochemical and morphological studies (152) and for investigating the neurotoxic effects of such compounds as acrylamide and hexachlorophene (154). Explants of brain tissue such as neonatal cerebellum have proved useful in the study of effects on myelination *in vitro* (155).

As yet, however, there has been relatively little experience of the application of tissue culture techniques in what may be termed routine neurotoxicology. Most of the neurotoxicological studies where they have been applied have been primarily concerned with mechanisms of pathogenesis using known toxicants – a task for which these techniques are particularly well suited. Toxicants can be administered to cultures in known pharmacological concentrations and come into direct contact with the target tissue without the influence of complicating factors such as metabolic transformation or the blood/brain barrier. In addition, secondary effects on the nervous system due to the possible influence of the toxicant on other systems (e.g. vascular, renal, digestive, endocrine or immune) are eliminated. Since metabolic conversion and other indirect effects are absent it is possible to use these techniques to determine whether a compound or one of its metabolites is responsible for its neurotoxic effects *in vivo*. For example, using organotypic CNS-PNS-muscle tissue culture, Spencer & Schaumburg (156) were able to demonstrate that the primary neurotoxic agent in n-hexane and methyl n-butyl ketone neuropathies is the metabolite 2,5-hexanedione.

The real strength, therefore, of tissue culture techniques in neurotoxicology is in the study of the mechanisms of neurotoxicity. The very factors that make tissue culture techniques valuable for this type of endeavour, however, limit their effectiveness as predictors of in vivo toxicity. Consequently, although it is possible to see a future for tissue culture methods in neurotoxicity testing, they can only be regarded as an adjunct to in vivo methods rather than a replacement, there being many types of neurotoxic phenomena that would not be detectable by these techniques.

A possible application of tissue culture methods, could be in preliminary screening. This could serve to allow early rejection of some types of neurotoxic compound before excessive effort and expenditure were invested in in vivo studies. In vitro studies could also help to yield information that could enable any necessary in vivo studies to be performed more effectively. As discussed in an earlier section of this report, an all-embracing neurotoxicity screening test based on a single structural model is not a realistic proposition. Thus, the future of tissue culture as a tool in neurotoxicity screening lies not in the development of elaborate culture systems that attempt to incorporate as much of the structural and functional complexity of the nervous system as possible, but in the use of several different systems, kept as simple as possible, geared to the answering of specific neurotoxicological questions. One can therefore envisage the use of cell cultures for identifying cell-type selective actions (e.g. (157)) and specific types of organotypic culture for studying specific types of neurotoxic effect in either developing or mature nervous tissue.

Culture of cerebellum from the newborn rat or mouse has proved an effective tool for studying developmental changes such as myelination and synaptogenesis. The advantage of studying development in culture is the availability of tissue for sequential microscopic observations and photographic recording, plus the ability to carry out biochemical studies on the tissue being observed morphologically (155).

A limiting factor of this type of culture system is the relatively small amount of tissue available for biochemistry. However, rotation-mediated aggregating cell cultures yield sufficient tissue to allow for extensive biochemical characterisation (158). Here, brains or parts of brains of neonatal rats are mechanically or enzymatically disassociated into single cells. The cell suspensions are inoculated into flasks where they re-aggregate into clusters and undergo morphological and biochemical differentiation resembling that found in vivo. Unlike other tissue culture systems cell-to-cell contacts are made in three dimensions. Although there is ample tissue for biochemical investigation, morphological investigations are more difficult since direct observations of living cells cannot be performed on the cultures because of their thickness. Each culture flask contains several thousand aggregates, which can be harvested sequentially for morphological examination. On the evidence of initial experiments (159-162), this technique has promise as a tool for evaluating developmental neurotoxicity. However, apart from studies with model compounds such as kainic acid (159), applications of this technique in neurotoxicology have, as yet, been limited.

Within the last decade, encouraging evidence has been accumulating concerning the effectiveness of organotypic cultures for evaluating the effects of chemicals that produce various types of neuropathological damage in the mature nervous system (155). Studies with metal compounds such as thallium salts (163,164), methyl mercury (165), triethyl tin (166), cadmium (167), aluminium (168), tellurium (155), anti-metabolites, and other organic compounds such as chloroquine (169) and 6-amino-nicotinamide have, on the whole, revealed a remarkable degree of conformity between the type and pattern of neuropathological change observed in the tissue culture and that observed in vivo. For instance, phenomena such as the neuro-fibrillary tangles produced in sensory neurones by aluminium and the vacuolation of myelin produced by triethyl tin can be reproduced in culture.

An organotypic system that has been used widely in experimental neurobiology is that composed of structurally and functionally coupled fetal mouse spinal cord, dorsal root ganglia and striated muscle. When mature, this complex displays both morphological and electrophysiological features typical of mammalian neuromuscular tissues in vivo (170,171). In recent years this system has been utilised to develop a tissue culture model of aliphatic hexacarbon neuropathy (172). This model has been found to replicate both the timing and the specific type of pathological changes of hexacarbon neuropathy in vivo and has been used to compare the neurotoxic potency of a variety of hexacarbons and their metabolites (173). This model can also reproduce the well known methyl ethyl ketone-induced potentiation of hexacarbon neuropathy (174).

On the basis of these findings it has been suggested (174) that simplified organotypic cultures such as explants of dorsal root ganglia could be used in screening for specific types of structural neurotoxicity. However, these authors identify further work that will have to be undertaken before these systems could be employed routinely:

a. simplification of maintenance procedures to reduce the costs and time involved;
b. the development of techniques for mass production of cultures to permit statistical analysis of data;

c. standardisation of nutrient media to minimise, as far as possible, both intralaboratory and interlaboratory culture variations;
d. validation of the simplified systems in a number of independent laboratories using a range of neurotoxins of well defined, but widely differing, properties.

Lower Vertebrate Models

The possible use of lower vertebrates as model systems for neurotoxicological research has been explored in recent years. In common with tissue culture, the main emphasis has been on their use for studies on mechanisms, although their application in neurotoxicity testing has been suggested in a number of publications.

A model system that received a certain amount of attention was the chick embryo and this has been employed quite extensively in teratological investigations. Its usefulness in the study of mechanisms of neurotoxicity has been illustrated by studies of lead neurotoxicity by Hirano & Kochen (175), but no detailed demonstration of the effectiveness of the chick embryo as a neurotoxicity screening tool appears to have been published.

A model system with apparently attractive possibilities is the *Xenopus* tadpole. This model has been characterised in some detail by Webster *et al.* (176). In many ways the *Xenopus* tadpole combines some of the advantages of tissue culture with some of the benefits of *in vivo* testing. Thus, substances can be introduced rapidly into the nervous system either by adding them to the growing medium or by injecting them subcutaneously, there being no demonstrable barrier akin to the blood/brain barrier. Behavioural responses can be studied, and much of the nervous system can be directly observed during growth and differentiation, since the epidermis of the tadpole is transparent. At the end of the dosing and observation period, whole mount preparations of the main areas of the nervous system can be prepared and examined for lesions using differential interference microscopy. To date, the main applications of this system have been in the investigation of myelin lesions produced by the cerebrospinal fluid from multiple sclerosis patients and the myelin lesions produced by hexachlorophene (177-179).

The *Xenopus* tadpole has been advocated as a potentially useful tool in neurotoxicity screening (176). However, as in the case of many of the tissue culture techniques, adoption of this method on any significant scale can occur only after sufficient validation studies have been performed in several laboratories using a wide range of neurotoxins.

Human Studies

Direct Studies

A theoretical alternative to live animal experimentation for the purpose of assessing toxic hazard to man is to study man himself but, for obvious reasons, this is not often a realistic option, except in special cases such as dermal toxicity. In the field of neurotoxicology, direct studies in humans are rarely possible except in special circumstances, such as in the context of clinical trials of new therapeutic agents. Thus, a clinical trial may be a way in which certain neurotoxic phenomena not readily detected in experimental animals (e.g. affective changes) can be detected. However, since human clinical trials are always preceded by rigorous animal testing, they can be regarded only as a supplement to animal testing and not as a replacement.

Epidemiological Studies

A great deal of neurotoxicological information can be gained from studies on humans unavoidably or accidentally exposed to chemicals. Epidemiological studies fall into two main categories; "searching for causes" or "searching for effects" (180). In the former case, outbreaks of neurotoxic disease are investigated and the chemical responsible is identified; in the latter case, the chemical is known, but its possible effects are not - exposure monitoring of workers and industrial hygiene come into this category.

It is salutary to consider how many of the well known environmental neurotoxins were first identified as the result of epidemiological studies rather than from animal tests; methyl n-butyl ketone is a good example (181). Furthermore, detailed studies of human cases of neurotoxic poisoning have given infinitely more relevant information than even the most careful and elegant animal tests. Thus, much of our current knowledge of methyl mercury neurotoxicity was obtained by clinical, biochemical, electrophysiological and pathological studies on humans exposed to the chemical in the notorious outbreaks of poisoning at Minamata Bay in the 1950s and in Iraq in 1971-2 (182-184). Similarly, it was study of post-mortem human material that revealed the nature of the neurotoxic lesion produced by organic tin (185). Further examples of the value of the study of human cases are given in a recent review by Le Quesne (186).

For obvious reasons, epidemiological studies cannot be regarded as a true alternative to neurotoxicity testing in animals. Nevertheless, by ensuring that the maximum neurotoxicological information is gained from incidents of accidental or unavoidable human exposure, the need for animal experimentation could be significantly reduced in future.

Since the human nervous system is rarely available for direct experimentation, neurobiologists have employed as surrogates a number of human tissues that are more readily available. Thus, for example, studies on the neurotransmitter serotonin have been carried out using blood platelets, and the ionic fluxes occurring in nerve endings have been modelled using red cell "ghosts". There is no evidence to date that such devices are of obvious value in neurotoxicity testing *per se*, but they could be relevant in certain specific studies of mechanism.

The use of *post-mortem* human tissue is of potential value if a biochemical test for neurotoxicity based on mechanism is available. The example of neurotoxic esterase assays conducted on human *post-mortem* tissue to predict the neurotoxic potential of organophosphates in man has already been cited.

SUMMARY AND CONCLUSIONS

1. The functional and structural complexity of the nervous system is reflected in the wide range of toxic actions that can be exerted upon it. These include such diverse phenomena as acute pharmacological effects, chronic structural and degenerative changes, interference with brain development, and effects on such "higher" mental functions as mood and memory. This diversity of neurotoxic end-point is accompanied by a multiplicity of potential mechanisms of neurotoxicity. For these reasons, it is impossible to conceive of a single, all-embracing "neurotoxicity test". Neurotoxicity testing strategies must, of necessity, involve both acute and chronic dosing regimens, involve several species, and preferably, both mature and immature individuals.

2. Apart from the inappropriately-named hen "demyelination" assay for organophosphate-induced delayed neurotoxicity, no neurotoxicity tests *per se* are specified by regulatory authorities, the tacit assumption being that many types of neurotoxic phenomena will be first detectable in the context of standard acute toxicity testing or during chronic feeding or inhalation studies. It cannot be assumed, however, that all types of neurotoxicity can be detected and characterised on the basis of routine acute and chronic toxicity tests in rodents. There will also be a need for more-specialised tests.

3. Animal tests have their limitations, particularly in view of the problem of extrapolating the data obtained to man. Some types of neurotoxic phenomena found in man are virtually impossible to detect using experimental animals. However, the option of performing neurotoxicity studies directly on man does not really exist, except in some specialised cases such as clinical trials of new therapeutic agents. However, epidemio-

logical studies have, in the past, contributed much to neurotoxicology.

4. Valid *in vitro* toxicological testing methods are based either on a detailed knowledge of the mechanism of the toxic action or on the employment of a good structural model possessing the essential characteristics of the target organ. In view of the many potential mechanisms of neurotoxicity and the fact that no model system could possibly approach the structural complexity of even a simple animal nervous system, it follows that there is no realistic prospect for the development of an *in vitro* test predictive of all *in vivo* manifestations of neurotoxicity. However, *in vitro* methods for detecting specific neurotoxic effects of compounds belonging to classes of chemicals whose mechanisms of action are understood and methods for detecting certain well-defined types of neurotoxic phenomena can be envisaged, and have been, and are being, developed.

5. Biochemical methods based on a knowledge of mechanism have considerable power in that they ultimately allow direct prediction of neurotoxicity to man. Furthermore, they have the potential to be performed entirely *in vitro*, possibly with *post-mortem* human tissue, thus eliminating the use of live animals. However, complete *in vitro* testing has a drawback in that it eliminates such critical factors to overall *in vivo* toxicity as absorption, metabolism, excretion, etc., and consequently to overcome this such methods are often performed *in vivo/in vitro*, (i.e. using tissue from animals dosed with the toxicant). However, even when not performed totally *in vitro*, such biochemical methods, because of their precision and predictive power, necessitate the use of far fewer animals than conventional *in vivo* methods. At present only one such method exists for predicting neurotoxicity of the structural type. This is the neurotoxic esterase assay for organophosphate-induced delayed neurotoxicity. This method has been exceptionally well validated and is preferable on both scientific and humanitarian grounds to the conventional *in vivo* hen "demyelination test" currently in use.

6. Because of their many scientific and humanitarian advantages, it is clearly desirable that, wherever possible, further alternative methods based on mechanism be developed. However, the difficulties in so doing must not be underestimated, particularly in the area of structural neurotoxicity. Since specific biochemical methods, although of considerable power, are limited in scope, the effort required for their development may be thought justified only in support of families of related compounds of sufficient economic importance. It is also necessary to appreciate that the development and validation of such methods may in itself require some measure of animal

experimentation, although this could, under some circumstances, be reduced by use of appropriate tissue culture methods or *in vitro* biochemical techniques.

7. Despite nervous tissue having been amongst the earliest tissue to be cultured, techniques for the culture of material of nervous origin are only now approaching the state of development where they could be said to be routine, and maintenance of such cultures still demands considerable specialised expertise. As yet there is relatively little experience of the application of tissue culture techniques in neurotoxicology. Those neurotoxicological studies where tissue culture techniques have been applied have been primarily concerned with the mechanisms of pathogenesis using known toxicants - a task for which these techniques are especially suitable. The very factors that make tissue cultures useful for the study of mechanisms, e.g. direct exposure of the toxicant to the target tissue, absence of complicating metabolic transformations, absence of blood/brain barrier, etc., limit their effectiveness as predictors of *in vivo* toxicity. Consequently, although tissue culture techniques could be potentially very useful as a preliminary screening tool (e.g. for development compounds), they will only be a valuable adjunct to *in vivo* testing, not a total replacement. Furthermore, there are many types of neurotoxicity (e.g. behavioural and functional disturbances) that presumably could not be detected by tissue culture methods.

8. The future of tissue culture as a tool in neurotoxicity testing lies not in the development of ultra-complex culture systems attempting to reproduce as much of the structural and functional complexity of the nervous system as possible, but in the use of as simplified a system as possible, geared to answering specific toxicological questions. This could entail the use of systems containing specific cellular elements of nervous tissue, thus enabling the relative sensitivity to the toxicant of each cell type to be assessed. On a more complex level, it could entail the use of organotypic cultures for the testing of specific types of neuropathological damage. Recent developments in the use of organotypic cultures for investigating chemically-induced peripheral neuropathy are particularly encouraging.

9. Lower vertebrate models such as the *Xenopus* tadpole combine some of the advantages of *in vivo* testing with some of the advantages of tissue culture, but their effectiveness as a potential neurotoxicity screening technique remains to be explored.

RECOMMENDATIONS

1. Since no single technique is capable of detecting all potential neurotoxic end-points, a multidisciplinary approach is necessary, and a structured, but flexible "scientific" approach tailored to the nature of the neurotoxic phenomenon under investigation is essential.

2. The number of animals used in neurotoxicity testing could be minimised if as much information relating to neurotoxicity as possible were derived from standard acute and long-term toxicity tests, thus avoiding unnecessary repetition. To achieve this, experimental protocols would have to be sufficiently flexible to allow specialised neurotoxicity detection techniques to be employed during these tests.

3. There will also be a need for more-specialised tests, and here the number of animals required should be reduced to a minimum by ensuring that all tests are designed and executed to the highest standards and with the most refined techniques, so that the maximum information is obtained from each animal used.

4. Epidemiological studies in man have been useful in the past and should be encouraged as an indirect way of reducing the requirement for animals in neurotoxicity investigations.

5. More effort should be put into the development of *in vitro* biochemical tests for certain well-defined types of neurotoxic phenomena.

6. Basic research should be encouraged on the culture of nervous tissues *in vitro*, so that rational judgement can be made concerning the potential of tissue cultures in neurotoxicity testing, including preliminary screening and the investigation of specific mechanisms of toxicity. Attempts should also be made to simplify culture systems as much as possible, and to reduce culture variability between different laboratories by the standardisation of methods and culture media. Straightforward methods should be sought to allow the inexpensive and reproducible production and maintenance of cultures in sufficient quantities to permit statistical analysis of data. Each potential technique should be independently validated in several laboratories using a wide range of neurotoxins.

7. Efforts should be encouraged to validate the use of lower vertebrate models, such as the *Xenopus* tadpole, as neurotoxicity screening techniques.

REFERENCES

1. Johnson, M.K. (1975). The delayed neuropathy caused by some organophosphorus esters: mechanism and challenge. CRC Critical Reviews of Toxicology 3, 289-316.
2. Bürki, H.R. (1979). Extrapyramidal side-effects. Pharmacology and Therapeutics 5, 525-534.
3. Schaumburg, H.H. & Spencer, P. (1976). Central and peripheral nervous system degeneration produced by pure n-hexane: an experimental study. Brain 99, 183-192.
4. Spencer, P.S. & Schaumburg, H.H. (1978). Distal axonopathy - one common type of neurotoxic lesion. Environmental Health Perspectives 26, 97-105.
5. Schaumburg, H.H. & Spencer, P. (1979). Toxic models of certain disorders of the nervous system - a teaching monograph. Neurotoxicology 1, 209-220.
6. Jacobs, J.M., Carmichael, N. & Cavanagh, J.B. (1975). Ultrastructural changes in the dorsal root and trigeminal ganglia of rats poisoned with methyl mercury. Neuropathology and Applied Toxicology 1, 321-337.
7. Cavanagh, J.B. (1973). Peripheral neuropathy caused by chemical agents. CRC Critical Reviews of Toxicology 2, 365-417.
8. Dobbing, J. (1974). The later development of the brain and its vulnerability. In "Scientific Foundations of Paediatrics" (ed. J.A. Davis & J. Dobbing), pp. 565-577. London: Heinemann.
9. Balazs, R. (1974). Influence of metabolic factors on brain development. British Medical Bulletin 30, 126-134.
10. Bondy, P.K. & Rosenberg, L.E. (1974). "Duncan's Diseases of Metabolism" 7th. edn. Philadelphia: Saunders.
11. Suzuki, K. (1980). Special vulnerabilities of the developing nervous system to toxic substances. In "Experimental and Clinical Neurotoxicology" (ed. P.S. Spencer & H.H. Schaumburg), pp. 48-61. Baltimore: Williams & Wilkins.
12. Hirono, I., Schibuya, C. & Hayashi, K. (1969). Induction of a cellular disorder with cycasin in newborn mice and hamsters. Proceedings of the Society for Experimental Biology and Medicine 131, 593.
13. Suzuki, K. & Zagoren, J.C. (1974). Degeneration of oligodendroglia in the central nervous system of rats treated with AY 9944 or triparanol. Laboratory Investigation 31, 503-509.
14. Pentschew, A. (1965). Morphology and morphogensis of lead encephalopathy. Acta Neuropathologia 5, 133-160.
15. Davies, D.R. (1963). Neurotoxicity of organophosphous compounds. In "Handbuch der Experimentellen Pharmakologie Erganswert" vol. XV, (ed. G.B. Koelle), pp. 860-882. Berlin: Springer-Verlag.
16. Raison, C.G. & Stanton, O.D. (1955). The schistosomicidal

activity of symmetrical diamino diphenoxyalkanes. British Journal of Pharmacology 10, 191-199.

17. Fisher, F. (1980). Neurotoxicology and government regulation of chemicals in the United States. In "Experimental and Clinical Neurotoxicology" (ed. P.S. Spencer & H.H. Schaumburg), pp. 874-882. Baltimore: Williams & Wilkins.
18. Jones, G. (1981). Toxicity requirements of the UK and EEC. In "Testing for Toxicity" (ed. J.W. Garrod), pp. 1-10. London: Taylor Francis.
19. Morton, D.M. (1981). Requirements for the toxicological testing of drugs in the USA, Canada, and Japan. In "Testing for Toxicity" (ed. J.W. Garrod), pp. 11-19. London: Taylor Francis.
20. Norton, S. (1977). Observational techniques in behavioural toxicology. In "Behavioural Toxicology: an Emerging Discipline" (ed. H. Zenick & L.W. Reiter), pp. 63-72 Research Triangle Park: US Environmental Protection Agency.
21. Irwin, S. (1964). Drug screening of new compounds in animals. In "Animals and Clinical Techniques in Drug Evaluation" (ed. J.H. Nodine & P.E. Siegler), pp. 36-55. Chicago: Year Book Medical Publishers.
22. Tilson, H.A. & Cabe, P.A. (1979). Studies on the neurobehavioural effects of polybrominated biphenyls in rats. Annals of the New York Academy of Sciences 320, 325-334.
23. Finger, F.W. (1972). Measuring behavioural activity. In "Methods in Psychobiology" (ed. R.D. Myers), pp. 1-25. New York: Academic Press.
24. Delini Stula, A., Radeke, E., Schlicht, G. & Hedwall, P.R. (1979). Detection of CNS-depressant properties of antihypertensives: validity of various test methods in rodents and estimation of therapeutic margin in hypertensive rats. Pharmacology and Therapeutics 5, 431-444.
25. Graham, R.C.B., Lu, F.C., & Allmark, M.G. (1975). Combined effect of tranquilizing drugs and alcohol on rats. Federation Proceedings 16, 302.
26. Kaplan, M.L. & Murphy, S.D. (1972). Effects of acrylamide on rotorod performance and sciatic nerve β-glucuronidase activity of rats. Toxicology & Applied Pharmacology 22, 259-268.
27. Dewar, A.J. (1980). Neurotoxicity testing - with particular reference to biochemical methods. In "Testing for Toxicity" (ed. J.W. Garrod), pp. 199-217. London: Taylor Francis.
28. Boissier, J. & Simon, P. (1960). L'utilisation du test de la traction (test de Julon-Courvoisier) pour l'etude des psycholeptiques. Therapie 15, 1171-1175.
29. Cabe, P.A. & Tilson, H.A. (1978). The hindlimb extensor response: a method for assessing motor dysfunction in rats. Pharmacology, Biochemistry and Behaviour 9, 133-138.
30. Tilson, H.A., Cabe, P.A., & Burne, T.A. (1980). Behavioural procedures for the assessment of neurotoxicity. In "Exper-

imental and Clinical Neurotoxicology" (ed. P.S. Spencer & H.H. Schaumburg), pp. 743-757. Baltimore: Williams & Wilkins.

31. Bhagat, B. & Wheeler, M. (1973). Effect of nicotine on the swimming endurance of rats. Neuropharmacology 12, 1161-1165.
32. Wallman, J. (1975). A simple technique using an optomotor response for visual psychophysical measurements in animals. Vision Research 15, 3-8.
33. Conquet, P.H., Tardieu, M. & Durand, G. (1979). Evaluation of ocular reflexes during toxicity studies. Pharmacology and Therapeutics 5, 585-591.
34. Marshall, J.F. (1975). Increased orientation to sensory stimuli following medial hypothalamic damage in rats. Brain Research 86, 373-387.
35. Sloane, S.A., Shea, S.L. Procter, M.M. & Dewsbury, D.A. (1978). Visual cliff performance in 10 species of muroid rodents. Animal Learning and Behaviour 6, 244-250.
36. Barlow, S.M., Knight, A.F. & Sullivan, F.M. (1978). Delay in postnatal growth and development of offspring produced by maternal restraint stress during pregnancy in the rat. Teratology 18, 211-218.
37. Baird, J.R.C. & Carter, A.J. (1979). Tests for effects of drugs on hearing and balance - screen for assessing the ototoxic potential of aminoglycoside antibiotics. Pharmacology and Therapeutics 5, 579-583.
38. Jansen, P.A.J., Niemegeers, C.J.E. & Dony, J.G.H. (1963). The inhibitory effect of fentanyl and other morphine-like analgesics on the warm water induced tail withdrawal reflex in rats. Drug Research 13, 502-509.
39. Fox, W.M. (1965). Reflex-ontogeny and behavioural development of the mouse. Animal Behaviour 13, 234-239.
40. Simonds, M.A. & Uretsky, N.J. (1970). Central effects of 6-hydroxydopamine on the body temperatures of the rat. British Journal of Pharmacology 40, 630-636.
41. Peters, G., Besseghir, K.P., Kasermann, H.P. & Peters-Haefeli, L. (1979). The effects of drugs on ingestive behaviour. Pharmacology and Therapeutics 5, 485-504.
42. Clark, R. (1966). A rapidly acquired avoidance response in rats. Psychoanalytical Science 6, 11-16.
43. Falk, J.L. (1970). The behavioural measurement of fine motor control effects of pharmacological agents. In "Readings in Behavioural Pharmacology" (ed. T. Thompson, R. Pickens & R.A. Heron), pp. 223-240. New York: Appleton-Century-Crofts.
44. Zenick, H., Padich, R., Tokarek, T. & Aragon, P. (1978). Influence of prenatal and postnatal lead exposure on discrimination learning in rats. Pharmacological Biochemistry and Behaviour 8, 347-356.
45. Chiba, S. & Ando, K. (1976). Effects of chronic administration of kanamycin on conditional suppression to auditory

stimulus in rats. Japanese Journal of Pharmacology 26, 419-425.
46. Maurissen, J.P.J. & Weiss, B. (1980). Vibration sensitivity as an index of somatosensory function. In "Experimental and Clinical Neurotoxicology" (ed. P.S. Spencer & H.H. Schaumburg), pp. 767-774. Baltimore: Williams & Wilkins.
47. Kodama, J., Fokoshima, M. & Sakata, T. (1978). Impaired taste discrimination against quinine following chronic administration of theophylline in rats. Physiology and Behaviour 20, 151-159.
48. Sobotka, T.J., Brodie, R.E. & Cook, M.P. (1975). Psychophysiologic effects of early lead exposure. Toxicology 5, 175-191.
49. Vorhees, C.V. (1974). Some behavioural effects of maternal hypervitominosis A in rats. Teratology 10, 269-273.
50. Vorhees, C.V., Brunner, R.L., McDaniel, C.R. & Butcher, R.E. (1978). The relationship of gestational age to vitamin A induced postnatal duplication. Teratology 17, 271-275.
51. Annau, Z. (1978). Electrical self-stimulation of the brain: a model for the behavioural evaluation of toxic agents. Environmental Health Perspectives 26, 59-67.
52. Ornstein, K. (1979). Drug evaluation by use of rewarding brain stimulation. Pharmacology and Therapeutics 5, 417-422.
53. Corsico, N. (1979). Proposed for an evaluation schedule of potential CNS activity of various agents. Pharmacology and Therapeutics 5, 427-429.
54. Stephan, F.K. & Nunez, A. (1977). Elimination of circadian rhythms in driving, activity, sleep and temperature by isolation of the suprachiasmatic nuclei. Behavioural Biology 20, 1-8.
55. Corne, S.J., Pickering, R. & Warner, B.T. (1963). A method for assessing the effect of drugs on the central action of 5-hydroxytryptamine. British Journal of Pharmacology 20, 106-112.
56. Chessin, M., Kramer, E.R. & Scott, C.C. (1975). Modifications of the pharmacology of reserpine and serotonin by iproniazid. Journal of Pharmacology and Experimental Therapeutics 119, 433-439.
57. Worms, P. & Lloyd, K.G. (1979). Predictability and specificity of behavioural screening tests for neuroleptics. Pharmacology and Therapeutics 5, 445-450.
58. Swain, H.H. (1979). The use of primates in screening dependence liability. Pharmacology and Therapeutics 5, 519-522.
59. Tilson, H.A. & Mitchell, C.L. (1981). Models for neurotoxicity. Reviews of Biochemical Toxicology 2, 265-294.
60. Tilson, H.A. & Cabe, P.A. (1978). Strategy for the assessment of neurobehavioural consequences of environmental

factors. Environmental Health Perspectives 26, 287-299.
61. Fowler, J.S.L., Brown, J.S. & Bell, H.A. (1979). The rat toxicity screen. Pharmacology and Therapeutics 5, 461-466.
62. Brimblecombe, R. (1979). Behavioural tests in acute and chronic toxicity studies. Pharmacology and Therapeutics 5, 413-415.
63. Martin, A.D. & Papworth, D.S. (1982). Assessment of mammalian toxicity of pesticides and other industrial chemicals - flexible guidelines or rigid protocols? Archives of Toxicology, supplement 5, 17-28.
64. Le Quesne, P.M. (1978). Clinical expression of neurotoxic injury and diagnostic use of electromyograph. Environmental Health Perspectives 26, 89-95.
65. Le Quesne, P.M. (1978). Neurophysiological investigation of sub-clinical and minimal toxic neuropathies. Muscle and Nerve 1, 392-395.
66. Seppalainen, A.M. (1978). Neurotoxicity of styrene in occupational and experimental exposure. Scandinavia Environment 4, supplement 2, 181-183.
67. Seppalainen, A.M. & Hernberg, S. (1972). Sensitive technique for detecting subclinical lead neuropathy. British Journal of Industrial Medicine 29, 443-450.
68. Saito, K. (1973). Electroencephalographic studies of petrol intoxication: comparison between non-leaded and leaded white petrol. British Journal of Industrial Medicine 30, 352-358.
69. Goudgold, J. & Eberstein, A. (1977). "Electrodiagnosis of Neuromuscular Diseases" 2nd edn., Baltimore: Williams & Wilkins.
70. Fullerton, P.M. & Barnes, J. (1966). Peripheral neuropathy in rats produced by acrylamide. British Journal of Industrial Medicine 23, 210-22.
71. Gillat, R.W. (1966). Applied electrophysiology in nerve and muscle disease. Proceedings of the Royal Society of Medicine 59, 989-993.
72. Fullerton, P.M. (1966). Chronic peripheral neuropathy by lead poisoning in guinea-pigs. Journal of Neuropathology and Experimental Neurology 25, 214-236.
73. De Jesus, C.P.V., Pleasure, D.E., Asbury, A.K. & Brown, M.J. (1978). Effects of methyl butyl ketone on peripheral nerves and its mechanism of action. Final Report Contract CDG 99-76-16. Cincinnati: National Institute for Occupational Safety & Health.
74. Mendell, J.R., Saida, K., Ganansia, M.F., Jackson, D.B., Weiss, H., Gardier, R.S., Chrisman, C., Allen, N., Couri, D., O'Neill, J., Marks, B. & Hetland, L. (1974). Toxic polyneuropathy produced by methyl n-butyl ketone. Science, New York 185, 787-789.
75. Johnson, B.L. (1980). Electrophysiological methods in neurotoxicity testing. In "Experimental and Clinical Neurotoxicology (ed. P.S. Spencer & H.H. Schaumburg), pp. 726-742. Baltimore: Williams & Wilkins.

76. Takeuchi, Y. & Hisanaga, N. (1977). The neurotoxicity of toluene: EEG changes in rats exposed to various concentrations. British Journal of Industrial Medicine 34, 314-320.
77. Liverani, S.L. & Schaeppi, U. (1979). Electroretinography as an indication of toxic retinopathy in dogs. Pharmacology and Therapeutics 5, 599-602.
78. Niemeyer, G. (1979). Electrophysiological testing of the function of the vertebrate retina. Pharmacology and Therapeutics 5, 593-597.
79. Glatt, A.F., Talaat, H.N. & Koella, W.P. (1979). Testing of peripheral nerve function in chronic experiments in rats. Pharmacology and Therapeutics 5, 539-543.
80. Narahashi, T. (1971). Mode of action of pyrethroids. Bulletin of the World Health Organisation 44, 337-345.
81. Narahashi, T. (1980). Nerve membrane as a target of environmental toxicants. In "Experimental and Clinical Neurotoxicology (ed. P.S. Spencer & H.H. Schaumburg), pp. 225-238. Baltimore: Williams & Wilkins.
82. Bercken, J. van der, Akkermans, L.M.A. & Zalm, J.M. van der. (1973). DDT-like action of allethrin in the sensory nervous system of Xenopus laevis. European Journal of Pharmacology 21, 95-106.
83. Wouters, W., Bercken, J. van der & Van Ginneken, A. (1977). Presynaptic action of the pyrethroid insecticide allethrin in the frog motor end-plate. European Journal of Pharmacology 43, 163-171.
84. Jaques, Y., Romey, G., Cavey, M.T., Kartolovski, B. & Lazdunski, M. (1980). Interaction of pyrethroids with the Na^+ channel in mammalian neuronal cells in culture. Biochimica et Biophysica Acta 600, 882-897.
85. Dayan, A.D. (1979). A morphologist's approach to detection and study of neurotoxicity. Pharmacology and Therapeutics 5, 571-577.
86. Sabatini, D.D., Bensch, K. & Barnett, R.J. (1963). Cytochemistry and electron microscopy. The preservation of cellular structure and enzymatic activity by aldehyde fixation. Journal of Cell Biology 17, 19-25.
87. Hayat, M.A. (1972). "Basic Electron Microscopy Techniques" New York: Von Nostrand Reinhold.
88. Spencer, P.S., Bischoff, M.C. & Schaumburg, H.H. (1980). Neuropathological methods for the detection of neurotoxic disease. In "Experimental and Clinical Neurotoxicology" (ed. P.S. Spencer & H.H. Schaumburg), pp. 743-757. Baltimore: Williams & Wilkins.
89. Dyck, P.J. & Lais, A.C. (1970). Electron microscopy of teased nerve fibres: method permitting examination of repeating structures of same fibre. Brain Research 23, 418-424.

90. Krinke, G. & Hess, R. (1981). The value of the fluorescence histochemistry of biogenic amines in neurotoxicology. Histochemical Journal 13, 849-863.
91. Hess, H.H. & Pope, A. (1972). Quantitative neurochemical histology. In "Handbook of Neurochemistry" (ed. A. Lajtha), vol. VII, pp. 289-327. New York: Plenum Press.
92. McMartin, D.M., Koestner, A. & Long, J.F. (1972). Enzyme activities associated with the demyelinating phase of Canine distemper. 1. β-glucuronidase, acid and neutral proteinases. Acta Neuropathologia, Berlin 22, 2275-287.
93. Bowen, D.M., Flack, R.O., Martin, R.O., Smith, C.B., White, P. & Davison, A.N. (1974). Biochemical studies on degenerative neurological disorders. 1. Acute experimental encephalitis. Journal of Neurochemistry 22, 1099-1107.
94. Rose, G.P., Dewar, A.J. & Stratford, I.J. (1980). A biochemical method for assessing the neurotoxic effects of hypoxic cell radiosensitizers: experience with misonidazole. British Journal of Cancer 42, 890-899.
95. Bowen, D.M. & Davison, A.N. (1976). Biochemistry of brain degeneration. In "Biochemistry and Neurological Disease" (ed. A.N. Davison), pp. 2-50. Oxford: Blackwell.
96. Garratini, S. & Samanin, R. (1977). Selective neurotoxicity of 6-hydroxydopamine. In "Neurotoxicology" (ed. L. Roizin, H. Shiraki & N. Grcevic), vol. I, pp. 15-23. New York: Raven Press.
97. Davison, A.N. & Dobbing, J. (1968). The developing brain. In "Applied Neurochemistry" (ed. A.N. Davison & J. Dobbing), pp. 253-286. Oxford. Blackwell.
98. Dobbing, J. (1968). Vulnerable periods in developing brain. In "Applied Neurochemistry" (ed. A.N. Davison & J. Dobbing), pp. 287-376. Oxford: Blackwell.
99. Dobbing, J. (1981). Nutritional growth restriction and the nervous system. In "Molecular Basis of Neuropathology" (ed. A.N. Davison & R.H.S. Thompson), pp. 221-233, London: Edward Arnold.
100. Balazs, R., Cocks, W.A., Eayrs, J.T. & Kovacs, S. (1971). Biochemical effects of thyroid hormones on the developing brain. In "Hormones and Development" (ed. M. Hamburgh & E.J.W. Barrington), pp. 357-359. New York: Appleton-Century-Crofts.
101. Chanda, R., Woodward, D.J. & Griffin, S. (1973). Cerebellar development in the rat after early postnatal damage by methylazoxmethanol: DNA, RNA and protein during recovery. Journal of Neurochemistry 21, 547-555.
102. Dudley, A.W., Chang, L.W., Dudley, M.A., Bowman, R.E. & Katz, J. (1977). Review of effects of chronic exposure to low levels of halothane. In "Neurotoxicology" (ed. L. Roizin, H. Shiraki, & N. Grcevic), pp 137-145. New York: Raven Press.
103. Konat, G. & Clausen, J. (1976). Triethyl lead hypomyelin-

ation in developing rat forebrain. Experimental Neurology 52, 124-133.

104. Konat, G. & Clausen, J. (1977). Triethyl lead-induced intoxication as an experimental model of hypomyelination. Proceedings of the International Society of Neurochemistry 6, 215.

105. Kurihara, T., Nussbaum, J.L. & Mandel, P. (1970). 2'3'-cyclic nucleotide-3'-phosphohydrolase in brains of mutant mice with deficient myelination. Journal of Neurochemistry 17, 993-997.

106. Nakhasi, H.L., Toews, A.D. & Horrocks, L.A. (1975). Effects of postnatal protein deficiency on the content and composition of myelin from brains of weanling rats. Brain Research 83, 176-179.

107. Blaker, W.D., Krigman, M.R., Thomas, D.J., Mushak, P. & Morell, P. (1981). Effect of triethyl tin on myelination in the developing rat. Journal of Neurochemistry 36, 44-52.

108. Rossiter, R.J. (1961). The chemistry of Wallerian degeneration. In "Chemical Pathology of the Nervous System" (ed. J. Folch-Pi), pp. 207-231. Oxford: Pergamon Press.

109. Dewar, A.J. & Moffett, B.J. (1979). Biochemical methods for detecting neurotoxicity - a short review. Pharmacology and Therapeutics 5, 545-562.

110. Hollinger, D.M. & Rossiter, R.J. (1952). Chemical studies of peripheral nerve during Wallerian degeneration. 5. β-glucuronidase. Biochemical Journal 52, 659-663.

111. McCaman, R.E. & Robins, E. (1959). Quantitative biochemical studies of Wallerian degeneration in the peripheral and central nervous systems. II. Twelve enzymes. Journal of Neurochemistry 5, 32-42.

112. Dewar, A.J., Moffett, B.J. & Rose, G.P. (1979). A biochemical approach to neurotoxicity testing. Abstracts of XIIIth International Congress of Biochemistry, Toronto, p. 550.

113. Zimmer, L., Johnson, P.C. & Carter, D.E. (1980). A comparison of biochemical, pathological or behavioural methods for the assessment of the effectiveness of treatment for methyl mercury poisoning in rats. Neurobehavioural Toxicology 2, 323-330.

114. Clarke, C., Davison, K.B. & Sheldon, P.W. (1982). Quantitative cytochemical assessment of the neurotoxicity of misonidazole in the mouse. British Journal of Cancer 45, 582-587.

115. Clarke, C., Davison, K.B., Sheldon, P.W. & Ahmed, I. (1982). Neurotoxicity of radiation sensitizers in the mouse. International Journal of Radiation Oncology and Biological Physics 8, 787-789.

116. Rose, G.P., Dewar, A.J. & Stratford, I.J. (1982). A biochemical neurotoxicity study to compare the neurotoxic potential of metronidazole, nitrofurantoin and miso-

nidazole. International Journal of Radiation Oncology and Biological Physics 8, 781-785.

117. Yates, C.M., Dewar, A.J., Wilson, H., Winterburn, A.K. & Reading, H.W. (1974). Histological and biochemical studies on the retina of a new strain of dystrophic rat. Experimental Eye Research 18, 119-133.

118. Dewar, A.J., Barron, G. & Yates, C.M. (1975). The effect of light deprivation on the progress of retinal degeneration in two strains of dystrophic rat. Experimental Eye Research 21, 507-514.

119. Dewar, A.J., Barron, G. & Reading, H.W. (1977). The effect of anti-inflammatory drugs on retinal dystrophy in the rat. Toxicology & Applied Pharmacology 42, 65-74.

120. Johnson, M.K. (1977). Improved assay of neurotoxic esterase for screening organophosphates for delayed neurotoxicity potential. Archives of Toxicology 37, 113-115.

121. Eto, M. (1974). "Organophosphorus Pesticides: Organic and Biological Chemistry". Cleveland: Chemical Rubber Company.

122. Johnson, M.K. (1969). The delayed neurotoxic effect of some organophosphorus compounds. Identification of the phosphorylation site as an esterase. Biochemical Journal 114, 711-717.

123. Richardson, R.J., Davis, C.S. & Johnson, M.K. (1979). Subcellular distribution of marker enzymes and of neurotoxic esterase in adult hen brain. Journal of Neurochemistry 32, 607-615.

124. Johnson, M.K. (1974). The primary biochemical lesion leading to the delayed neurotoxic effects of some organophosphorus esters. Journal of Neurochemistry 23, 785-789.

125. Clothier, B. & Johnson, M.K. (1979). Rapid ageing of neurotoxic esterase after inhibition by di-isopropyl phosphorofluoridate. Biochemical Journal 177, 549-558.

126. Johnson, M.K. (1981). Initiation of organophosphorus neurotoxicity. Toxicology & Applied Pharmacology 61, 480-481.

127. Johnson, M.K. & Lotti, M. (1980). Delayed neurotoxicity caused by chronic feeding of organophosphates requires a high point of inhibition of neurotoxic esterase. Toxicology Letters 5, 99-102.

128. Lotti, M. & Johnson, M.K. (1978). Neurotoxicity of organophosphorus pesticides. Predictions can be based on in vitro studies with hen and human enzymes. Archives of Toxicology 41, 215-221.

129. Lotti, M. & Johnson, M.K. (1980). Neurotoxic esterase in human nervous tissue. Journal of Neurochemistry 34, 747-749.

130. Crow, T.J., Deakin, J.F.W. & Longden, A. (1975). Do antipsychotic drugs act by dopamine receptor blockade in the nucleus accumbens? British Journal of Pharmacology 55, 295-296.

131. Cattebini, F., Galli, C.L., Groppetti, A. & Racagni, G.

(1979). Significance of neurochemical parameters in the pre-clinical evaluation of neuroleptic drugs. Pharmacology and Therapeutics 5, 563-570.

132. Clement-Cormier, Y.C., Kebabian, H.W., Petzold, G.L. & Greengard, P. (1974). Dopamine-sensitive adenylate cyclase in mammalian brain: a possible site of action of anti-psychotic drugs. Proceedings of the National Academy of Sciences, USA 71, 1113-1117.

133. Dewar, A.J. (1978). Neurochemistry. In "Companion to Psychiatric Studies" (ed. A.D. Forrest, J.W. Affleck & A.K. Zealey), 2nd edn., pp. 91-108. Edinburgh: Churchill-Livingstone.

134. Sokoloff, L., Reivich, M., Kennedy, C., Des Roisiers, M.H., Patlak, C.S., Pettigrew, K.D., Sakurada, O. & Shinohara, M. (1977). The 14C-deoxyglucose method for the measurement of local cerebral glucose utilisation: theory, procedure and normal values in the conscious and anaesthetized albino rat. Journal of Neurochemistry 28, 897-916.

135. Sokoloff, L. (1981). The deoxyglucose method for the measurement of local glucose utilisation and the mapping of local functional activity in the central nervous system. International Reviews of Neurobiology 22, 287-333.

136. Sharpe, F.R., Kauer, J.S. & Shepherd, G.M. (1975). Local sites of activity-related glucose metabolism in rat olfactory bulb during olfactory stimulation. Brain Research 98, 596-600.

137. Wolfson, L.I. & Brown, L. (1976). Glucose utilisation and dopamine agonists. Abstracts of the Society for Neuro-science 2, 510.

138. Schoental, R. & Cavanagh, J.B. (1977). Mechanisms involved in the "dying-back" process; an hypothesis implicating co-enzymes. Neuropathology and Experimental Neurobiology 3, 143-147.

139. Spencer, P.S., Sabri, M.I., Schaumburg, H.H. & Moore, C.L. (1979). Does a defect in energy metabolism in the nerve fibre cause axonal degeneration in polyneuropathies? Annals of Neurology 5, 501-506.

140. Sabri, M.I. & Spencer, P.S. (1980). Toxic distal axon-opathy: biochemical studies and hypothetical mechanisms. In "Experimental and Clinical Neurotoxicology" (ed. P.S. Spencer & H.H. Shaumburg), pp. 206-219. Baltimore: Williams & Wilkins.

141. Graham, D.G. (1980). Hexane neuropathy: a proposal for the pathogenesis of a hazard of occupational exposure and inhalant abuse. Chemical-Biological Interactions 32, 339-345.

142. Pant, H.C. & Gainer, S. (1980). Properties of calcium-activated proteases in squid axoplasm which selectively degrades neurofilament proteins. Journal of Neurobiology 11, 1-12.

143. Cavanagh, J.B. (1982). The pattern of recovery of axons in the nervous system of rats following 2,5-hexanediol intoxication: a question of rheology? Neuropathology and Applied Neurobiology 8, 19-34.
144. Sabri, M.I. & Spencer, P.S. (1979). Developing a test for axonal neurotoxins of environmental significance. Transactions of the American Society of Neurochemistry 10, 63.
145. Cavanagh, J.B. (1979). The "dying-back" process. A common denomination in many naturally occurring and toxic neuropathies. Archives of Pathology and Laboratory Medicine 103, 659-664.
146. Cooper, J.R., Bloom, S. & Roth, T.R.H. (1978). "The Biochemical Basis of Neuropharmacology". Oxford: University Press.
147. Bradford, H.F. (1975). Isolated nerve terminals as an *in vitro* preparation for the study of dynamic aspects of transmitter metabolism and release. In "Handbook of Psychopharmacology" (ed. L.L. Iversen, S.D. Iversen & S.H. Snyder), vol. I, pp. 191-252. New York: Plenum Press.
148. Damstra, T.E. & Bondy, S.C. (1980). Neurochemical assay system for assessing toxicity. In "Experimental and Clinical Neurotoxicology" (ed. P.S. Spencer & H.H. Schaumburg), pp. 820-833. Baltimore: Williams & Wilkins.
149. Bondy, S.C., Anderson, C.L., Harrington, M.E. & Prasad, K.N. (1979). The effects of organic and inorganic lead and mercury on neurotransmitter high affinity transport and release mechanisms. Environmental Research 19, 102-111.
150. Massari, V.J., Tizabi, Y. & Sanders-Bush, E. (1978). Evaluation of the neurotoxic effects of p-chloroamphetamine: a histological and biochemical study. Neuropharmacology 17, 541-548.
151. Bondy, S.C. (1982). Neurotransmitter binding interactions as a screen for neurotoxicity. In "Mechanisms of Actions of Neurotoxic Substances" (ed. K.N. Prasad & A. Vernadakis), pp. 25-50. New York: Raven Press.
152. Richelson, E. (1975). Tissue culture of the nervous system: applications in neurochemistry and pyschopharmacology. In "Handbook of Psychopharmacology" (ed. L.L. Iversen, S.D. Iversen & S.H. Snyder), vol. I, pp. 101-136. New York: Plenum Press.
153. Kasuya, M. (1972). Effects of inorganic, aryl, alkyl and other mercury compounds on the outgrowth of cells and fibres from dorsal root ganglia in tissue culture. Toxicology & Applied Pharmacology 23, 136-146.
154. Heilbronn, E. & Walum, E. (1979). Tissue cultured neuronal cell lines as test systems for toxic compounds. Abstracts of the International Congress on Neurotoxicology, Varese, p. 79.
155. Yonezawa, T., Burnstein, M.B. & Peterson, E.R. (1980). Organotypic cultures of nerve tissue as a model system for

neurotoxicological investigation and screening. In "Experimental and Clinical Neurotoxicology" (ed. P.S. Spencer & H.H. Schaumburg), pp. 788-802. Baltimore: Williams & Wilkins.

156. Spencer, P.S. & Schaumburg, H.H. (1975). Experimental neuropathy produced by 2,5-hexanediol, a major metabolite of the neurotoxic industrial solvent methyl n-butyl ketone. Journal of Neurology, Neurosurgery and Psychiatry 38, 771-775.
157. Heilbronn, E. (1981). Cell cultures; an alternative in toxicology? - with special reference to the nervous system. Acta Pharmacologia et Toxicologia 49, 31.
158. Trapp, B.D. & Richelson, E. (1980). Usefulness for neurotoxicology of rotation-mediated aggregating cell cultures. In "Experimental and Clinical Neurotoxicology" (ed. P.S. Spencer & H.H. Schaumburg), pp. 803-819. Baltimore: Williams & Wilkins.
159. Honegger, P. & Richelson, E. (1976). Biochemical differentiation of mechanically disassociated mammalian brain in aggregating cell culture. Brain Research 109, 335-354.
160. Honegger, P. & Richelson, E. (1977). Biochemical differentiation of aggregating cell cultures of different foetal rat brain regions. Brain Research 133, 329-339.
161. Honegger, P. & Richelson, E. (1977). Kainic acid alters neurochemical development in foetal rat brain aggregating cell cultures. Brain Research 138, 580-584.
162. Honegger, P. & Richelson, E. (1979). Neurotransmitter synthesis, storage and release by aggregating cell cultures of rat brain. Brain Research 162, 89-101.
163. Spencer, P.S., Peterson, E.R., Madrid, R. & Raine, C.S. (1973). Effects of thallium on neuronal mitochondria in organotypic cord-ganglion-muscle combination cultures. Journal of Cell Biology 58, 79-95.
164. Yonezawa, T., Tanaka, J. & Okabe, H. (1977). Study on the neurotoxic effects of thallium. Journal of Toxicological Science 2, 111-117.
165. Kim, S.U.(1971). Neurotoxic effects of alkyl mercury compounds on myelinating cultures of mouse cerebellum. Experimental Neurology 32, 237-246.
166. Graham, D.I., Kim, S.U., Gonatas, N.K. & Gugotte, L. (1975). The neurotoxic effects of triethyl tin sulphate on myelinating cultures of mouse spinal cord. Journal of Neuropathology and Experimental Neurology 34, 401-412.
167. Tischner, K.H. & Schroeder, J.M. (1972). The effect of cadmium chloride on organotypic cultures of rat sensory ganglia. Journal of Neurological Science 16, 383-399.
168. Seil, F.J. & Lampert, P.W. (1969). Neurofibrillary spheroids reduced by aluminium phosphate in dorsal root ganglia neurons *in vitro*. Journal of Neuropathology and Experimental Neurology 28, 74-85.

169. Tischner, K.H. & Fisher, H. (1975). Uptake of tritium-labelled chloroquine into organised cultures of rat spinal ganglia. An electron microscope autoradiographic study. Acta Neuropathologia 32, 353-357.

170. Peterson, E.R. & Crain, S.M. (1972). Regeneration and innervation in cultures of adult mammalian skeletal muscle coupled with foetal rodent spinal cord. Experimental Neurology 36, 136-159.

171. Raine, C.S. (1973). Ultrastructural application of cultured nervous system tissue to neuropathology. Progress in Neuropathology 11, 27-68.

172. Veronesi, B. (1980). "An Organotypic Model of Hexacarbon 'Dying-back' Neuropathy", Ph.D. Thesis. New York: Albert Einstein College of Medicine.

173. Veronesi, B. & Spencer, P.S. (1982). A tissue culture model of sub-chronic aliphatic hexacarbon neuropathy - implications for neurotoxicity screening. Toxicology & Applied Pharmacology (in press).

174. Veronesi, B., Lington, A. & Spencer, P.S. (1982). A tissue culture model of methyl ethyl ketone-induced potentiation of sub-chronic aliphatic hexacarbon neurotoxicity. Toxicology & Applied Pharmacology (in press).

175. Hirano, A. & Kochen, J.A. (1973). Neurotoxic effects of lead in the chick embryo. Morphological studies. Laboratory Investigations 29, 659-668.

176. Webster, H. de F., Trapp, B.D. & Cullen, M.J. (1980). Xenopus tadpole: a useful model for studying cellular effects of neurotoxic compounds. In "Experimental and Clinical Neurotoxicology" (ed. P.S. Spencer & H.H. Schaumburg), pp. 775-787. Baltimore: Williams & Wilkins.

177. Tabira, T., Webster, H. de F. & Wray, S.H. (1976). Multiple sclerosis cerebrospinal fluid produces myelin lesions in tadpole optic nerve. New England Journal of Medicine 295, 644-649.

178. Tabira, T., Webster, H. de F. & Wray, S.H. (1977). In vitro test for myelinotoxicity of cerebrospinal fluid. Brain Research 120, 103-112.

179 Webster, H. de F., Ulsamer, A.G. & O'Connell, M.F (1974). Hexachlorophene-induced myelin lesions in the developing nervous system of Xenopus tadpoles: morphological and biochemical observations. Journal of Neuropathology and Experimental Neurology 33, 114-163.

180. Friedlander, B.R & Hearne, F.T. (1980). Epidemiologic considerations in studying neurotoxic disorders. In "Experimental and Clinical Neurotoxicology" (ed. P.S. Spencer & H.H. Schaumburg), pp. 650-662. Baltimore: Williams & Wilkins.

181. Billmaier, D., Yee, H.T., Allen, N., Craft, B., Williams, N., Epstein, S. & Fontaine, R. (1974). Peripheral neuropathy in a coated fabrics plant. Occupational Medicine 16, 665-671.

182. Bakir, F., Damluji, S.F. & Amin-Zaki, L. (1973) Methyl mercury poisoning in Iraq. Science, New York 181, 230-241.
183. Clarkson, T.W., Smith, J.C., Marsh, D.O. & Turner, M.D. (1975). A review of dose-response relationships resulting from human exposure to methyl mercury compounds. In "Heavy Metals in the Aquatic Environment" (ed. P.A. Krenkel), pp. 11-12. Oxford: Pergamon Press.
184. Le Quesne, P.M., Damluji, S.F. & Rustan, H. (1974). Electrophysiological studies of peripheral nerves in patients with organic mercury poisoning. Journal of Neurology, Neurosurgery and Psychiatry 37, 333-339.
185. Gruner, J.E. (1958). Lesions du nevraxe secondaires a l'ingestion d'ethyl-etain (Stalinon). Revue de Neurologie, Paris 98, 109-116.
186. Le Quesne, P.M. (1981). Toxic substances and the nervous system: the role of clinical observation. Journal of Neurology, Neurosurgery and Psychiatry 44, 1-8.
187. Cavanagh, J.B. & Nolan, C.C. (1982). Selective loss of Purkinje cells from the rat cerebellum caused by acrylamide and the responses of β-glucuronidase and β-galactosidase. Acta Neuropathologia, Berlin 58, 210-214.

Neurotoxicity Testing: Some Observations

H. W. READING

It is difficult to add anything to Dr Dewar's excellent review of neurotoxicity testing. I can only act as the Devil's Advocate in stressing some of the difficulties involved in using alternatives to animals which have occurred in my own experience.

Extensive animal testing of new drugs will not in itself ensure that all possible neurotoxic effects will be discerned. A particular case which illustrates this was presented by the diaminodiphenoxyalkanes, drugs which were very effective schistosomicidal agents for the treatment of bilharzia. These drugs, which were developed in the 1950s were of immense therapeutic and economic potential for tropical and semi-tropical countries, especially the underdeveloped territories of the Third World. Unfortunately, they produced in humans a specific neurotoxicity in the retinal photoreceptors, the result being cellular degeneration and blindness (1). This was not seen in animal testing, and from what we now know about their mode of action (2) would not have been detected in tests on actual organs or cell cultures. Their neurotoxicity depends on the integrity of the system for the regeneration of visual pigment. Interference with this sets in motion a train of events which eventually ends in the release of lysosomal enzymes from the pigment epithelium, bringing about digestion of the visual cells (3). Such a train of events, of course, requires an intact retina *in situ* in the eye, with all the necessary blood supply and transport mechanisms.

This leads to the problem of using human subjects as an alternative to animals in neurotoxicity testing. It has already been stated that this possibility is to some extent theoretical. However, I would point out that the final indication of the neurotoxicity of a drug can only be obtained after administration to humans. A substantial proportion of my own research has been directed toward a search for peripheral models of CNS tissue components. Many other workers have addressed themselves to this problem, which is fraught with difficulties and pitfalls, especially concerned with data interpretation. My colleagues and I in Edinburgh have been interested in the mode of action of lithium, major tranquillisers and antidepressants in affective illness. We have used as neuronal models, blood cells and platelets from patients who have received drug treatment.

The platelet might be regarded as a useful model of the monoaminergic neurone, since they possess common receptors, especially those for serotonin (4). However, the action of antidepressants and major tranquillisers on platelets does not always mimic actions on neuronal receptors. For example, the neuroleptic agent, haloperidol, which inhibits dopamine activation of adenylate cyclase in neuronal membranes such as synaptosomes, will not do so in platelets. Both lithium and haloperidol are effective agents in the treatment of affective illness, and in certain intractable cases have been administered together, with useful therapeutic results. However, such medication has sometimes produced severe neurological disorders. We attempted to investigate this toxic action using platelet aggregation and Ca^{2+} release as measures of platelet function. We found that haloperidol actually acted as an antagonist to lithium on these platelet functions (6). It appeared that the two therapeutic agents act antagonistically on the same or similar receptors on the platelet membrane. It is difficult to explain from these *in vitro* results how potentiation of a toxic effect occurs *in vivo* in humans.

Another well-recognised effect of neuroleptics lies in their action on the mammotrophs of the anterior pituitary in affecting prolactin secretion, an effect obviously impossible to assess using platelets or blood cells as models. A further aspect of this problem concerns patients with unipolar depression, who as a group showed a significant reduction in $Na^{+}.K^{+}$.ATPase activity in their erythrocyte membranes. The level of activity returns to normal on recovery or remission of symptoms, and is independent of drug therapy (7). Platelets from such patients do not show these changes (8). It is hard to reconcile red cell and platelet membrane differences, since the platelet is considered as a good model for the neurone. On the other hand, encouraging results are emerging from work on cultured lymphocytes taken from patients and families with a history of manic depressive illness. It appears that a defect in a specific receptor (β-adrenergic) can be identified in relation to the illness (9).

Concerning tissue culture as an alternative to experimental animals for neurotoxicity testing, culture of cells from the peripheral nervous system is certainly well advanced, and such cells in culture can be reasonably well-characterised with their respective neurotransmitters. However, the situation is nowhere near as advanced with CNS tissue and the outgrowth of the brain, the retina. In these cases, one can maintain organ cultures from either fetal or adult tissues for comparatively short periods, but not on a scale which could be considered adequate for routine toxicity testing. The cell culture approach to routine neurotoxicity testing of new drugs would require cell culture on a relatively large scale. At present, CNS material is cultured as monolayers, but the identification of cell types is equivocal. Intersynaptic connections between cells can be established, but characterisation of cells with different neurotransmitters is very difficult. In addition, differentiation processes, which are an essential part of the development of the CNS, can only be seen in primary cultures which are of limited life and scale. The large-scale production of cells required for neurotoxicity testing, as mentioned above, would require the use of transformed cells, a process involving the introduction of viral material, in itself a potentially dangerous operation, especially as in some cases a Simian virus is used. Such large-scale production of cells for culture precludes the selection of differentiated specific transmitter cell types. It would be essential to use identified neurones and glial cells to test the action of neurotoxic drugs *in vitro*. It would appear that the technical difficulties involved preclude such material being used for neurotoxicity testing in the foreseeable future. Such observations indicate that we are a long way from using human peripheral cells as models for CNS function.

My colleagues in Edinburgh have had extensive experience in using human *post-mortem* brain material for biochemical investigations of the toxic effects of compounds and of disease states. The problems of this approach are many and varied;

complexities of source material, differences in post-mortem conditions, inadequate medical histories, storage, possible unrecognised disease states, legal and ethical difficulties, consent from families, etc. However, this approach offers distinct advantages if the mechanisms of expected or suspected neurotoxic properties of new drugs are known. Such material can be used for certain biochemical assays after prolonged post-mortem storage with little deterioration in activities.

In conclusion, I would submit that there is undoubtedly a case for a drastic reduction in the numbers of animals used in routine toxicity testing and that the ever increasing burden of the cost of breeding and maintaining experimental animals will help bring this about, along with the introduction of alternative testing techniques. At the same time, we must remember that no drug is without some form of undesirable side-effect, which may be regarded as a toxic action, and all such actions must be investigated fully before a decision on the balance between advantage and disadvantage can be made. It is worth noting as an example, that long-term administration of the phenothiazines produces unwanted movement disorders, but their introduction and prolonged use have immeasurably improved the atmosphere and well-being of both patients and staff in psychiatric hospitals over the last twenty years.

REFERENCES

1. Arden, G.B. & Fojas, M.R. (1962). The mode of action of the diaminodiphenoxyalkanes and related compounds in the retina. Vision Research 2, 163-174.
2. Reading, H.W. (1970). Effects of a retinotoxic phenoxyalkane on the visual cycle in rabbit retina. Biochemical Pharmacology 19, 1307-1313.
3. Dewar, A.J., & Reading, H.W. (1975). The biochemical aspects of Retinitis Pigmentosa. International Journal of Biochemistry 6, 615-641.
4. Sneddon, J.M. (1973). Blood platelets as a model for monoamine-containing neurones. In "Progress in Neurobiology" (ed. G.A. Kerkut & J.W. Phillips), vol. I, pp. 153-198. Oxford: Pergamon Press.
5. Loudon, J.B. & Waring, H. (1976). Toxic reactions to lithium and haloperidol. Lancet ii, 1088.
6. Reading, H.W. & Rosie, R. (1979). Effects of lithium and haloperidol on blood platelet function. Biochemical Society Transactions 7, 933-934.
7. Hesketh, J.E., Loudon, J.B., Reading, H.W. & Glen, A.I.M. (1978). The effect of lithium treatment on erythrocyte membrane ATPase activities and erythrocyte ion content. British Journal of Pharmacology 5, 323-329.
8. Scott, M., Reading, H.W. & Loudon, J.B. (1979). Studies on

human blood platelets in affective disorders. Psychopharmacology 60, 131-135.
9. Wright, A.F., Crichton, D.N., Loudon, J.B., Morton, J.E.N. & Steel, M. (1982). β-Adrenoceptor-binding defects in cell lines from families with manic depressive disorder. Annals of Genetics (in press).

The Integrative Approach

ROBERT HESS, G. KRINKE
and J. SCHAEPPI

The most outstanding feature of evolution is the development of the nervous system, and it has reached the highest degree of structural and functional complexity in man. Its complexity, only part of which is understood, renders the nervous system particularly vulnerable. Consequently, the pathophysiological mechanisms of only a few out of a large variety of neurological diseases produced by neurotoxic agents are just beginning to be perceived. Most neurotoxins affect specific regions of the central or peripheral nervous system, producing particular patterns of functional derangement. Of particular concern to the toxicologist are those agents which produce irreversible structural changes. By contrast, the actions exerted on the nervous system by medicaments are not considered hazardous, as overt behavioural effects are produced which are assumed to be reversible.

Given a fundamental similarity of the nervous system within the mammalian species, the potential deleterious effects of neurotoxic chemicals on man can be predicted or verified in the laboratory animal. Much too often, accidental, occupational or drug-induced neuropathy has been identified in man and has later been reproduced in animals, instead of producing the evidence first in animals and introducing the appropriate preventive measures. Hexacarbon neuropathy is one recent example in point (1).

It is our experience that neurotoxicity can and should be assessed through customary acute and subchronic testing in laboratory animals (2). The prerequisite, however, is an experimental design appropriate to identifying target organ toxicity; e.g. as delayed neurotoxicity is a slow process, it would be improper arbitrarily to restrict the duration of the post-treatment observation period following exposure, as has been suggested (3). Repeated (subchronic) exposure of a small number of animals to a chemical at sublethal dose-levels is usually adequate to reveal neurotoxicity. Induced neurotoxicity with acute onset is associated with marked changes of behaviour and of the highly integrated neuromotor functions. The effects are evident from observation of spontaneous behaviour and they may be further assessed semi-quantitatively by neurological examination.

However, neurotoxicity which develops chronically and insiduously in the course of protracted treatment may occur without overt behavioural changes. Loss of neural function is then masked by overall adaptation of the residual neural tissue, in spite of the presence of often extensive neural lesions (4). Specific neurological and electrodiagnostic tests allow the detection of lost function in specific neural tracts and systems (5), which would then serve as a guide for the subsequent histopathological evaluation.

Once neurotoxicity is identified (Table I), the effect needs to be characterised with the aim of evaluating its risk potential using more specific assay procedures (Table II).

Table I

Laboratory Animal Studies in Neurotoxicity

Purposes

1. Identification of neurotoxicity in customary acute, subchronic or reproductive toxicity tests

2. Multidisciplinary characterisation of neurotoxicity by functional/morphological/biochemical methods

3. Evaluation of safety with regard to actual means and levels of (human) exposure

Limitations

1. Limited choice of animal species

2. Lack of human cerebral abilities, e.g.
   - cortical representation of skilled motor functions
   - audio-vocal communication
   - formation and verbal expression of abstract concepts

As functional tests estimate the total available capacity of the neural tissue, they are not suited to assessment of the extent of structural changes possibly confined to a few tissue components; the use of contemporary neuropathological techniques is, therefore, considered essential for defining the nature of a given neurotoxic disease in the animal model (6). In fact, the most useful system for classifying neurotoxicity is based on the morphological identification of the cellular target sites (7).

It is concluded that observations on the intact animal are indispensable for deciding whether neurotoxicity is present or absent, and to characterise neuropathy when it occurs. Although the animal model obviously is limited by the rudimentary development of certain higher cortical functions present only in the human brain (Table II), it is nonetheless a reliable predictor of neurotoxicity in man. At the present time there is no evidence that any toxic chemical might exert a unique effect upon this particular human capability.

Table II

Multidisciplinary Approach to Neurotoxicity Testing

Observation of general behaviour

Neurological examination

Electrodiagnostics

Specific behavioural tests

Pharmacokinetics, metabolism, regulatory barriers (blood-brain/blood-nerve)

Organ/tissue distribution studies

Neuropathology:
- light microscopy, histochemistry, electron microscopy, morphometry

For certain specific purposes it may be advantageous to employ systems less complex than the integrated nervous system; tissue culture methods are being developed for studying cellular physiology, neurogenesis and synaptogenesis, or for monitoring the direct effects of active substances, including toxins, on neuronal or glial cells *in vitro* (8,9). The obvious limitation of these systems is their restriction to certain types of cell or to the particular culture conditions, which do not take into

Type of Test	Use/Advantage	Disadvantage for Neurotoxicity Testing
Electrophysiology		
Molluscs, arthropods, lower vertebrates	Single neuron physiology	Limited specificity
Biochemical methods		
Biochemical markers	Mechanisms relating to known toxicants	Mechanisms elaborated *in vivo*
Neurotransmitter/receptor studies		No structural correlate
Neurotoxic esterase	Neurotoxicity screening	Restricted to OP-neurotoxicity
Binding sites	*in vivo/in vitro*	
Tissue culture techniques		
Organotypic cultures: Embryonic tissue; cord-ganglion-muscle	Study of action of known toxicants; as adjunct of *in vivo* testing in developmental neurobiology	Restricted to selective cell types Low level of organisation Deficient in biotransformation capacity
Aggregating cultures		
Cultures of single cells		

Table III In Vitro Testing Methods for Neurotoxicity

account either transport across biological barriers, biotransformation, or the failure of all sorts of physiological mechanisms supporting the nervous system in vivo (Table III). Therefore, caution is necessary before assuming that effects occurring in vitro are identical to those which would be observed in the intact organism. Furthermore, certain in vitro systems are more appropriate for the study of one particular mechanism than others. At present, there is no single system or set of systems imaginable which could be used as a general predictive screen for neurotoxicity.

Table IV

Limitation of Studies in Man

Retrospective epidemiological studies:

Exposure:
- dose-level usually too low for producing well-defined symptoms and signs
- dose-level usually uncertain, eventually unknown
- to more than one toxic agent
- obscured by pre-existing or concomitant condition or disease

Pathology:
- post-mortem changes preclude optimal methodology
- biopsy studies rarely feasible (peripheral neuropathies)

Prospective studies:

- unethical with agents likely to produce irreversible effects

There are a number of well-known examples to illustrate the considerable value of laboratory animal studies for predicting neurotoxicity in man (7). The following recent example refers to certain alkyl tin compounds reported to induce neurobehavioural toxicity (10). Trimethyl tin, an intermediate in certain industrial processes, causes brain damage affecting primarily the limbic system (11). In rats, following an acute sublethal dose of 7-8mg/kg of $(CH_3)_3SnCl$, neuropathological changes are first observed in the hippocampus, affecting selectively the end blade region ((12,13), Krinke & Hess, in preparation); the behavioural sequelae are distinctive and consist of hyperactivity, tremor, aggressive mode, and spontaneous seizures. The same syndrome, including amnesia, disorientation, EEG changes and signs of cerebellar dysfunction, has been observed in workers accidentally exposed to trimethyl tin (14,15). This example is cited in proposing that the optimum strategy of predictive neurotoxicity testing should be to determine, in a multidisciplinary manner, whether neurobehavioural changes and neuropathology, would occur in a limited number of animals properly treated and observed. The only other alternative to identify a neurotoxin would be to observe the effects directly in humans. Studies on man impose severe limitations (Table IV). In fact, there is no alternative to studies on animals if the human experiment of placing people at unnecessary risk is to be avoided. The neurotoxicologist bears a heavy responsibility to prevent long-lasting and cruel suffering which is imposed by induced neurological disease.

REFERENCES

1. Spencer, P.S., Couri, D. & Schaumburg, H.H. (1980). n-Hexane and methyl n-butyl ketone. In "Experimental and Clinical Neurotoxicology" (ed. P.S. Spencer & H.H. Schaumburg), pp. 456-475. Baltimore: Williams & Wilkins.
2. Schaeppi, U. & Hess, R. (1982). What can specific behavioural testing procedures contribute to the assessment of neurotoxicity in laboratory animals? Agents and Actions (in press).
3. Fowler, J.S.L., Brown, J.S. & Bell, H.A. (1979). The rat toxicity screen. Pharmacology and Therapeutics 5, 461-466.
4. Schaeppi, U. & Krinke, G. (1982). Pyridoxine neuropathy: correlation of functional tests and neuropathology in beagle dogs treated with large doses of vitamin B6. Agents and Actions 12, 575-582.
5. Schaeppi, U., Teste, M. & Siegenthaler, U. (1982). Sensory and motor maximum nerve conduction velocity in the peripheral and central nervous system of the beagle dog. Agents and Actions 12, 566-574.
6. Krinke, G., Thomann, P. & Hess, R. (1980) Experimental toxic models of neurological disease. In "Animal Models of Neurological Disease" (ed. F.C. Rose & P.O. Behan), pp. 110-122. Tunbridge: Pitman.
7. Spencer, P.S. & Schaumburg, H.H. (1980). Classification of neurotoxic disease: a morphological approach. In "Experimental and Clinical Neurotoxicology" (ed. P.S. Spencer & H.H. Schaumburg), pp. 92-99. Baltimore: Williams & Wilkins.
8. Dimpfel, W. (1980). Rat nerve cell cultures in pharmacology and toxicology. Archives of Toxicology 44, 55-62.
9. Pfeiffer, S.W. (ed.) (1982). "Neuroscience Approached Through Cell Culture". Boca Raton, Fla.: CRC Press.
10. Kimbrough, R. (1976). Toxicity and health effects of selected organo tin compounds: a review. Environmental Health Perspectives 14, 51-56.
11. Brown, A.W., Aldridge, W.N., Street, B.W. & Verschoyle, R.D. (1979). The behavioural and neuropathologic sequelae of

intoxication by trimethyl tin compounds. American Journal of Pathology 97, 59-82.
12. Bouldin, T.W., Goines, N.D., Bagnell, C.R. & Krigman, M.R.: Pathogenesis of trimethyl tin neuronal toxicity. Ultrastructure and cytochemical observations. American Journal of Pathology 104, 237-249.
13. Dyer, R.S., Walsh, T.J., Wonderlin, W.F. & Bercegay, M. (1982). The trimethyl syndrome in rats. Neurobehavioural Toxicology and Teratology 4, 127-133.
14. Ross, W.D., Emmett, E.A., Steiner, J. & Tureen, R. (1981). Neurotoxic effects of occupational exposure to organo tins. American Journal of Psychiatry 138, 1092-1095.
15. Besser, R., Krämer, G., Hopf, H.C., & Rey, C. (1982). Trimethyl tin intoxication in man: clinical aspects and EEG in six cases. In "Proceedings of the International Congress of Clinical Toxicology", Snowmass, Colorado, USA; August 9-13, 1982.

Human Accidents

NIGEL LEGG

Neurotoxic accidents in man are natural experiments, providing information which could not be obtained in any other way. The results are often tragic in personal or social terms, and if only to prevent a recurrence of similar tragedies they should be studied as fully as possible. In such experiments, the main investigative tool is observation rather than intervention, but attempts at treatment, which have to be carried out on the scantiest of guidelines, can also provide valuable information. Such natural experiments are open-ended, and very unlike the specificity of many laboratory research projects, which are designed to answer one or two questions with a definite yes or no. Nevertheless, it is this very non-specificity which widens the potential use of these experiments, and makes their careful observation so necessary.

The illness known as the "Toxic Oil Syndrome" in Spain is a recent toxicological accident which illustrates these situations. It began in May 1981 with a widespread epidemic of a diffuse clinical syndrome. The features included fever, headaches, cough, rashes and myalgia. The myalgia worsened, and patients developed thrombocytopenia, thromboembolism, pulmonary hypertension, peripheral neuropathy and a soft tissue syndrome akin to scleroderma. Many became profoundly wasted, partly because of dysphagia and inadequate nutrition and partly through neurogenic muscle atrophy, possibly due to anterior horn cell damage. The disorder is still evolving, and fresh symptoms and signs have appeared more than a year after the onset in the survivors. These now include myoclonic jerks, muscle spasms, pseudomyotonia and tremor. More than 370 people have died and many thousands are thought to have been affected. No treatment has been conclusively shown to alter the course of the disease.

Initially, the syndrome, which had many inflammatory features, was thought to be infective. Six weeks after the outbreak it was found to be related to the consumption of rapeseed oil which had been modified and sold as cheap olive oil. The chemical and physical processes employed in modifying it could not be fully established. Once the connection had been found, the oil was taken off the market, the Government bought in unused stocks to prevent further consumption, and no further cases appeared.

It is still too soon to draw any conclusions about the nature of the toxic agent or the manner in which it has produced damage. Animal toxicity tests have been performed with samples of presumably abnormal oil, but no illnesses have been produced. Observation of the clinical features and correlations between these and the physiological and pathological data are still going on.

It is obvious from the diffuse nature of the lesions and the wide range of clinical syndromes that this is a very important poison, and lessons may well be drawn from this experience which have relevance to many disease processes. Within the realm of neurological disease we know that it has influenced muscles and peripheral nerves, producing an intensely fibrotic reaction in the latter, and it may well have damaged anterior horn cells as well. Thus, it may have lessons, at present still hidden, for an understanding not only of certain muscle and nerve disorders, but also motor neurone disease. These lessons should be uncovered when full clinical studies have been completed.

General Discussion

A. N. WORDEN

Rapporteur

Dr Le QUESNE said that she felt that Professor Hess was somewhat optimistic in suggesting that available methods might be enough to pick up all neurotoxic effects. Substances such as the organic solvent perhexeline were picked up in man and there were many instances, such as arsenic neuropathy, for which there was not a good animal model. Sensory neuropathies were very difficult to detect in animals and one had to rely on human screening and early warning systems and to develop these to the maximum extent. The exploitation of accidents had been measured and this was an area into which we had to put a great deal of effort, because the data emerging, for instance from the methyl mercury episode in Iraq, had been of enormous value: we now knew more about human threshold levels of toxicity, the levels that were toxic to the fetus and all aspects of fetal toxicity. At the moment there was really no likelihood of these accidents not happening because the majority of human toxic problems arose in this way, as with the organophosphates such as dipterex, in which delayed neuropathy was well established in man and yet was virtually impossible to produce in hens. For this particular organophosphate the threshold for delayed neuropathy was lower in man than in the hen. When one was talking about simple screening procedures for neurotoxicity, man was of course an absolutely ideal subject because the screening procedures for neurotoxicity were simple: a very good clinical history and very good neurological examination were really all that was necessary. Neurotoxicologists devoted an excessive amount of effort to detecting minimal changes in a highly variable human population and trying to draw presumed neurotoxic effects out of the amorphous human background that were very often not real effects. Too much effort was put into this aspect when our techniques for detection were not really adequate. We were not prepared to accept toxic complications of drugs. A mortality rate of 50% for operations might be acceptable, yet we were not prepared to accept any mortality from the use of drugs.

Dr Ruth CLAYTON said that one could use only primary cultures.

It was, in effect, much easier to get large amounts of primary cultures under standardised conditions than was generally recognised. How many tests were there which neurotoxicologists felt ought to be performed that were not susceptible to miniaturisation because of, for example, binding? Many enzyme assays similarly did not require material in bulk, but what percentage could be regarded as unsuitable in principle for miniaturisation?

Dr DEWAR apologised for having had to abbreviate considerably his remarks on tissue culture. For qualitative investigations to determine whether or not a material were toxic, he saw no reason why one could not utilise only a very small amount of material. He referred to the work of Peter Spencer on the use of organotypic culture for looking at hexacarbons. Much work had been done to rank these compounds for their neurotoxic potential. The workers concerned would themselves acknowledge that before such a procedure could be used as a screening test, as distinct from its use in a scientific investigation, there would be a need to produce the system on a slightly larger scale and to do this reproducibly. If one was talking about a screen in which many compounds were going to be put through, very little tissue might be needed for each compound. The question of metabolites had been mentioned and the fact was that in some instances the metabolite was more toxic than the parent compound.

Dr READING said that, so far as behavioural testing was concerned, perhaps the only way was to look in man himself. He was concerned that concentrations of a drug in contact with cell cultures were probably not going to show the toxic effects that they would in man, lithium being a case in point. A concentration of 1 million molar was not a toxic, but a therapeutic, concentration. If the concentration were increased to 1.4 million molar, the patient became very ill indeed. That was not a kind of effect that was likely to be found with the aid of tissue cultures.

Dr A. GOLDBERG complimented Dr Dewar for describing the most important concept of development within the areas of alternatives to testing, that of mechanisms. He firmly believed that if the mechanism were understood it would be possible to design toxicity tests more appropriately. He felt that one had to go a step further and to take a look at the test and the alternatives to it and at the same time to separate this from the development of research for the tests. These were two different processes and two different sets of thinking. He enquired about the separation of our thinking concerning new compounds and families of compounds and the formulations that had previously existed. In the area of human experience, for example in Minimata Bay or in Iraq with methyl mercury, or in Michigan with the polybiphenyls, these were treated as accidents. If one examined the data retrospectively, however, it could be seen that, though they were indeed accidents, they could have been prevented. In most cases there was a simple explanation, such as the faulty labelling of packages.

Inhalation Toxicity

D. G. CLARK

This chapter does not contain the deliberations of a FRAME Working Party, but, since inhalation is such an important topic, Dr Brown and I have agreed that we will present the information in a Working Party format. Dr Brown has therefore surveyed the alternatives to animal inhalation experiments in his paper, and I have then presented our conclusions and recommendations.

It is worthwhile stressing just why inhalation toxicity is so important: breathing is mandatory. Of all the routes of entry into the body, it is the one least able to be controlled. One can avoid taking pills, avoid splashes on the skin and refrain from drinking toxic chemicals. But we cannot control what we breathe. The potential for toxic insult via breathing is enormous. A man working 8 hours/day, 5 days/week for 45 years will inhale 30 million litres of his workplace air. Each and every one of us will inhale over 250 million litres of air as we pass from the cradle to the grave. This air may be contaminated with gases, vapours, fumes, aerosols, dusts, smogs, smokes and fibres. Exposure may be either inadvertent, because it is part of our workplace or general environment, or deliberate, as in the case of cigarette smoking, glue sniffing or the inhalation of therapeutic drugs. All the contaminated air passes into the lungs, which contain delicate tissues designed to facilitate the passage of respiratory gases to and from the bloodstream. Thus, contaminated air not only poses a toxic threat to the body, but also a direct toxic threat to the lungs themselves.

The necessity to test chemicals for their capacity to be toxic by inhalation is obvious, yet to test them using the classical toxicological approach of animal models is the most technically-complex, difficult and expensive area of all toxicology. The cost of a 2-year inhalation study, for example, is now in the region of £250,000. In addition to the scientific and ethical pressures to develop alternatives to classical inhalation toxicity methods, there is thus a major financial pressure. But any alternatives will have to give information at least as good as that provided by existing methods. As there is no alternative to breathing, there can be no compromise of reduced standards for testing chemicals for their inhalation toxicity.

Inhalation Toxicology

R. C. BROWN and ALAN POOLE

INTRODUCTION

Exposure to airborne toxic substances is a widespread phenomenon; air pollution from natural or industrial sources and the self-inflicted or passive exposure to tobacco smoke all constitute a risk to human health. Although the study of this type of hazard in general is the subject of this paper, the expertise of the authors is in the area of particulate hazards, so most of our examples are drawn from that field. We hope, however, that many of our comments apply equally to work aimed at the evaluation of the risks posed by hazardous gases and vapours.

HUMAN STUDIES

Human exposure to inhaled toxic gases, fumes and aerosols (of fluids or particulates) has long been recognised as a source of danger to health and even life. In some well-established cases a danger was recognised when sufficient humans had suffered and then precautions could be taken to avoid, or protect against, the risk. Miners in the 2nd century used bags, sacks or bladders to protect themselves against dust (1), while Agricola (2) advocated the 5-day week in which "Prudent miners burn the piles of wood (to break rock) on Friday and then do not descend again before Monday.... and in the meantime the poisonous fumes pass away". Although this crude "epidemiological" approach to risk evaluation and avoidance has been refined only slightly during the ensuing centuries, studies of well-defined groups exposed to clear risks and with rare pathological conditions have enabled the recognition of the hazard arising from the inhalation of a wide range of substances.

The evaluation of risk has, however, proved more difficult when the potential hazard is widespread, ill-defined and suspected of increasing the incidence of already-common conditions. This is well illustrated by the controversy surrounding the hazards of lead in petrol and by the time taken for the recognition of cigarette smoking as a cause of pulmonary disease.

The study of defined occupational groups working with a particular agent, using lung function tests and X-ray examination, has led to the view that inhalation risks are part of occupational medicine, the general public only being involved in exceptional cases, such as exposure to volcanic ash or industrial chemicals released in accidents. However, the increasing demand for the pre-emptive evaluation of toxic risks and the need for more studies of the mechanisms by which known toxicants exert these effects have led to the development of inhalation toxicology as a recognised but ill-defined specialist area, in which both industrial and environmental hazards can be evaluated in non-human systems.

ANIMAL STUDIES

The lungs are merely one route by which toxic agents can enter the body, and it is clear that data from all types of toxicological investigation are of value in assessing any inhalation risk. However, the lung is not only a route of entry but also an important target organ, and agents having an immediate effect, such as corrosive or irritant gases and those which are not cleared from the lung, will exert a toxic effect at the site of entry, either immediately or during their prolonged residence. It is therefore essential that some agents be tested by exposing animals directly to an atmosphere containing the suspect compound or product. The generation of such atmospheres is technically demanding: exposing animals but not laboratory staff to an agent in a similar form to that likely to be encountered, in practice adds to the technical difficulties, and hence to the costs of inhalation studies. Nevertheless, this must be regarded as the most realistic method of modelling human exposure to airborne toxicants (see, for example, (3)), and the techniques needed for the exposure of many animal species have been devised. However, the costs and technical problems encountered in using such techniques preclude their widespread application.

Attempts to simplify animal exposure have frequently involved the direct instillation of materials into the lung via the trachea. Such methods produce a patchy and uneven distribution of the instilled material, as is illustrated in Table I. In a further experiment, rats were dosed with silica, the lungs removed after some days, and the SiO^2 content estimated. Of 36 rats examined, 9 had no silica remaining in their lungs, and the content of the remainder varied considerably. Thus, while this method may enable range-finding experiments to be carried out, the variability and abnormal distribution of instilled material means that large numbers of animals would have to be used in definitive experiments using this route of administration.

Table 1

Mean extents and ranges of fibrosis (%)

	LL	RUL	RML	RLL
1 week (10)	75 (10-90)	5 (5-20)	6.5 (5-40)	12 (5-60)
2 week (10)	72 (0-90)	1.1 (0-5)	5.5 (0-50)	11 (0-50)
4 week (4)	73 (20-100)	23 (0-70)	16 (0-80)	35 (0-100)
10 week (5)	89 (80-90)	44 (10-70)		50 (20-80)

A group of male Sprague-Dawley rats were given 25mg quartz (DQ12) by intratracheal instillation in 0.5ml saline. A specially constructed fibre optic endoscope was used and all instillations were carried out by an experienced operator. The lungs were removed, fixed and examined by standard techniques. The area of fibrosis was estimated as a percentage of the total section area and this extent is given as the mean and range for each group of animals. LL = left lung; RUL = right upper lobe; RML = right middle lobe; RLL = right lower lobe. The figure in brackets after the exposure time is the number of rats in each group. As can be seen, the left lung is affected more than the right lung and the right lower lobe more than the middle and upper lobes.

MATHEMATICAL MODELLING

Since only particles of limited size can be inhaled, a great deal of effort has been expended on calculating and measuring the size of these "respirable particles". While such considerations do not apply to gases or vapours, one obvious way of avoiding any hazard from solid particles or from fluid droplets is to ensure that they are too large to penetrate into the respiratory regions of the lung. Such particles will impinge on the mucous membranes of the nose or upper respiratory tract and be cleared from there by the mucociliary escalator. Products or processes could therefore be designed so as to avoid the generation of respirable aerosols. Thus, while large particles may still present a toxic hazard, this will be no different to that posed by their ingestion or direct irritancy.

A substantial volume of animal experimentation has suggested that only fibres of certain shapes and dimensions are responsible for any carcinogenic activity (4,5). Hence, fibrous dusts exhibit another size-dependent property which might enable the design of inherently harmless products.

While it is possible to design a "safe" product, its manufacture at an economic price may prove difficult. Nevertheless, information about which particle sizes are respirable or pathogenic can be used as an aid to selecting the least hazardous material or process from a range of alternatives.

IN VITRO STUDIES

The numerous references to the application of tissue culture to lung research makes it impractical to discuss and precis all the approaches and techniques. We can, however, describe some studies and comment on the application of such investigations to understanding the processes resulting from toxic injury to that organ.

Studies with Cells of the Immune System

The necessity for having a system to clear the lung of bacteria, viruses and dusts inhaled together with air is self evident (and the lung is now well-recognised as an immunologically important organ). There are many immunocompetent cells present in the lungs - macrophages, plasma cells, lymphocytes and mast cells, but their role in immunological surveillance will not be discussed here (for review, see (6)).

Various toxicants can interact with and damage macrophages and phagocytic leukocytes. This may cause an impairment of the immune system, resulting in conditions such as silico-tuberculosis, in which silica reduces resistance to mycobacteria (see (7)). Among other results from such interactions are the release of various inflammatory mediators and the production of free radicals from oxygen; these latter have been implicated as an important source of cellular injury (8). Free radicals may also cause the direct oxidation of xenobiotics, leading to the formation of active metabolites, and have also been implicated in lung injury resulting from exposure to paraquat, bleomycin and 12-0-tetradecanoyl-phorbol-13-acetate (TPA) (9-11). Investigations in this and other laboratories have demonstrated that the *in vitro* exposure of macrophages to pathogenic dusts results in the accumulation of malonaldehyde; this is frequently used as an indication of lipid peroxidation caused by free radical reactions (for review, see (12)).

Cytotoxicity and Morphological Investigations

In general, experiments concerned solely with the toxicity of agents towards cultured cells have not been of great use in mechanistic or predictive studies. However, a number of authors have found that the toxicity of various mineral dusts towards macrophages or macrophage-like cell lines correlated with the fibrogenic activity of those dusts *in vivo*. Mineral dusts have been subjected to particularly intense study in such tissue culture systems, and, while fibrous dusts are toxic towards both macrophages and fibroblasts, silica seems to be toxic only towards the former (13). The size of the fibres causing cell death *in vitro* is similar to that of those causing tumours *in vivo*, so the study of mineral dust cytotoxicity has been advocated as a preliminary screen for potentially pathogenic dusts (14-16).

The effects of various agents on the morphology and cellular composition of organ cultures have been studied by a number of investigators. The toxic effects of metals (17) and asbestos (18) on cultured human fetal lung have been reported. Evans *et al.* (17) concluded that embryonic lung could be useful in studying species-specific morphological reactions to a variety of agents. A number of authors, notably Mossman (19,20), have reported on the use of tracheal explants in studies of particulate toxicants.

Biochemical Investigations

Cytotoxic assays have had a limited success, but if progress is to be made it is essential that alterations in specific cellular activities are used as end-points. For example, lysosomal and cell sap enzyme release may provide an empirical test for fibrogenic agents, but is unlikely to provide an explanation for the role of macrophages in the development of fibrosis. By studying biochemical changes in cell and organ culture, it might prove possible to develop screens for toxic materials based on a sound knowledge of mechanism, or at least on credible hypotheses.

In an attempt to explain the biochemical processes involved in dust-induced pulmonary disease, Richards and his co-authors (21-23) postulated a direct effect of dust on lung fibroblasts. Using cultures of fibroblasts treated with dusts *in vitro*, they investigated changes in such parameters as the synthesis of DNA, collagen, and total protein, and on the basis of their observations suggested that such cultures might provide an *in vitro* model for studying pulmonary fibrosis.

Other authors (24-26) have suggested that a specific fibrogenic factor (i.e. one capable of exerting a stimulant effect on fibroblasts) might be released from damaged macrophages. Thus, in order to model the fibrogenic process *in vitro*, it would be essential to use cultures of both macrophages and fibroblasts. However, it may be unnecessary to postulate a specific factor, since collagen synthesis could result from a common inflammatory response, mediated by one or more of the substances known to be released from damaged cells. In this laboratory, we have been investigating the release of arachidonic acid metabolites from macrophage cultures treated with a variety of toxic substances (see Table II), we believe that this or similar activities could underlie the development of fibrosis.

Table II

Release of ^{3}H from P388D1 Cells Pretreated with Labelled Arachidonic Acid

Treatment	% of total tritium in medium (mean ± standard error)
control	3.9 + 0.2
TPA 0.1µg/ml	9.2 + 0.6
crocidolite (blue asbestos)	
80µg/ml	7.3 + 0.9
160µg/ml	12.5 + 0.8
320µg/ml	17.9 + 0.3
crocidolite 320µg/ml + indomethacin 15µg/ml	7.3 + 0.15

The macrophage-like cell line, P388D1, was grown to near confluence in 24-well multiwell dishes. The cells were then incubated with ^{3}H-arachidonic acid for 24 hours, washed and exposed to TPA or crocidolite for a further 24 hours. The medium was removed, centrifuged, and an aliquot counted in the scintillation counter, the cell layer was lysed and an aliquot of the resulting suspension similarly counted. The proportion of tritium released into the medium is given above. The addition of inflammatory agents to these cultures caused the increased release of radio-label which parallel experiments have shown to be located mainly in prostaglandins; this is confirmed by the inhibitory effect of indomethacin, a known inhibitor of cycloxygenase. This type of system can distinguish between inflammatory and non-inflammatory agents rapidly and at little cost. Primary macrophages behave in a similar fashion.

At the moment, there is insufficient information about the disease process in vivo to enable its accurate modelling in vitro. A great deal more work is necessary both in animals and in tissue culture before any system can provide anything other than an empirical test for agents causing lung damage.

Although much effort has been expended in studies on xenobiotic metabolism in the liver, there is a dearth of information on similar processes operating in the lung. However, because the lung is such a prominent target organ for carcinogens and various drugs, this omission is rapidly being corrected. All the common methods of studying such metabolism (microsomes, tissue slices, perfused organ and tissue culture) are being used and each has advantages and disadvantages (27). Pulmonary drug metabolism has been reviewed a number of times (9,28). In vitro studies of particular note are those of Cohen and his co-workers, who have used cultured tracheal cells (29) and short-term organ culture (30,31). Wiebel et al. (32) reported that the human epithelial type II cell line, A549, had some functional drug metabolism, so this cell line appears to have some potential for use in further investigations.

Clearly cell lines or short-term cell and organ cultures have some limitations which can only be overcome by the development of improved methods for the isolation and maintenance of relatively pure populations of differentiated lung cells. This would offer great scope for further investigations in pulmonary toxicology. Also, the study of cultures containing mixtures of differing, but defined, cell types might enable the analysis of cellular interactions in the development of pulmonary lesions.

CONCLUSION

It is now well established that the lung is much more than a ventilatory organ. It has been shown to be capable of synthesising, releasing and degrading a large number of biological mediators, as well as possessing a whole range of drug-metabolising enzymes (33). The heterogeneity of the lung makes an integrated in vivo investigation of these processes impractical and complicates the evaluation of the hazards posed by agents likely to have a deleterious effect on pulmonary function. Agents which affect one function may predispose the lung to damage from a second insult, and such synergistic effects are known in various human lung diseases, such as lung cancer in asbestos workers and uranium miners who also smoke cigarettes. The impracticability (mainly for financial reasons) of developing animal models for the study of synergism necessitates using both animals and alternatives in the study of pulmonary toxicology.

ACKNOWLEDGEMENTS

The authors wish to thank Dr J.C. Wagner and Dr J.H. Edwards for their help with the experiment reported in Table I, and Mrs J. Bolan for typing the manuscript.

REFERENCES

1. Legge, R.T. (1936). History of industrial medicine and occupational diseases. Industrial Medicine and Surgery 5, 30-45.
2. Agricola, G. (1556). "De Re Mettalica" (translated by Hoover, H.C. & Hoover, L.H., 1950), 638 pp. New York: Dover Publications.
3. Wagner, J.C. & Berry, G. (1973). Information obtained from animal experiments. In "Biological Effects of Asbestos" (ed. P. Bogovski, J.C. Gibson, V. Tinbrell & J.C. Wagner), pp. 85-88. Lyon: International Agency for Research on Cancer.
4. Stanton, M.F. & Layard, M. (1978). The carcinogenicity of fibrous minerals. In "Definitions and Measurement Methods", Workshop on Asbestos (ed. C.C. Gravatt, P.D. La Fleur & K.F.J. Heinreich), pp. 143-152. Washington: National Measurement Laboratory.
5. Wagner, J.C., Berry, G. & Pooley, F.D. (1980). Carcinogenesis and mineral fibres. British Medical Bulletin 36, 53-56.
6. Bienenstock, J., McDermott, M.R. & Befus, A.D. (1982). The significance of bronchus-associated lymphoid tissue. Bulletin European de Physiopathologie Respiratoire 18, 153-177.
7. Cole, L.G. (1948). "Lung Dust Lesions (Pneumoconiosis) versus Tuberculosis". 424 pp. White Plains, NY: American Medical Films.
8. Weiss, S.J. & Lobuglio, A.F. (1982). Biology of diseases. Phagocyte-generated oxygen metabolites and cellular injury. Laboratory Investigations 47, 5-18.
9. Boyd, M.R. (1980). Biochemical mechanisms in chemical-induced lung injury: roles of metabolic activation. Critical Reviews in Toxicology 7, 103-176.
10. Galvan, L., Huang, C.H., Prestayko, A.W., Stort, J.T., Evans, H.E. & Crooke, S.T. (1981). Inhibition of bleomycin-induced DNA breakage by superoxide dismutase. Cancer Research 41, 5103-5106.
11. Johnson, K.J. & Ward, P.A. (1982). Acute and progressive lung injury after contact with phorbol myristate acetate. American Journal of Pathology 107, 29-35.

12. Fantone, J.C. & Ward, P.A. (1982). Role of oxygen-derived free radicals and metabolites in leukocyte dependent inflammatory reactions. American Journal of Pathology 107, 397-418.
13. Brown, R.C., Gormley, I.P., Chamberlain, M. & Davies, R. (eds.) (1980). "The In Vitro Effects of Mineral Dusts". 373 pp. London: Academic Press.
14. Brown, R.C., Chamberlain, M., Griffiths, D.M. & Timbrell, N. (1978). The effect of fibre size on the in vitro biological activity of three types of amphibole asbestos. International Journal of Cancer 22, 721-727.
15. Chamberlain, M. & Brown, R.C. (1978). Cytotoxic effects of asbestos and other mineral dusts in tissue culture cell lines. British Journal of Experimental Pathology 59, 183-189.
16. Davies, R. (1980). The effect of dust on enzyme release from macrophages. In "The In Vitro Effects of Mineral Dusts" (ed. R.C. Brown, I.P. Gormley, M. Chamberlain & R. Davies), pp. 67-74. London: Academic Press.
17. Evans, P.H., Rajan, K.T. & Webb, M. (1981). The toxic effects of metal dusts on human foetal lungs in vitro. In "Culture Techniques - Applicability for Studies on Prenatal Differentiation and Toxicity" (ed. D. Neubert & H.J. Merker), pp. 319-323. Berlin: Walter de Gruyter.
18. Rajan, K.T. & Evans, P.H. (1973). Experimental methods - organ culture. In "Biological Effects of Asbestos" (ed. P. Bogovski, J.C. Gibson, V. Tinbrell & J.C. Wagner), pp. 94-98. Lyon: International Agency for Research on Cancer.
19. Mossman, B.T., Adler, K.B. & Craighead, J.E. (1980). Cytotoxic and proliferative changes in tracheal organ cultures after exposure to mineral dusts. In "The In Vitro Effects of Mineral Dusts" (ed. R.C. Brown, I.P. Gormley, M. Chamberlain & R. Davies), pp. 241-250. London: Academic Press.
20. Mossman, B.T. & Craighead, J.E. (1981). Mechanisms of asbestos carcinogenesis. Environmental Research 25, 269-280.
21. Richards, R.J., Wusterman, F.S. & Dodgson, K.S. (1971). The direct effects of dusts on lung fibroblast growth in vitro. Life Sciences 10, 1149-1154.
22. Richards, R.J. & Morris, T.G. (1973). Collagen and mucopolysaccharide production in growing lung fibroblasts exposed to chrysotile asbestos. Life Sciences 12, 441-451.
23. Richards, R.J. & Wusterman, F.S. (1974). The effects of silica dust and alveolar macrophages on lung fibroblast growth in vitro. Life Sciences 14, 355-364.
24. Heppleston, A.G. & Styles, J.A. (1967). Activity of a macrophage factor in collagen formation by silica. Nature, London 214, 521-522.
25. DeLustro, F. & LeRoy, E.C. (1982). Characterization of the release of human monocyte regulators of fibroblast proliferation. Journal of the Reticuloendothelial Society 31, 295-305.

26. Elias, J.A., Rossman, M.D. & Daniele, R.P. (1982). Inhibition of human lung fibroblast growth by mononuclear cells. American Review of Respiratory Disease 125, 701-705.
27. Fry, J.R. & Bridges, J.W. (1977). The metabolism of xenobiotics in cell suspension and cell cultures. In "Progress in Drug Metabolism" (ed. J.W. Bridges & L. Chasseaud), vol. II, pp. 71-118. London: Wiley.
28. Remmer, H. (1974). Pulmonary drug-metabolism enzymes. In "Lung Metabolism" (ed. A.E. Junod & R. de Haller), pp. 137-158. London: Academic Press.
29. Cohen, G.H., Marchok, A.C., Nettesheim, P., Steele, V.E., Nelson, F., Huang, F. & Selkirk, J.K. (1979). Comparative metabolism of benzo(a)pyrene in organ and cell cultures derived from rat trachea. Cancer Research 39 1980-1984.
30. Cohen, A.M., Haws, S.M., Moore, B.P. & Bridges, J.W. (1976). Benzo(a)pyrene-3-yl hydrogen sulphate. A major ethyl acetate-extractable metabolite of benzo(a)pyrene in human, hamster and rat lung cultures. Biochemical Pharmacology 25, 2561-2570.
31. Cohen, G.H. & Moore, B.P. (1977). The metabolism of benzo(a) pyrene, 7,8, dihydro-7-8-dihydroxy benzo(a)pyrene and 9-10-dihydro-9-10 dihydroxybenzo(a)pyrene by short-term organ cultures of hamster lung. Biochemical Pharmacology 26, 1481-1487.
32. Wiebel, F.J., Lambiotte, M., Summer, R.H. & Wolff, T. (1980). Established cell cultures as model systems for carcinogen metabolism. In "Carcinogenesis - Fundamental Mechanisms and Environmental Effects" (ed. B. Pullman, P.O.P. Ts'O & H. Gelboin), pp. 347-361. Amsterdam: Reidel.
33. Junod, A.F. & de Haller, R. (eds.) (1975). "Lung Metabolism" 501 pp. London: Academic Press.

Recommendations

D. G. CLARK and R. C. BROWN

We have four recommendations on inhalation toxicology:

1. We strongly recommend that the first stage of any inhalation toxicity investigation is organ culture - of the brain. Without

doubt, cultivating the human brain to think is the best substitute for animal experiments. The question that must be asked at the outset is: are inhalation studies needed at all?

Dr Brown has described the mathematical and physical models that can be used to predict where particles will deposit in the respiratory tract. If the chemical to be tested contains particles too large to be inhaled, then there is no need for any inhalation studies. If the particles are of such a size that they impact in the nostrils, the inhalation toxicity reduces to one of local irritation of the nostrils and of swallowing of the chemical. A feeding study may therefore be more appropriate than an inhalation study.

Another question that should be asked is: has the work been done before? A literature search can provide valuable information. The advent of computer literature searches has now simplified this procedure to such a point that they should be automatically undertaken before any experiments are considered. A note of warning should be sounded, however, in that much of the old toxicological work in the literature is of uncertain quality. Details are often insufficient to equate the work with modern toxicological practices, and the exact chemical composition of the sample is often in doubt.

The molecular structure and physical properties of chemicals leading to certain types of toxic responses are well established in some areas of inhalation toxicology. One example would be the physical properties known to be associated with glue sniffing toxicity. An alert, enquiring human brain, well primed with up-to-date scientific knowledge, can often eliminate some of the almost-reflex toxicological testing, by relating the new chemical to known structures and properties.

2. Our second recommendation is that where good alternatives exist, they should be used. In particular, several in vitro methods are now available for the study of lung fibrosis, and these should be considered instead of long-term inhalation experiments.

3. If animal experiments are inevitable, the most appropriate test using the minimum number of animals should be used. Although many toxicologists are constrained by the international guidelines and regulations under which they must operate, there is still scope for the intelligent application of simple tests. Examples of this approach would be the use of intra-tracheal injection instead of inhalation exposure and the use of the inhalation hazard test instead of the inhalation LD50.

4. Finally, we recommend more research to validate promising in vitro tests, recognising the dilemma that in validating these tests more animals will be used in the short-term in order to reduce the numbers used in the long-term. The ideal situation,

of course, would be for us to agree which chemicals should be used in any validation programme, so that the tests could be compared one with another, rather than each test being validated with one, often restricted, group of chemicals.

General Discussion

A. N. WORDEN

Rapporteur

Mr D. SWANSTON asked for comments on the value of intra-tracheal and intra-pleural injections in reducing the number of animals. Dr BROWN replied that these methods would be recommended in pilot studies to reduce the need to undertake inhalation experiments later. However, such techniques were not complete substitutes for inhalation, since the deposition following intra-tracheal injection was different to that following inhalation and the local necrosis that often occurs was not seen with inhalation exposure.

Ms Sheila SILCOCK asked whether the screening tests described were applicable to irritant gases or only to dust problems? Dr CLARK said that some of the tests described, such as the macrophage culture technique and intra-tracheal injection, were particularly useful for dusts, but that there were also very reliable short-term tests for irritant gases. In particular, the Alarie mouse sensory irritation test had been validated and calibrated so that the results of a single five minute exposure can be directly extrapolated to longer-term effects in man.

Professor R. HESS asked for views on the suggestion that one may extrapolate from oral toxicity studies to inhalation studies using some form of conversion factor. Dr CLARK replied that this was a topic which was being discussed in the EEC at the present time, and that data on the rat LD50s and LC50s of a range of chemicals were being collected in order that this comparison could be made. He thought it required a large leap of imagination to go from one to the other with confidence. With certain chemicals or groups of chemicals, one could say that toxicity was toxicity and that a high or low toxicity chemical would be of high or low toxicity whether injected intravenously, orally-dosed or inhaled. In these cases, an oral LD50 value could give valuable information on possible inhalation toxicity. But inhalation toxicity had other unique problems in that a chemical could be lethal purely by an irritant action on the lungs, whereas it was very unlikely that an oral chemical could be lethal because it had an irritant action on the mouth or stomach.

Dr Janet MASSEY asked for an opinion on experiments where the animal was dosed and the macrophages taken for study in culture. Dr BROWN replied that such combined in vivo/in vitro tests, where the animal was dosed and the macrophages collected by broncho-alveolar lavage, were used extensively and could give very valuable information on both the acute and chronic effects of chemicals on the lungs.

Testing for Cutaneous Toxicity

RONALD MARKS

It is not only topically applied medicaments, cosmetics or toiletries that may cause damage to the skin; all materials that are destined for some type of skin contact are a potential source of injury. Growing awareness of this fact has prompted a search for tests that can predict toxicity to the skin accurately and conveniently.

The aim in this paper is to review the available methods for the prediction of acute toxicity from substances that by design will contact the skin. It is not intended to discuss the potentially serious problems of long-term toxicity and carcinogenicity or the difficult questions that sometimes arise from absorption of substances into the body via the skin.

TYPES OF SKIN DISORDER ENCOUNTERED

The skin disorder that most frequently results from exposure to a toxic material is eczema (dermatitis). Eczema represents a particular pattern of inflammation in the epidermis. A material may cause this reaction by being directly irritant to the skin, by evoking a cell-mediated delayed hypersensitivity response (allergic contact dermatitis) or by interacting with light energy to cause a photocontact dermatitis.

Other types of toxic reaction to the skin from environmentally encountered substances include the sensation of stinging or burning without visible skin change at one end of the scale to severe erosion of the skin at the other. It also includes "contact" urticaria, depigmentation and hyperpigmentation, and follicular reactions with the development of acne-type lesions.

While all these disorders are important, it seems practical to devote most of this paper to irritancy, which is responsible for the bulk of the problems encountered. It should be realised that "irritancy" is a blanket term to cover all toxic reactions in the skin after application of materials to the skin that result in eczematous inflammation.

TEST SYSTEMS FOR DETERMINATION OF IRRITANCY

Animal Testing In Vivo

Animal tests are conducted either on the skin or in the eye. Ocular testing is based on the test described by Draize and subsequently modified on many occasions (1,2). Apart from any suggestion that ocular testing is unpleasant aesthetically and of doubtful ethical propriety, there have been genuine doubts as to its reproducibility and usefulness as a predictive system. Objective evaluation of the rabbit eye test by a variety of techniques including tonometry and measurement of corneal thickness has been recommended to add precision (3). However, these do not enhance the accuracy of the predictive information sufficiently and I believe that the basic problem of ocular testing is the choice of the eye as the substrate tissue.

Epicutaneous testing of the skin of small mammals such as rats, guinea-pigs, rabbits and mice also has problems. Although there are clear and obvious similarities in the way that human and animal skins behave, there are important differences in their structure and physiology which influence their reactivity. Although the core cell of the epidermis is similar in all mammalian skins, there are differences in the granular cells and in the biochemistry of keratinisation between species which imply a functional significance. There are also differences in melanin production and distribution, and in the distribution, relative sizes and function of hair follicles and sweat glands, as well as in the overall structure of the dermis and its vasculature.

These variations between species could well influence the results of testing for irritancy. First, the pattern of percutaneous penetration may differ, allowing different concentrations of material to contact different areas of the skin at different times. Secondly, the reactivity of skin differs, which may give misleading information with regard to the effect in man and may also fail to correctly rank order or distinguish substances whose toxicity is similar. Kligman (4) makes the point that the dose-response relationship for irritants is very flat in animal skin, so that discriminative ability is very low. He further states that animal testing is of little value for mild irritants. Indeed, when formal comparisons have been made between rabbit and human skin for irritancy, poor relationships have been found (5,6), although some studies have demonstrated a good correlation between results in animals and man (7).

Epicutaneous Toxicity Testing in Man

There are clear advantages to the testing of substances on man. In the first place, there is less difficulty in extrapolating the results of such testing directly to its intended use, and, secondly, the overall reliability is likely to be improved. However, there are precautions and difficulties which must be recognised.

Test Panel

The ethics of such testing has been questioned. Indeed, there are some countries in which it is very difficult to perform simple epicutaneous toxicity tests in human volunteer subjects - yet the regulatory bodies of the same countries require such tests to be made before allowing registration of the product!

Aside from the questions of ethics, there are also practical problems. The first concerns the number of subjects in such a test. The number required should depend on the discriminative ability of the test system for the range of toxicities to be tested, and the representative nature of the test panel in terms of the population to be exposed to the material. At present, there is no accepted formula which will indicate the numbers needed and this probably explains some of the variability in test results between different laboratories.

The question of the composition of the test panel has to be taken seriously. Some years ago, we were asked to examine the percutaneous absorption of a topical corticosteroid. The topical product was a "reformulation" and was a gel. It had been tested by repeat insult patch testing in Mexico. We applied it under occlusion for 12 hours per day over areas of the back and arms in a test panel in Cardiff - and produced severe irritation of the skin in everyone tested. The only conclusion that can be drawn is that the dark-complexioned subjects of Mexico were much hardier than the fair-skinned, light-eyed Celtic population that we sampled in Wales.

Black-skinned individuals have a denser and thicker stratum corneum (8) and it appears that they are less easily irritated and sensitised than caucasian subjects (9). Recently a classification has emerged of reactivity to ultraviolet light (UVL), as the Boston classification (Table I). A similar classification for irritancy would be very useful, and a suggested scheme is outlined in Table II. Kligman (4) believes that UVL sensitivity and susceptibility to irritation go hand-in-hand. However, this may not always be the case. For example, in a recent study (10) we have characterised the reactivity of both normal and psoriatic subjects to anthralin and found a poor relationship between minimal irritancy dose and UVL sensitivity (Table III).

Skin reactivity also changes with age. Grove *et al.* (11) showed that there was a decreased blister-formation time in elderly subjects with an ammonium hydroxide technique, and they equated this with increased susceptibility to irritation. Decreased immunological responsiveness and decreased rates of wound healing have also been noted in elderly subjects, and clearly these factors would influence the appearance of skin reactions in epicutaneous toxicity testing. Our own work has shown that both structural and functional changes occur in the epidermis and stratum corneum with increasing age. Epidermal cells shrink in volume (12), corneocytes increase in area (13,14), and changes occur in water loss, intracorneal cohesion and percorneal penetration (15).

Table I

Boston Classification of Sensitivity to Ultraviolet Light

Classification	Description
I	Always burns, never tans
II	Always burns, sometimes tans
III	Sometimes burns, always tans
IV	Never burns, always tans
V	Mediterranean type
VI	Black types

Table II

A Possible Classification of Susceptibility to Environmentally Determined Dermatitis

Classification	Description	Investigative finding
I	Frequent dermatitis in past	Reacts strongly to reagent*
II	Some dermatitis in past	Reacts moderately to reagent*
III	"Sensitive" skin only	Reacts moderately to reagent*
IV	Normal skin	Reacts weakly to reagent*
V	Normal skin	No reaction to reagent*

[*Either 5% sodium lauryl sulphate or ammonium hydroxide (1:1 aqueous solution)]

Table III

Relationship Between Minimal Irritancy Dose for Anthralin (MID50) and Sensitivity to Ultraviolet Light, Determined as Minimal Erythema Dose (MED) for Normal Subjects and Psoriatics

Group	Correlation coefficient	Significance
Controls (40)	0.15	N.S.
Psoriatics (40)	0.10	N.S.

At the other end of the age scale, there is much less data. It seems that a baby's skin is more-easily irritated than that of an adult. However, in general, children are less easily sensitised than older age-groups, and considerable caution is required in extrapolating a test result to the likely effects in small children. For these reasons, it is obvious that the age of the test panel must be stated and preferably standardised. Furthermore, the age of the test panel should bear some relationship to the age of the intended user groups for the project in question. Interestingly, the sex composition of a test panel does not appear to influence the results (16).

The reactivity of skin may vary with season and with ambient environmental conditions; these factors should be stated, as they may well alter a test result. The anatomical site used for testing is also of importance. Feldman & Maibach (17) showed that there was regional variation in the percutaneous penetration of labelled hydrocortisone, and there are many other region-dependent physiological variables in skin function which may influence the toxicity of applied materials, including rates of sweat and sebum production, desquamation and blood supply. Recently, we examined the "stinging" properties of topical preparations containing lactic acid and found that the sensation of stinging varied markedly with body site (Table IV).

Table IV

Regional Differences in Sensation of Stinging Elicited by Open Application of a Lactic Acid Containing Preparation in 24 Normal Human Volunteers Aged 20-30

Cheeks	Chest	Neck	Arms
41	2	47	5

The figures represent total scores for 24 subjects who evaluated the "stinging" due to the preparations applied twice daily for one week, on a 0-3 scale for each site.

Technical Considerations

The next factor to be considered in human toxicity testing is the actual technique employed. For weak or potentially moderately irritant substances a "repeat insult patch test" protocol is usually employed (6). The patches are kept in contact with the skin for 48 hour periods and then renewed at the same sites. Between 5 and 10 repeat applications are usually made to the same sites but the choice of the exact number appears to be completely arbitrary and decided according to the experience of the investigator and the tolerance of the test panel. It is important that the patch is occlusive to maximise the penetration. A variety of designs of occlusive dressing have evolved and our gratitude is due to the International Contact Dermatitis research group for their careful evaluation of the various dressings available. A small chamber made of inert material (aluminium) on an adhesive paper backing, such as the Finn chamber, is probably best.

A case has been made for compromising the test area by lightly scarifying it either by scratching with a 30 gauge needle, by an abrading instrument (18) or by repeatedly stripping off the horny layer with adhesive tape. These procedures remove the barrier of the stratum corneum and reveal the basic irritancy of the material in question to the epidermis and underlying tissues. Application of 20% aluminium chloride to scarified skin will cause irritation and pustulation, but will cause no reaction on intact skin - application of a deodorant to a "shaved" axilla will confirm this phenomenon in those who have some doubts. Whether a "compromised skin" type of test should be used or not depends on the particular question being asked of the experiment.

"Use" Tests

The ultimate test of safety as far as irritancy is concerned for any product is the number of problems experienced when it is in use. Even when the individual components of a product appear to have low irritancy in some form of repeat insult patch test, it is prudent to test the complete product. The cumulated minor irritancies of the individual substances can summate to cause unpredicted skin reactions. This is especially the case if one of the substances included in the preparation enhances the penetration of the others. Of equal relevance to the testing of the complete product is testing to simulate the actual conditions of use. Such tests throw up unsuspected answers. Frosch (19) describes chamber tests with 8% soap solutions and standardised washing tests of the antecubital fossae and face to determine the potential irritancy of soaps. They rated the reactions on a 0-4 scale for erythema, discomfort and scaling, and a 0-3 scale for fissuring on the eighth day of the tests. To the surprise of all concerned, the syndets showed as much irritancy as some of the older alkaline groups.

Under some circumstances, it is virtually impossible to characterise the irritancy of materials adequately in the conditions in which they will be used. We encountered this type of problem in the evaluation of the irritancy of adhesive dressings destined to hold stoma appliances in place (20). The peristomal skin is a notorious source of discomfort and distress for patients with an ileostomy, as the skin is almost continuously bathed in irritant bowel content. Some 70% of ileostomy patients experience some type of peristomal skin reaction in a five-year period. The protocol that we adopted used both daily and weekly renewal of the adhesive materials for a total of 3 weeks on either side of the abdominal wall of healthy subjects. Irritancy was assessed from the cumulated scores for the test panel, each individual score being based on a 7-point arbitrary scale. We tested seven materials and found that there were clear differences between the products - differences which accorded with clinical observation.

Evaluation of the Test Site - Clinical

Evaluation can be either clinical or instrumental. It is usual practice to wait at least 15 minutes after removal of the test patches before inspecting and assessing areas for erythema under good lighting. It is also customary to grade the intensity of reaction on an arbitrary scale. If this procedure is adopted, it is important to ensure that the scoring is reproducible and the scale wide enough to give adequate sensitivity. However, Wooding & Kligman (21) made a strong case for bringing cutaneous toxicity testing into line with other types of toxicity testing by determining the minimal irritancy dose or minimal irritancy time for 50% (MID50 or MIT50). There is much sense to this approach from the standardisation viewpoint, provided that the type of response evoked is identical within the test panel and that when MID50 or MIT50 doses for different substances are being compared, standardised conditions are employed in each test and the materials in question evoke exactly the same type of reaction.

Evaluation of the Test Site - Instrumental

There is some loss of precision from the subjective assessment of erythema in the determination of the threshold of irritancy. The problem becomes even more critical when coloured substances or black skins are being evaluated. This problem is most dramatically encountered when assessing the irritancy of anthralin.

Clearly, visual inspection is inadequate and some other technique is required. Mustakallio (22) used thermography to detect the increased skin temperature of skin reactions due to anthralin, and Kersey et al. (23) employed skin-fold calipers to measure the local oedema after application of the same substance. It should be noted that, although oedema and increased blood flow are both features of the inflammatory process, they do not necessarily occur in the same time sequence or indeed occur equally in all irritant reactions. Clinical observation and measurements taken using skin contact thermometry, skin-fold calipers and ultrasound skin thickness determination have persuaded us that skin thickness measurements are less sensitive parameters in anthralin irritancy than the temperature (T. Kingston, P.J. Dykes & R. Marks, in preparation). We used the rise in skin temperature as the measure of irritancy and took as the minimal irritancy dose that concentration of anthralin required to raise the temperature of the test site 0.5°C above the untreated peripheral zone.

As mentioned above, when oedema or infiltration are important components of a particular toxicity, then measurements of dermal thickness can be made using either skin-fold calipers or ultrasound. Our group have used both these methods to evaluate a particular form of toxicity - the skin thinning effect from the use of topical corticosteroids (24-26). Harpenden skin-fold calipers employed using the "minimal possible pinch" technique can measure the dermal thinning, but are not sufficiently accurate. We now prefer an ultrasound device employing a 50 megahertz transducer to measure dermal thickness. This technique has now been developed to the point that epidermal thickness can also be measured, and we believe that this non-invasive assessment may well have increasing application in toxicological assessment (P. Payne & R. Marks, in preparation).

Some substances have a particular drying effect on the horny layer and cause scaling without much inflammation. As part of our programme of exploration of measurement of skin reactivity, we have evaluated two methods for measurement of changes in the skin surface. The first relies on the production of hard positive replicas of the skin surface and the measurement of the skin contour of these by a stylus in an instrument known as a surfometer (27). This technique is perfectly adequate for measuring the surface swelling effect from emollients but is inadequate for assessment of scaling. To measure scaling, we have used a macrophotographic scanning densitometric method (28-29). In this technique, the negatives of macrophotographs of the skin sites are scanned in a scanning densitometer and the resulting traces assessed quantitatively. This provides a useful measure of scaling and it is believed that when the method has been further developed to make it a one-step procedure with instantaneous read-out it will be a practical and useful tool.

TESTING FOR SENSITISATION

Animal Tests

The use of animals for the detection of potential sensitisers in man rests on less shaky ground than the use of animals for predictive testing for irritancy. Draize (30) published the first test employing guinea-pigs. Subsequently, a more sensitive test has been used - the guinea-pig maximisation test (31). In this technique, intradermal injections are given with and without Freund's complete adjuvant or by topical application to two groups of approximately 20 guinea-pigs (test and control groups). There seems to be good correlation of the results obtained in this way with clinical experience. This area has been well reviewed by Bronaugh & Maibach (33).

Human Tests

The protocol for an experiment to detect sensitisation using human subjects should include a gap after the period of initial exposure with subsequent retesting at a long enough time interval for any immunological changes to have taken place. A commonly employed protocol is reapplication of the test material 3 times per week for 2 weeks, and then application of the challenge dose at a separate site after a further 7 days, with reading of the result 48 hours later - some 15 minutes after removal of the dressing - with a further inspection 24 hours later.

The prediction of the sensitising potential of a substance is in some ways more straightforward and in others more difficult. Theoretically, everyone will be affected by an irritant if enough exposure is given. Sensitisation will only occur in a comparatively small proportion of those exposed. For this reason, the major difficulty is the number of subjects in the test panel. A material that sensitises only 0.1% of the population of users of a hand cream will cause unpleasant dermatitis in 1 in 1000 and should be considered dangerous on this account. To detect this, it may be necessary to test more than 1000 subjects - clearly not a practical proposition.

One way of improving the chances of picking up a sensitiser is to ensure good penetration by stripping off the stratum corneum at the test sites or by applying 5% sodium lauryl sulphate beforehand (so-called "maximisation tests"). Another way in which it is theoretically possible to enhance the chances of detecting a potential sensitiser is to include a group of very easily sensitised subjects in the test panel. Ethical considerations aside, this must remain outside the realms of practical toxicology, as it is not yet possible to identify such a group with confidence.

Testing for sensitisation will remain one of the more unsatisfactory aspects of cutaneous toxicology until more practical and accurate methods are devised.

TESTING FOR PHOTOTOXICITY

The essence of testing for phototoxicity is the application of the test material under occlusion and subsequent irradiation with artificial UVL. It is important that non-irradiated control patches are also assessed so as to be able to distinguish plain irritant or allergic responses from the light-determined reactions. The exact protocol varies with the experience and preference of the investigator and the properties of the particular material under investigation. In the photomaximisation test of Kaidbey & Kligman (34), five repeat exposures and irradiations are given. The initial UV irradiation contains both UVB and the non-erythematogenic UVA, but subsequent challenge doses of UVL consist of UVA alone as this is the waveband that causes the bulk of the phototoxic reactions. The vehicle employed is also of great importance. Marzulli & Maibach (35) showed that reactions to Bergapten were greater when 70% alcohol was used than when 90% alcohol was employed.

A variety of *in vivo* animal tests for the detection of phototoxicity or photosensitisation have also been described.

IN VITRO TESTING FOR CUTANEOUS TOXICITY

The difficulties of using man or other experimental animals for *in vivo* toxicity testing include: ethical considerations, limitation of the range of toxicity that can be tested, variability of the response, susceptibility to artefacts with relatively small technical deviations, and high cost in resources (time and money).

There would be major advantages in having reliable *in vitro* tests with which to assess toxicity to the skin. Save in the area of phototoxicity, progress to this end has been slow and uncertain. Three *in vitro* tests were used to assess the phototoxic potential of various fragrance materials by Addo *et al.* (36):

a. *Candida killing test* (39). Cultures of *Candida utilis* on sabouraud dextrose agar with filter-paper discs containing the test substance were either irradiated with UVA ($1.2 mW/cm^2$) or UVB for 24 hours or kept in the dark. Phototoxicity was demonstrated by clear zones around the discs.
b. *Photohaemolysis* (38). Ninety-nine ml of human washed RBCs suspended in barbitone buffer and 1ml of test substance diluted in alcohol were divided into 5ml aliquots in

Petri dishes and were then irradiated with UVA (or UVB) for periods of up to 3 hours. After centrifugation, the released haemoglobin in the supernatant was determined as cyanmethaemoglobin using Drabkin's solution and spectrophotometric assessment.

c. Photo-oxidation (39). Material diluted in alcohol added to 0.61mM L-histidine monochloride monohydrate in 0.01mM sodium phosphate buffer, pH 7.4. The solutions were irradiated with UVA or UVB for 2-3 hours and the histidine that had not been split at the imidazole ring was estimated in a Pauly reaction.

The *Candida* test appears to indicate phototoxicity of the type characterised by activity against DNA, such as is observed with the psoralens. An erythematous reaction with a prolonged latent period after the photopatch tests is typical clinically. Positive photohaemolysis tests are indicators of substances which attack cell membranes, typified by pitch or anthraquinone-based dyes or protoporphyrin. Immediate erythema with smarting and oedema are found in photopatch tests with this type of reaction.

The photo-oxidation of histidine may give an indication of potential photoallergy from the test substance, as it seems that the formation of oxidised protein accounts for the antigenic stimulation in some instances.

Table V

Cell Killing Effect of Anthralin and Anthralin Metabolites in Cell Culture

Addition to culture	Keratinocytes per dish ($x10^5$)* mean + s.d.
Control (ethyl acetate only)	4.23 x 0.82
Anthralin (3×10^{-6}M in ethyl acetate)	2.53 x 0.67
Anthralin dimer (3×10^{-6}M in ethyl acetate)	2.43 x 0.41
Danthron (3×10^{-6}M in ethyl acetate)	4.62 x 0.99

[*The keratinocytes were obtained from pig ears. The exposure to the anthralin was continuous for 3 days.]

Progress in the *in vitro* detection of phototoxicity has not been mirrored by the development of useful *in vitro* tests for the detection of irritancy and potential sensitisers. There have been some studies on whole skin in chambers in which the release of enzymes from the skin into the medium has been measured, but this has so far proved unreliable in our hands. In any case, the technique is limited by the supply of human skin. Considerable progress has been made in techniques of culture of adult human keratinocytes, since the description of the irradiated 3T3 feeder layer technique by Rheinwald & Green (40). These would seem to be ideal for the assessment of toxicity and it is disappointing that so little work seems to have been reported using this type of system. Our own studies with adult human and pig keratinocytes have been confined to the investigation of anthralin toxicity, but many further studies are planned (Table V).

CONCLUSIONS

We live in an imperfect world in which progress of any kind is slow and often made only by compromise. The current state of cutaneous toxicity testing leaves much to be desired, with questions, problems and inconsistencies outweighing answers. However, it now seems certain that for substances of low and medium toxicity, in vivo testing in man is preferable to animal testing procedures. To make this human testing more reliable, and in order that the results may be compared at different times and between different laboratories, standardisation of the whole procedure is required. The development of objective measurement techniques would greatly improve the precision of human testing.

Where substances of unknown toxicity or potentially high toxicity are involved, some preliminary animal tests may still be required, although these may be replaced in the future by in vitro tests. There is an urgent need for the development of such in vitro tests. They would serve as screening tests and also supplement some of the testing now performed in man. However, it seems likely that "use" tests in man will always be needed.

REFERENCES

1. Draize, J.H., Woodard, G. & Calvery, H.O. (1944). Method for the study of irritation and toxicity of substances applied topically to the skin and mucous membranes. Journal of Pharmacology and Experimental Therapeutics 82, 377-389.
2. Code of Federal Regulation. (1973). Tests for eye irritants. Title 16, Section 1500.42.
3. Heywood, R. & James, R.W. (1978). Towards objectivity in the assessment of eye irritation. Journal of the Society of Cosmetic Chemists 29, 25-29.
4. Kligman, A.M. (1982). Assessment of mild irritants. In "Principles of Cosmetics for the Dermatologist" (ed. P.

Frost & S.N. Horwitz), pp. 265-273. St. Louis: Mosby.
5. Weil, C.S. & Scala, R.A. (1971). Study of intra- and inter-laboratory variability in the results of rabbit eye and skin irritation tests. Toxicology & Applied Pharmacology 19, 276-360.
6. Philips, L., Steinberg, M., Maibach, H.I. & Akers, W.A. (1972). A comparison of rabbit and human skin response to certain irritants. Toxicology & Applied Pharmacology 21, 369-382.
7. Steinberg, M., Akers, W.A., Weeks, M.H., McCreesh, A.H. & Maibach, H.I. (1975). A comparison of test techniques based on rabbit and human skin responses to irritants with recommendations regarding the evaluation of mildly to moderately irritating compounds. In "Animal Models in Dermatology". (ed. H. Maibach), pp. 1-11. Edinburgh: Churchill-Livingstone.
8. Weigand, D.A., Haygood, C. & Gaylor, J.R. (1974). Cell layer and density of negro and caucasian stratum corneum. Journal of Investigative Dermatology 62, 563-568.
9. Weigand, D.A. & Gaylor, J.R. (1974). Irritant reaction in negro and caucasian skin. Southern Medical Journal 67, 548-551.
10. Kingston, T. & Marks, R. (1983). Irritant reactions to dithranol in normal subjects and psoriatic patients. British Journal of Dermatology 108, 307-313.
11. Grove, G.L., Duncan, S. & Kligman, A.M. (1982). Effect of ageing on the blistering of human skin with ammonium hydroxide. British Journal of Dermatology 107, 393-400.
12. Marks, R. (1981). Measurement of biological ageing in human epidermis. British Journal of Dermatology 104, 627-633.
13. Marks, R., Lawson, A. & Nicholls, S. (1983). Age related changes in stratum corneum structure and function. In "Stratum Corneum" (ed. R. Marks & G. Plewig), pp.175-180. Berlin: Springer-Verlag.
14. Plewig, G., Scheuber, E., Reuter, B. & Waidelich, W. (1983). Thickness of corneocytes. In "Stratum Corneum" (ed. R. Marks & G. Plewig), pp. 171-174. Berlin: Springer-Verlag.
15. Marks, R., Black, D. & Hatzis, J. (1982). Characterisation of the effects of ageing on the stratum corneum. Proceedings of the 12th Congress of the IFSCC, Paris, 1982.
16. Björnberg, A. (1975). Skin reactions to primary irritants in men and women. Acta Dermatoverner, Stockholm 55, 191-194.
17. Feldman, R. & Maibach, H. (1967). Regional variation in percutaneous penetration of hydrocortisone in man. Journal of Investigative Dermatology 48, 181-186.
18. Haley, T. & Hunziger, J. (1974). Instrument for producing standardized skin abrasion. Journal of Pharmacological Science 63, 106.
19. Frosch, P.J. (1982). Irritancy of soaps and detergent bars. In "Principles of Cosmetics for the Dermatologist" (ed. P.

Frost & S.N. Horwitz), pp. 5-12. St. Louis: Mosby.
20. Marks, R., Evans, E. & Clarke, T.K. (1978). The effects on normal skin of adhesives from stoma appliances. Current Medical Research 5, 720-725.
21. Kligman, A.M. & Wooding, W.M. (1967). A method for the measurement and evaluation of irritants on human skin. Journal of Investigative Dermatology 49, 78-94.
22. Mustakallio, K.K. (1979). Irritation and staining by dithranol (anthralin) and related compounds. 1. Estimation with chamber testing and contact thermography. Acta Dermato-Venerologica (suppl. 85) 59, 125-132.
23. Kersey, P., Chapman, P., Rogers, S., Rawlins, M. & Shuster, S. (1981). The inflammatory response to anthralin and its relation to aryl hydrocarbon hydroxylase. British Journal of Dermatology (suppl. 20) 105, 64-67.
24. Dykes, P.J & Marks, R. (1979). An appraisal of the methods used in the assessment of atrophy from topical corticosteroids. British Journal of Dermatology 101, 599-609.
25. Tan, C.Y. Marks, R. & Payne, P. (1981). Comparison of xeroradiographic and ultrasound detection of corticosteroid induced dermal thinning. Journal of Investigative Dermatology 76, 126-128.
26. Dykes, P.J., Francis, A.J. & Marks, R. (1976). Measurement of dermal thickness with the Harpenden skin-fold caliper. Archives of Dermatological Research 256, 261-263.
27. Nicholls, S., King, C.S. & Marks, R. (1978). Short-term effects of emollients and a bath oil on the stratum corneum. Journal of the Society of Cosmetic Chemists 29, 617-624.
28. Marshall, R. & Marks, R. (1983). Assessments of skin surface by scanning densitometry of macrophotographs. Clinical and Experimental Dermatology 8, 121-127.
29. Marshall, R.J. & Marks, R. (1982). Examination of skin surface roughness with a macrophotographic scanning densitometric technique. Bioengineering and the Skin 3, 153-154.
30. Draize, J.H. (1955). Dermal toxicity. Food Drug Cosmetic Law Journal 10, 722.
31. Magnussen, B. & Kligman, A.M. (1969). The identification of contact allergens by animal assay. The guinea-pig maximization test. Journal of Investigative Dermatology 52, 268-276.
32. Kligman, A.M. (1966). The identification of contact allergens by human assay. III. The maximization test. A procedure for screening and rating contact sensitizers. Journal of Investigative Dermatology 47, 393-409.
33. Bronaugh, R.L. & Maibach, H.I. (1982). Primary irritant, allergic contact, phototoxic, and photoallergic reactions to cosmetics and tests to identify problem products. In "Principles of Cosmetics for the Dermatologist" (ed. P. Frost & S.N. Horwitz), pp. 223-243. St. Louis: Mosby.
34. Kaidbey, K.H. & Kligman, A.M. (1980). Photomaximization test for identifying photoallergic contact sensitizers. Contact

Dermatitis 6, 161-169.
35. Marzulli, F.N. & Maibach, H.I. (1970). Perfume phototoxicity. Journal of the Society of Cosmetic Chemists 21, 685-689.
36. Addo, H.A., Ferguson, J., Johnson, B.E. & Frain-Bell, W. (1982). The relationship between exposure to fragrance materials and persistent light reaction in the photosensitivity dermatitis with actinic reticuloid syndrome. British Journal of Dermatology 107, 261-274.
37. Kagan, J., Gabriel, R. & Reed, S.A. (1980). Alpha-terthienyl, a non-photodynamic phototoxic compound. Photochemistry and Photobiology 31, 465-469.
38. Frain-Bell, W., Hetherington, A. & Johnson, B.E. (1979). Contact allergic sensitivity to chrysanthemum and the photosensitivity dermatitis and actinic reticuloid. British Journal of Dermatology 101, 491-501.
39. Weil, L. (1965). On the mechanism of the photo-oxidation of amino acids sensitized by methylene blue. Archives of Biochemistry and Biophysics 110, 57-68.
40. Rheinwald, J.G. & Green, H. (1975). Serial cultivation of strains of human epidermal keratinocytes: the formation of keratinizing colonies from single cells. Cell 6, 331-343.

Skin Phototoxicity in Man

A. R. YOUNG

A skin phototoxin may be described as a substance that will induce a reaction only in the presence of ultraviolet or visible radiation. For practical purposes, this is the 290-800nm waveband of the electromagnetic spectrum. Phototoxins may be produced as a consequence of metabolic disorders, e.g. porphyrins, or may be administered orally as drugs (side-effects), e.g. chlorpromazine, or may be applied to the skin as in fragrances or treatments for various skin diseases, e.g. tar products. A phototoxic response may be acute, e.g. inflammation, which may be direct or immunologically mediated (photoallergy), or may be long-term, e.g. skin cancer (photocarcinogenesis). Substances administered orally may undergo liver metabolism and thus the photoactive compound in the skin may be chemically different from a possibly non-photoactive parent compound. The important consideration is, of course, the substance in the skin. Substances applied directly to the skin are much less likely to undergo metabolism.

At present, animals, often hairless mice, are routinely used to evaluate possible phototoxicity in new compounds. The methods used are expensive, time-consuming, and not always appropriate for prediction in man. The interests of FRAME, and indeed of the pharmaceutical and fragrance industries, would be met if reliable and predictive in vitro methods could be developed.

Daniels (1) proposed a simple method using yeast for phototoxicity screening. In essence, the method relies on growth inhibition of yeast on agar, in the presence of both the compound of interest and ultraviolet radiation, and is suitable for dose-response studies (2). Daniels reported good correlations with substances that normally cause phototoxicity by topical contact, e.g. psoralens which are the active agents in some plants that cause phytophotodermatitis, anthracene and tar derivatives. However, substances known clinically to be phototoxic when administered orally gave mixed results, with several false negatives. Recently, Weinberg & Springer (3) have used a modified version of the Daniels test to investigate phototoxicity with fragrance substances. They obtained very good correlations with yeast growth inhibition and acute, non-photoallergic, phototoxicity. These data suggest that the yeast method is suitable for assessing acute phototoxicity in topically applied substances; possibly, where metabolic activation by liver enzymes is not necessary for phototoxicity. It would be interesting to carry out studies in which known, orally delivered, phototoxins were incubated in a liver homogenate prior to the yeast test. The relationship between the Daniels test and photoallergens has not been systematically examined.

Incidently, it should be noted that whereas 8-methoxy-psoralen and anthracene cause acute phototoxicity in mouse and man, and give positive results with the Daniels test, only 8-methoxypsoralen is a photocarcinogen (4). These limited data suggest that acute phototoxicity is not a predictive indicator of photocarcinogenicity.

REFERENCES

1. Daniels, F. (1965). A simple microbiological method for demonstrating phototoxic compounds. Journal of Investigative Dermatology 44, 259-263
2. Young, A.R. & Barth, J. (1982). Comparative studies on the photosensitizing potency of 5-methoxypsoralen and 8-methoxypsoralen as measured by cytolysis in Paramecium caudatum and Tetrahymena pyriformis, and growth inhibition and survival in Candida albicans. Photochemistry and Photobiology 35, 83-88.

3. Weinberg, E.H. & Springer, S.T. (1981). The evaluation in vitro of fragrance materials for phototoxic activity. Journal of the Society of Cosmetic Chemists 32, 303-315.
4. Forbes, P.D., Davies, R.E. & Urbach, F. (1976). Phototoxicity and photocarcinogenesis: comparative effects of anthracene and 8-methoxypsoralen in the skin of mice. Food Drug Cosmetic Toxicology 14, 303-306.

Dermal Toxicity

J. M. FACCINI and J. P. GUILLOT

TEST FOR THE DETERMINATION OF THE INDEX OF PRIMARY CUTANEOUS IRRITATION IN THE RABBIT

Objective

This method is used to determine the primary irritation resulting from the application of a test substance. Primary irritants are those substances which, with a single application, cause an inflammatory cutaneous orthoergic reaction. The reaction is localised at the point of contact and appears within 24 hours of application.

The irritation depends upon the test substance, its concentration and the length of time it remains in contact with the skin.

Experimental Protocol

Experimental Animals and Skin Preparations

Six male albino New Zealand white rabbits are used for each trial. The rabbits are clipped with a fine toothed electric clipper to bare a skin surface of 14cm x 14cm (the cutting height = 0.05mm); thus a precise cut can be achieved without irritating the skin mechanically. The animals are left to rest for 24 hours and then only those with perfectly healthy skin are chosen for the test.

As legislation requires that the test should also be made on abraded skin, a stillette of the type used for human skin vaccinations is used to make superficial incisions on the epidermis of the right flank only. These incisions are superficial and should not damage the dermis.

Application of the Test Substance

Two sterile hydrophilic, four-layered gauze pads, 2cm square, are placed on the skin of the rabbits. One of the pads is attached to the right flank, which has been scarified, and the other to the left, intact side. The liquid product is then applied at a rate of 0.5ml per area, pad and animal. These impregnated gauze squares are kept in contact with the skin by a patch consisting of a central disc of 22mm diameter with a surrounding adhesive hypoallergenic, perforated plaster, 10mm wide.

Finally, an adhesive tape 6cm wide is wound around the animal to complete the fixing of the patches. Care is taken so that the respiratory and abdominal movements of the animals are not restricted.

Evaluation of Primary Cutaneous Irritation

After 23 hours of contact with the skin, the patches are removed. One hour later, the primary irritation index is evaluated and the animals are then put back into their individual cages. Forty-eight hours later, a second reading is made to determine the extent of any recovery (the two readings are performed 24 and 72 hours, respectively, after the application of the substance).

Readings are made of both the scarified and non-scarified zones following the scale of scores proposed by the "Journal Officiel de la Republique Française", as shown below:

Erythematous (and scar) lesions:

No erythema	0
Very slight erythema (barely perceptible)	1
Well-defined erythema	2
Erythema very marked	3
Severe erythema, crimson red, with slight eschar formation (injuries in depth)	4

Oedematous lesions:

No oedema	0
Very slight oedema (barely perceptible)	1
Slight oedema (edges of area well-defined by definite raising)	2
Moderate oedema (area raised approximately 1mm)	3
Severe oedema (raised more than 1mm and extending beyond area of application)	4

Potential Alternative Methods

As this test is simply one of primary irritation, it could hopefully be replaced by in vitro techniques using cell or organ cultures. Cultures of epithelial cells seem to be an obvious approach that is currently under trial. However, the problem with this method is that although it may give an indication of a toxic cellular reaction, it does not reproduce the in vivo situation. The reaction of the skin to a chemical irritant is complex, involving blood vessels, nerves, local hormones and circulating inflammatory cells, and is dependent on the barrier function of the epidermis. It is likely that such barrier function will be better assessed by organ culture, perhaps using skin taken from human cadavers.

The use of human volunteers, therefore, remains the most plausible alternative at present and for the immediate future. Nevertheless, some form of limited screening, perhaps using smaller numbers of animals, is still necessary to evaluate the potential toxicity of a new chemical; with the hope that, eventually, this screening could be replaced by in vitro methods. Despite the fact that people are ready to volunteer for such studies, there must be careful control by ethical committees. Such committees should, obviously, comprise members who are, by virtue of a toxicological training, capable of assessing any potential risk. In point of fact, current French law forbids the use of volunteers and, for this reason, as well as those cited above, the rabbit remains the mainstay of dermal toxicity in France. At the IFT the maximum use of all animals is made: the skin is undamaged by the clipping procedure, and since the test substance often provokes no reaction, the animals can, after a suitable rest period, be used again, a maximum of three times in all, providing the previous tests were negative.

The test described above is for primary irritation, only involving one application of the test substance. For products such as medicinal creams, for example, that are destined for chronic use, tests need to be performed to assess potential toxicity resulting from repeated dermal application for periods of between 1 and 3 months on average. Any eventual systemic toxicity will depend on cutaneous absorption and metabolism. Furthermore, the risks attendant upon the use of human subjects without prior animal toxicity tests are, in some respects, of the same order as those that would be associated with similar compounds administered orally. There are, at present, no in vitro alternatives.

EVALUATION OF THE SENSITISING POTENTIAL OF A TEST SUBSTANCE BY TOPICAL APPLICATION IN ALBINO GUINEA-PIGS

Experimental Procedure

The method used at the IFT is a modification of the method of Magnussen & Kligman (1).

Preliminary Study

A sensitisation test cannot be performed if pathological, orthoergic skin reactions result from a single application of the test substance (just as it is, or at the maximum concentration envisaged for use) to shaven guinea-pig skin. In cases where this type of reaction is noted, the maximum concentration which does not cause a reaction is determined by applying two different doses of concentrations of the test substance to each of four guinea-pigs.

The quantity or concentration chosen will only be used for the challenge test. The induction is always done with the product as such at a dose of 0.5ml per animal in case of a liquid or viscous compound and 0.5g for a powder or paste.

Determination of Sensitising Potential

Animals. Twenty albino Hartley guinea-pigs (10 males and 10 females, weighing between 300g and 400g at the start of the trial) are used.

Induction. Induction comprises 10 topical applications of the test substance using occlusive patches and 2 intradermal injections of Freund's complete adjuvant. On the Monday of each week, the treatment region - immediately behind the right shoulder blade - is clipped. On days 1 and 10 the guinea-pigs receive an intradermal injection of 0.1ml of Freund's complete adjuvant diluted to 50% in sterile isotonic saline. The two injection sites should be as close as possible to the centre of the area clipped. The test substance is applied 3 times per week, at 2 day intervals, for 3 weeks and once at the start of the 4th week.

The application site is just above the injection site. The product is applied at 0.5ml per animal under a patch test during 48 hours. The 10th and final occlusive patch is removed on day 24, after 48 hours of contact with the skin.

Suspension of treatment. Treatment is suspended from days 24 to 35 inclusive, i.e. for a period of 12 days. This is the time lapse necessary for the organism to produce an immunological response.

Challenge reaction. On day 36 all the guinea-pigs are clipped to bare an area of skin on the left flank of the abdomen, a region which has never before been treated; 0.5ml of test substance (or dose or concentration previously chosen) is applied to this site using an occlusive patch. It stays in contact with the skin for 48 hours under the same experimental conditions as the patches used for induction and is removed on day 38.

Evaluation of sensitising reactions. Readings are made of the challenge site 1,6,24 and 48 hours after the removal of the occlusive patch. The intensity of erythema and oedema are scored using the following scales. Any other anomalies are also noted, e.g. vesicles, thickening of skin, dryness, focal reactions (reactivation of induction site).

Erythema:

No erythema	0
Slight erythema (hardly visible)	1
Evident erythema	2
Marked erythema	3
Severe erythema (crimson-red) with slight scar formation (profound lesions)	4

Oedema:

No oedema	0
Very slight oedema (hardly visible)	1
Oedematous zone well defined (swelling apparent)	2
Moderate oedema (about 1mm thick)	3
Severe oedema (thickness greater than 1mm) covering the whole of the treated area or more	4

A histological examination of the skin is conducted where a lesion is noted macroscopically or in the case of a doubtful reaction.

Expression of results. Macroscopic and histological examinations are conducted "blind". Results are positive if one or more animals show a macroscopic skin reaction which is confirmed histologically as a sensitisation reaction. Results are negative if no animals show evident macroscopic reactions or if the histological examination does not confirm the macroscopic reading. Results are doubtful if an evident macroscopic reaction is found, but the origin of this reaction cannot be determined histologically.

Potential Alternative Methods

Sensitisation reactions are the result of an allergic state

(more precisely a state of delayed hypersensitivity) and result from immunological mechanisms.

The incidence and intensity of reactions depend upon: the allergenic potential of the test substance; the individual susceptibility of the subject (controlled by genetic factors); the mode of exposure of the hapten, particularly the frequency and duration of contacts.

Since only a small percentage of subjects may become sensitised, it is essential to have experimental conditions which favour the maximum induction of an allergy.

Taking into account the restriction of the number of animals used (20 guinea-pigs) the result obtained must be reliable enough to forecast the possible risks of the test substance when used by man. This is achieved by the use of an occlusive patch to increase hydration and permeability of the stratum corneum, together with use of Freund's complete adjuvant to maximise the immunological reaction. This provides a method with sufficient sensitivity to detect both weak and strong allergens.

It is, therefore, a highly artificial, but nevertheless, effective test due to the susceptibility of the guinea-pig to allergens. It is difficult to imagine an *in vitro* test, even in the distant future, capable of replacing this method. Once again, a more realistic hope lies with man. The problem is that hypersensitivity is a low incidence phenomenon. The guinea-pig is rendered more sensitive by the use of Freund's adjuvant, which "maximises" the reaction. The use of similar methods in man would be extremely dangerous. The possibility of dispensing with this test in the guinea-pig will rely on a more profound understanding of cell-mediated hypersensitivity. It is now known that several T-lymphocyte subsets exist, and new types of immunoglobulins are continually being discovered. It will probably be as a result of a greater understanding and recognition of atopy in man that the need for performing this currently essential test in the guinea-pig will eventually be obviated.

REFERENCE

1. Magnussen, B., & Kligman, A. (1969). The identification of contact allergens by animal assay. The maximization test. Journal of Investigative Dermatology 52, 268-276.

General Discussion

N. J. VAN ABBÉ

Rapporteur

Professor GLOXHUBER asked what should be done to study the skin irritancy of an entirely new chemical. Professor MARKS said that it would be totally wrong to use human subjects initially; until satisfactory in vitro tests were available, animal testing had to be used.

Dr Gill LANGLEY enquired whether Dr Young had information on the mechanism underlying the yeast test. Dr YOUNG said that it was not known how yeasts were inactivated by photosensitisers, but he thought that DNA binding might be involved, though the initial damage appeared to be to the cell membrane. He also noted that the mechanism of human photosensitisation was unknown. Mr VAN ABBÉ commented that, in his view, it was not always essential to understand the mechanism involved in a new test method, and cited the Ames test as an example.

Mr J. MIDDLETON asked about the possible emergence of in vitro methods for predicting skin sensitising potential, but Professor MARKS did not know of any promising approaches of this kind. Dr JOHNSON thought this was a long way off, but that much could be achieved by studying chemical structure in predicting likely sensitising potential. Dr FACCINI felt that consideration of structure could certainly reduce the numbers of animals needed. In answer to a query from Professor Marks, Dr FACCINI noted that the French regulations which prohibited the use of human volunteers involved a political decision, but he felt that views expressed by the FRAME Toxicity Committee would help to formulate opinion in Europe.

Eye Irritancy Testing

D. W. SWANSTON

INTRODUCTION

In the field of toxicological testing for hazard evaluation, eye irritancy testing has long attracted both scientific and lay comment. This has at times led not only to vigorous debate, but also to much confusion over the aims, validity and necessity for eye testing in animals and, as a procedure in product safety clearance and operator hazard evaluation, it has tended to become set apart from other toxicological methods on subjective rather than scientific grounds.

There are three criticisms of the estimation of eye hazard in animals:

a. The use of living animals for scientific experiments is wrong in principle, and animals should, and can, be readily replaced by non-animal alternatives such as *in vitro* tests.
b. In some circumstances testing in animals may be required but areas exist where the justification for such tests is doubtful or non-existent, such as the testing of cosmetics, household products or pesticides; this is an aspect of a wider philosophy which questions the continuing development of such items when a satisfactory range of products already exists. This is a popular misconception which fails to take into account that products or compounds may "wear out", for example, through increasing biological or microbiological resistance to a pesticide or antibiotic, or doubts about the undesirable effects of a product only becoming apparent

after more general use. Erroneously, eye testing is also often portrayed as involving only the safety clearance of cosmetics and allied products by rigorous animal techniques. The industry concerned has been, and continues to be, an innovator in scientific aspects of eye testing, as is shown by the large investment in the search for alternatives to the Draize test. This has had a significant effect in the direction of such research, since cosmetics companies not unnaturally pursue research on materials relevant to their products. Thus, a major proportion of the research has involved surface-active agents.

c. Present procedures for eye testing are not sufficiently predictive for man or are artificially severe and discriminate poorly between substances of varying irritant potential; this is the scientific criticism which is considered in this report.

It is the object of this report to review the present position of eye irritancy testing both *in vitro* and *in vivo*, and to examine the feasibility of replacing whole animal studies by *in vitro* or isolated-organ methods and, failing this, to suggest improvements in the present *in vivo* approach. Thus, subjective non-scientific considerations have been set aside, while bearing in mind the conditions of the Cruelty to Animals Act of 1876, which require, wherever possible, the limitation or elimination of pain during animal experimentation; the Home Office now urges licensees to consider the development and use of non-animal alternative techniques in an effort to restrict the number of animals used.

At present, the method of evaluating potential eye hazard by animal testing is dominated by the Draize test approach, which, in spite of controversy over many years, has remained largely unaltered in principle during the four decades since it was introduced (1). A modification was introduced by Draize in 1959 (2), whereby a series of 9 rabbits received 0.1ml of test substance in one eye only. The treated eyes of 3 rabbits remained unwashed, while the eyes of the other 2 groups were irrigated with 20ml of warm water for 2 and 4 seconds respectively, after the instillation of the test material, the eyes being examined and scored for irritant effects at 1, 2, 3, 4 and 7 days after treatment, or as long as any injury persisted. After simple arithmetical weighting, the numerical scores for corneal, iridal and conjunctival irritation were summed to give a single numerical value indicating degree of irritancy on a scale with a maximum value of 110. An expanded Draize procedure requiring up to 18 rabbits was introduced four years later (3). Briefly stated, 0.1ml or 0.1g of test substance is introduced in one eye of each of 6 rabbits, and the response is observed at 24, 48 and 72 hours. If 4/6 animals reach the criteria for a positive reaction, the test as a whole is considered positive, but 2/6 or 3/6 individual positive responses require a second test on 6 animals, which is considered as a positive irritant result if 3 or more animals show the required degree of reaction. In the event of less than 3 individual positive responses in the second test, a third group of 6 animals is tested, the substances being adjudged positive eye irritants if one or more animals show a positive reaction.

In order to assess the value of both in vitro and in vivo eye irritancy testing in predicting potential hazard, it is profitable to examine the process of eye irritation against which the relevance of any new methodology can then be judged.

CHEMICAL IRRITATION OF THE EYE - MECHANISMS

According to Duke-Elder (4), there are three important factors which determine the damaging effects of chemicals in the eye:

a. intimacy and duration of contact;
b. physical properties which determine its penetrability;
c. chemical reactivity with the tissues of the eye.

The most important physical characteristic determining the extent of a reaction is considered to be an ability to penetrate corneal tissue.

Intimacy and Duration of Contact

Intimacy of contact of a test substance with the eye is increased by surface activity and, in ophthalmology, substances such as polyvinyl alcohol are added to eye drop formulations to form a film over the surface of the eye and enhance contact of the therapeutic agent with the ocular membranes. In experimental chemical irritation, the importance of concentration and residence time in the eye have been shown by the influence of eye irrigation on the subsequent degree of irritation produced (5). In practice, the time during which irrigation may be of benefit is often very brief, especially with reactive chemicals. Davies et al. (6), using sodium lauryl sulphate, found little subsequent benefit to washed eyes over unwashed eyes if irrigation was delayed for more than 20 seconds after contamination with the chemical.

Penetration Across the Cornea

The permeability of the cornea to substances placed upon it is determined by their physical properties, including ionisation, partition coefficient, and tonicity. The permeability with poorly-dissociated compounds is related to changes effected by pH on the degree of dissociation (7). Non-polar and highly surface-active agents, and substances which are miscible or soluble in both oil and water, pass across the epithelium with much greater facility than across the exposed stroma. The affinity of the vehicle is important, as polar compounds in water and non-polar compounds in oil are preferentially retained in their vehicles and then penetrate the cornea only slowly (8).

Tonicity affects corneal permeability. Bathing solutions of NaCl ranging from 0.9 - 10.0% do not increase corneal permeability, but solutions hypotonic to 0.9% NaCl do, reaching a maximum with 0.4% NaCl, when the permeability is increased 10-fold relative to that for 0.9% NaCl. Endothelial permeability is, however, increased by hypertonic solutions (7).

Experiments in rabbits with pilocarpine have shown that ocular permeability can vary with age, the penetration through the corneas of 20-day-old animals being twice that of 60-day-old subjects (9). Noxious substances which penetrate into and across the cornea may react in the tissue, inflicting much damage, or on gaining entry to the anterior chamber cause injury to the delicate internal structures therein. The significance of tissue penetration to eye injury, especially with an active compound, can be shown by considering a well-known substance, namely, ammonia. Although not a chemically strong base like the caustic alkalis, ammonia is one of the most dangerous compounds to the eye, as it passes through the cornea with ease because of its partition characteristics and small molecular size. On gaining access to the anterior chamber, the hydroxide formed in the aqueous humour fully exposes structures such as the iris, lens and ciliary body to the devastating effect of active hydroxyl. It is not surprising that, in addition to a serious keratitis, internal inflammation occurs, provoking cataract, uveitis and acute glaucoma. Clinical eye effects of ammonia have been graphically described (10).

Chemical Reactivity with Eye Tissue

The cornea is tolerant to acids or bases within a pH range of about 3 to 11, beyond which damage occurs, alkali burns being more destructive than those from acid (11,12). However, the severity of injury by acids seems to be related to the protein affinity of the anion, and this property may then cause acid injury to occur at a less extreme (higher) pH than suggested above (13). Carboxylic acids such as acetic acid are not particularly "strong" acids in the chemical sense, compared to the highly dissociated mineral acids, yet are capable of inflicting severe injury to tissues. Conversely, recent work by York et al. (14) suggests that the pH threshold for corneal damage by a base may be as high as 12.5-13.0, although this might be modified in the presence of other substances such as surfactants. The potential for corneal injury by metal cations has been found to correlate with the degree of tissue binding and protein denaturation shown by the cation (15). Thus, the affinity for protein, as well as extremes of hydrogen ion concentration, is a major factor for tissue-damaging potential, as evidenced by the eye-damaging capabilities of cationic dyes and surfactants.

Tissue injury, especially in the eye, can also arise as a result of inhibition of enzyme systems, leading to metabolic disturbance and destabilisation of tissue integrity through sulphydryl (-SH) group oxidation or binding action - an effect typical of some of the old lachrymatory or vesicant war gases. For example, many of the lachrymators or "tear gases" have been found to irreversibly bind -SH groups, leading to inhibition of thiol-dependent enzyme systems (16). Lewisite or β-chloro-vinyl dichloroarsine, a typical representative of the arsenical vesicants or blistering agents, inactivates -SH groups by binding, leading to inhibition of pyruvate oxidase. However, this binding was found to be reversed by a dithiol compound, British Anti Lewisite (BAL) or dimercaptopropanol, which competed with the arsenical, freeing the -SH groups and dramatically restoring tissue integrity and function to normality (17,18). The mustard gas group typified by "mustard" itself, b,b'-dichloroethyl sulphide, are powerfully vesicant and inhibit hexokinase, but apparently not through -SH inactivation. Hexokinase was considered to be an important factor in irritancy, and a correspondence was demonstrated between vesicant action and <u>in vitro</u> inhibition of yeast hexokinase (19).

The most significant effect of "mustard", and substances such as dimethyl sulphate and nitrogen mustards (alkyl chloroethyl-amines), is the ability to damage tissues as a result of alkylation of enzymes and proteins, causing inhibition or denaturation and, in the case of nucleic acids, the formation of cross-links between adjacent strands of DNA. This leads to failure of cell replication and a consequent manifestation of cytotoxicity. The noxious effect of such processes on tissue is characterised by a silent phase of several hours after contact, followed by serious progressive damage often following a protracted course.

CHEMICAL IRRITATION OF THE EYE - BIOLOGICAL RESPONSES

When superficially irritating materials enter the eye, the response is limited to blinking, lachrymation and conjunctival reddening, accompanied perhaps by a little conjunctival oedema (chemosis). More-vigorous irritation may result in sustained lid closure, copious lachrymal discharge, significant conjunctival congestion and swelling and, where the cornea is involved, mild stromal swelling or superficial epithelial necrosis. Marked irritation is characterised by an intensification of any of the foregoing effects, plus conjunctival necrosis and reddening and swelling of the lids (blepharitis). The cornea may become cloudy or even opaque, either as a result of denaturation injury to the epithelium and perhaps involvement of Bowman's membrane, or to the occurrence of marked stromal oedema, with damage perhaps penetrating to Descemet's membrane or the endothelium, which may delay or impair final healing. As mentioned above, substances penetrating the cornea to gain access to the anterior chamber can cause damage to the lens and produce a uveitis involving iris and ciliary body and a rise in the intraocular pressure. If corneal anaesthesia occurs, this is usually a serious sign, indicating destruction of corneal nerve endings and suggesting a noxious effect on tissue viability.

Certain compounds cause eye irritation via an indirect route involving prostaglandins, which may catalyse or potentiate the effect of inflammatory mediators such as bradykinin or histamine. Applied separately to the rabbit eye, neither histamine nor prostaglandin PGE_1 cause any significant effect of conjunctival swelling and reddening. However, histamine/PGE_1 mixtures combined in ratios of up to 200:1 have been found to cause severe conjunctival swelling and congestion, indicating a pronounced potentiating effect of PGE_1 on histamine. Surprisingly, intracameral injections of histamine are ineffective, while PGE_1 similarly injected in very low doses causes the increase in protein content of the aqueous humour and the dose-related rises in intraocular pressure seen after marked eye irritation. In contrast to external application, PGE_1 does not potentiate histamine action within the eye where inflammation appears to be solely the result of PGE_1 release (20). One of the external effects of histamine on the eye is to reduce the adhesiveness of the corneal epithelium (21). Prostaglandins are released following various types of eye injury, either physical of chemical, among the latter being the application of strong alkali to the cornea (22).

Rises in intraocular pressure and protein content of the aqueous humour are typical of those produced by compounds such as nitrogen mustard, which may not act as a direct irritant, but requires an intact nervous pathway for its effect, stimulation of the sensory fibres in the cornea releasing a mediator and producing an inflammatory reaction as a consequence of a specific transmitter-receptor mechanism for one of the mediator substances released (23,24). This mechanism almost certainly involves prostaglandins and prostaglandin-potentiated histamine as previously mentioned, and it is of relevance that the instillation of antazoline, an antihistamine, can reverse the rise in conjunctival temperature and thus congestion in the rabbit eye caused by the instillation of mustard oil (25).

Following corneal injury, healing takes place by migration of cells into the injured or denuded epithelial areas, and if the injury extends to the limbus, then the conjunctival cells may participate with, in pigmented eyes, migration of a line of pigment cells into the cornea itself (26,27). Certain injuries may cause neovascularisation of the cornea, i.e. invasion by blood vessels, spreading in from the limbal plexus. This response to corneal irritation is more common in laboratory animals such as the rabbit, than in man, where it is more often seen as a result of disease or, perhaps, corneal graft. Neovascularisation was assumed to be simply a consequence of corneal oedema; however, it appears that oedema alone is not a sufficient stimulus, but requires the presence of a vessel-stimulating factor liberated from damaged tissue to initiate the process (28). Where damage is sufficient to involve not only the epithelium but also the underlying Bowman's membrane, resolution of injury may never be complete, and some degree of corneal opacity or scarring may remain. Deeper penetrating chemical burns of the cornea, involving the innermost layers and perhaps the appearance of the compound in the aqueous humour, not only damage the superficial layers, but experimental studies of alkali burns of the cornea using electron microscopy have revealed that the end-result of healing after such injury is a transformation of corneal epithelium to conjunctival epithelium at the periphery of the cornea. In addition, the endothelium also shows cellular necrosis which, if allowed to persist (through lack of remedial measures), slows the rate of regeneration, which leads to overstimulation of the repair process and the formation of a retrocorneal membrane, a condition which in man is pathological (29). Nevertheless, corneal epithelium does possess very considerable powers of regeneration, and even quite marked denaturation injury, provided it remains superficial with no involvement of the deeper layers, can eventually heal with surprisingly little effect.

EYE IRRITANCY TEST SYSTEMS

In Vitro

The liberation of histamine or serotonin from mast cells has been used as an index of irritant potential. Rat peritoneal mast cells are labelled with 5-OH tryptophan which is metabolised in the mast cell to 5-OH tryptamine (serotonin). The cells are then treated with a test substance whose irritant potential is gauged by its ability to provoke serotonin release from the mast cells as indicated by radioactivity in free solution. The irritant potency is derived by comparing the test data with that for sodium dodecyl sulphate using a computer model to compare the dose-response curves (30). A good correlation between in vivo and in vitro results using single surfactants has been demonstrated. Mixtures and multiple formulations were not screened unless all the individual components satisfied the requirements of the model, but where they did, a 100% correlation was obtained. The test may not be appropriate for those compounds which have not been found to fit the requirements of the model. The Rat Mast Cell Assay was considered to be a cheap, repeatable technique for eliminating testing of severe eye irritants, and although animal tissue was required, one rat supplied sufficient material for tests equivalent to the use of 48 animals in normal in vivo procedures. It was not seen as a test model for ocular irritation.

The use of acid-soluble collagen/glycosaminoglycan solution as a model for corneal protein has been investigated, whereby the heat precipitation of such solutions might serve as an indication of potential to produce corneal opacity. This work is at an early stage and requires extensive validation by known corneal opacifacients and non-opacifacients (S.J. Williams, personal communication).

Human buccal scrapings have been employed as indicators of irritancy (31). Cells are suspended in synthetic saliva, mixed with the test surfactant, and examined after a 10-15 minute contact by means of phase-contrast microscopy, and the proportion of cells lacking viable nuclei used to give an index of potential irritancy. Using a series of purified alkyl sulphates, results have been obtained which correlate with those found by testing in the rabbit eye (32). However, it was felt that, useful though the test was in screening, it was still essential to have a test system which would take into account the many factors influencing eye irritation, not least corneal penetrating ability. The composition of the suspension medium appears to be a very critical factor, requiring further investigation.

Scaife (33) has given details of a method for quantifying the effects of purified detergents on cultured cells, has compared the results to findings elsewhere in the literature, and has also related the results to data obtained by the same materials in the rabbit eye. Fluorescein diacetate is added to cells in culture as an indicator of intact and damaged cells (34). Cells are freely permeable to this non-fluorescent compound, which under the action of non-specific esterases, liberates fluorescein which only diffuses slowly out of intact cells; these cells thus fluoresce green. The damaged cells can be indicated by treating with ethidium bromide, which stains both RNA and DNA red. This, together with loss of fluorescein by diffusion, makes the damaged cells appear red. The red staining of DNA and RNA in the intact cells is swamped by the green fluorescence. The relative proportions of red and green cells after exposure to a test compound gives a measure of cytotoxic and, by inference, irritant potential to tissue. With the surfactants tested, carbon chain length, critical micelle-forming concentration, and degree of ethoxylation were found to have an important influence. Correlation of *in vitro* with *in vivo* potency was found in some series; on the other hand, inverse correlations were sometimes obtained, suggesting that the mechanism of surfactant irritation in the eye is not straightforward and is probably complicated by the hydrophobic and hydrophilic characteristics of the layers of the cornea and their differing sensitivity to ions. It has been pointed out that although correlation of the *in vitro* results with those obtained in the rabbit eye may have been uncertain, the detergent concentrations *in vitro* were more akin to those which would occur in the human eye in practice, as opposed to the higher concentrations used experimentally in the rabbit eye test, and thus might offer useful guidance to possible effects in human eyes. It was concluded that the fluorescein diacetate test was economic and relatively simple, but the requirements for both a simple and reliable *in vitro* test had not been fulfilled. Nonetheless, the test formed a basis for further investigations, and it would be useful to study formulations of surfactants, e.g. shampoos, rather than single detergents, considering at the same time solubility and penetration effects.

Simons tested three shampoo formulations for their cytotoxicity to an established line of mouse embryo cells, cell viability following a 48-hour exposure to the test compound being assessed by counting the number of viable cells remaining. The test ranked the shampoos in the same order as the Draize test (35). Analysis of the data indicated that the test could distinguish major from minor irritants, but lacked discrimination in the intermediate areas. However, with modifications, the test could provide a useful basis for *in vitro* irritancy screening.

The chick embryo as a "half-way house" alternative to whole mature animals is under examination as a possible model for irritancy. The vascular chorioallantoic membrane has features that are said to confer some of the benefits of working with a whole animal (36).

Tests using isolated organs may be similarly described as hybrid *in vitro/in vivo* techniques and are "alternatives" in that they do not use the whole sentient animal model. These types of model form the basis of much standard pharmacology and include the guinea-pig ileum technique and isolated heart preparations. One such technique using the enucleated rabbit eye has been developed as a test system for irritant potential (37), and further details of the technique and its validation with chemicals of varying irritant potential have been presented by York *et al.* (14). The enucleated eye is immobilised in a non-deforming clamp within a temperature controlled humidified chamber and periodically moistened by superfusion with saline. After treatment with test materials, the cornea is examined by slit-lamp biomicroscopy during a 4-hour period for corneal change or damage and corneal thickness is measured. On the basis of the results obtained, the test is suggested as a valid model for irritancy, being sufficiently reliable to screen out severe irritants and serve as a satisfactory method for testing shampoos. The results with various irritant chemicals broadly agree with published observations. It is suggested that *in vivo* testing would be needed where this test yielded a slight or negligible result, but the effect *in vivo* would not be expected to be severe. The test would not take account of conjunctival irritation or duration of corneal healing.

Kastner & Frotsch (38) examined 16 anionic surfactants by two *in vitro* and three *in vivo* tests (including the Draize test) and compared the results with those obtained on human skin. Most results correlated with the human findings, with the exception of the *in vitro* haemolytic activity test.

Prottey & Ferguson (39) have tested soaps and detergents for irritancy by penetration through guinea-pig skin, keratin denaturation in human callus, ability to extract amino acids from guinea-pig skin, and histamine release from mast cells, comparing these effects with the irritant effects on rat skin *in vivo*. Although a test of skin irritancy, the principles might be applied to eye irritation. None of the tests ranked the surfactants in the order indicated by the rat skin *in vivo* results, and it was felt that this cast doubt on all of these procedures in the estimation of irritant potential. The main difficulty was seen as simulating the testing of the whole animal in the face of the complex interactions existing *in vivo*. It should be noted here that it is not known whether the correlation would have been different had the results been compared to human rather than rat skin test data.

In Vivo (Animal) Systems

Models

The albino rabbit is virtually the universal species for ocular irritancy testing, since it is easily obtained, not over-expensive, tractable, and possesses a large eye and a large corneal area relative to the total surface of the eyeball. The lack of pigment allows inflammatory reactions to be easily observed. The lachrymal apparatus differs from that of man, since well-developed Harderian gland as well as a lachrymal gland is present. The maximum volume of a bland solution that can just be accommodated in the eye in the absence of any eye movement such as blinking is about 0.08ml.

Primate eyes are anatomically closer to man than those of the rabbit; in, for example, their pigmentation and lachrymal apparatus. With primates, however, drawbacks such as expense, availability or temperament, have now largely precluded their consideration as models for eye hazard evaluation.

Species Variation in Irritant Response

No single animal species has been found to model exactly for the human eye either in anatomical terms or in response to irritation. The sensitivity of the cornea varies with species, and Hellauer (40) found the following decreasing orders of sensitivity: ox, man, rabbit, dog, cat. Two sensory irritants, CR and CS, were tested in solution in the eyes of man, guinea-pig and rabbit, and the median sensory irritant threshold concentration (TC50) determined for each of the three species by a blink test. From this, for CR, the rabbit eye was estimated to be 90 times and the guinea-pig eye 40 times less sensitive than that of man, while, for CS, the relative values were 18 for rabbit and 6 for guinea-pig (41,42). The rabbit eye has also been found to have a low irritant sensitivity to certain soaps (43). The nictitating membrane, although viewed as a possible trap for test substances, does not, when surgically removed, affect the healing rate of a damaged cornea and is not considered a major factor in difference of response between species (44). Lachrymal discharge in response to irritation is serous (clear and watery) in man and primates, and while initially serous in the rabbit, within 24 hours of irritation the discharge becomes milky from Harderian gland admixture (26).

A point of difference between the eyes of primates or humans and the albino rabbit eye is pigment. It is not clear whether this constitutes a factor in irritant response. When 70% isopropanol was tested in rabbit eyes there was no difference in the degree of iritis between pigmented and unpigmented rabbits (45). This was a small experiment, presumably carried out by the standard Draize technique. It is established that melanin pigment granules are a calcium reservoir in the vertebrate eye, calcium being one of the elements essential for membrane conductance. The marked lack of calcium in the albino eye may be connected with the poor visual acuity in such subjects (46). Melanin is also highly active in binding chemical substances such as polycyclic aromatics, especially those containing fused rings (47). Although it is not apparent what influence, if any, the presence or absence of eye pigment might have on irritant response, it is a fact that the albino eye does differ in some physiological aspects from the normal pigmented eye.

The central corneal thicknesses of man, monkey and dog are similar at 0.51, 0.52 and 0.55mm, respectively, the cat being the thickest at 0.62 and the rabbit the thinnest at 0.37mm (48). The rabbit aqueous humour has a pH of 8.2, compared to the 7.1 in humans, suggesting less buffering reserve in the rabbit with respect to controlling hydroxyl ion concentration (49). This, together with the thinner cornea when compared to monkey and man, might partly explain the susceptibility of the rabbit eye to iris inflammation. The limbal areas of the albino rabbit eye are more extensively vascularised than in the pigmented primate eye and seem to be related to the predisposition of the rabbit cornea to neovascularisation after relatively minor injury, especially where the whole eye is flooded with material, as in the Draize technique (44).

Corneal penetration rates have been studied in the excised corneas of various animal species, namely, man, dog, monkey, rabbit and swine, using 70% isopropyl alcohol, DMSO, 10% acetic acid, and diethyl cresyl phosphate. Although the penetration rate for animals was sometimes higher or lower relative to man, there was little to choose between the species overall, with the rabbit seemingly showing the best average approximation to man (48). The situation might differ in the dynamic in vivo situation.

Beckley (50) tested a liquid detergent in the eyes of humans, monkey, dog and rabbit. The Draize technique was used for animals and multiple instillation in humans. The human subjects sometimes developed a mild conjunctivitis, but no corneal or iris involvement occurred. In the animal species, the monkey was least affected, but nevertheless showed a mild keratitis not seen in man. Corneal effects were most severe in the dog, whereas in the rabbit conjunctival and iridal effects predominated and eye changes persisted the longest.

A soap suspension and a detergent household cleaner formulation caused irritation when tested in the eyes of man, monkey and rabbit by the Draize procedure using both macroscopic and biomicroscopic examination. The results were used to categorise the two materials into "accept", "accept with caution" and "probably injurious to human eyes". The monkey results correctly placed the compounds in the "accept with caution" category, which equated with the effects actually observed in the humans, but the rabbit underscored with the soap and overscored with the detergent solution (51).

Technical Considerations

Of the two most commonly used species in eye testing, the monkey appears to be a better predictor with respect to irritancy in man than the rabbit. It may be that the rabbit eye overreacts as a result of gross contamination of the eye, as stimulation of the conjunctivae and the richly vascular limbal plexus promotes neovascularisation and more-consistent results seem to accrue when test material is placed on the eye rather than in the conjunctival sac. Where a cup aspirator has been used to control application and limit contamination to the cornea, the results in rabbits have been more akin to those of the monkey (44). This method has been used elsewhere to give more uniform and reproducible Draize scores (52). In the same study, viscous irritant solutions were tested by the normal Draize technique. The resulting scattered corneal lesions were seen as an indication of non-uniformity of exposure by the method and a cause of eye-to-eye variability when testing viscous solutions by conventional instillation into the conjunctival sac. Bucher et al. (53) have condemned the quantification of corneal damage by area affected as unscientific.

The validity of large volumes (0.1ml) relative to eye capacity has been questioned as an unrealistically gross contamination. When dichloromethane was instilled into rabbits eyes at volumes of 0.1ml or 0.01ml, the effect on lids and conjunctivae was similar, but the duration of effects with the smaller volume was reduced from 11 to 4 days. Keratitis was present, but with the smaller volume was less marked and persistent, the duration of the effects falling from 14 to 4 days. Neovascularisation occurred with the higher volume only. The magnitude of corneal thickness change was less with 0.01ml (54). Nevertheless, the hazard assessment of dichloromethane as an eye irritant was not materially changed by the reduction in volume.

A major investigation into the effects of volume on irritant response has been carried out using Draize-type rabbit tests and instillation volumes of irritant test materials of 0.1, 0.03, 0.01 and 0.003ml (55). This was prompted by the suggestion of the NAS 1138 Committee in 1977 (56) that a smaller dose than 0.1 ml or 0.1g could appreciably reduce the response of eyes of test animals to a range more consistent with human experience. Of the range of volumes, 0.01ml gave the best separation of irritant materials. In the same investigation, the effect of group size on the precision of the test was studied, and it was found that by increasing numbers up to a group size of 6 animals, a marked benefit in precision resulted; increasing the group size to 9 or 12 yielded little further benefit when set against the increase in animal numbers. When human experience of the various irritants tested was graded according to the NAS Evaluative Criteria for Ocular Irritancy (56), namely, lack of significant effect, moderate, substantial, or severe irritation, these criteria, applied to the rabbit test using 0.01ml volumes, best predicted the actual published human experience. Evaluation of irritancy grading in terms of days to clear was suggested, with a standard observation period of lesions of up to 21 days where necessary.

Williams et al. (57) tested 7 compounds varying from mild to marked irritancy by the Draize technique, but using a volume of 0.01ml, all compounds having been previously evaluated using the standard volume of 0.1ml. Although a dose-volume effect was seen, the rank correlation of irritancy was not changed. Thus, reducing the volume of test material moderated the response without compromising test sensitivity. Some materials showing a degree of irritancy at 0.1ml were not detected at 0.01ml, but it was felt that in these cases even if irritant effects did occur in humans, they would be such as to be of little significance.

Several techniques have been applied to quantify or better demonstrate changes arising from ocular irritation. Corneal thickness has been considered a useful quantitative measurement that correlates well with Draize scores (58). The technique is attractive in that it is genuinely quantitative and also non-invasive, measurements being made optically by a slit-lamp biomicroscopic attachment. The subjective Draize score has been compared to several objective procedures, namely, corneal thickness measurement, evaluation of corneal and conjunctival water content, and conjunctival and aqueous humour concentrations of a dye bound to plasma proteins after intravenous injection. Several solvents were used as test materials. It was concluded that corneal thickness measurement should be used as an additional technique to the standard Draize method (59). However, caution has been sounded about its reproducibility in a more widespread and varied context of use (N. Van Abbé, 1981, personal communication). Careful technique is essential, for if the slit-lamp beam does not exactly bisect the corneal vertex, significant variability in readings can occur. Furthermore, the correlation of corneal thickness with Draize scores does not necessarily hold in terms of individual animals and difficulties can arise where only a discrete portion of the cornea is irritated as opposed to a diffuse effect.

Dose-related rises in intraocular pressure have been found following chemical irritation of the eye (60) and the application of the measurement of such rises to both systemic and local effects in the eye considered in detail (61). The applanation technique is non-invasive, but usually requires application of local anaesthetic to eliminate the corneal reflex when contact is made between the cornea and the probe. The technique is basically simple, but requires skill and care on the part of the operator, and any technique involving correct contact of a probe to a living membrane is bound to contain significant inherent technical errors. Such errors require the acceptance of differences of up to 3-4mm Hg, and on a normal intraocular pressure range of 16-20mm Hg would represent an error of 20% (62,63). All tonometers based on the applanation method are likely to be affected to a greater or lesser degree by corneal oedema tending to modify the true deformation resistance of the cornea. Hand-held tonometers do not seem to be particularly affected in this respect (61-63), but an apparent inverse relationship between corneal oedema and intraocular pressure has been observed using a pneumatic tonometer, where manifestations of ocular hypotension exactly mirrored rises in corneal thickness. This was considered to be a measuring artefact where the apparent required degree of corneal flattening (applanation) was achieved with less force due to lowered deformation resistance of a hydrated, thickened cornea.

Examination by slit-lamp biomicroscopy is a versatile and useful method of detecting corneal injury. There are several techniques of illumination, each showing certain anatomical structures to particular advantage. Staining with dyes such as fluorescein, neutral red, alcian blue or rose bengal can differentiate between viable and necrotic corneal cells and demonstrate ulceration, epithelial loss, etc. (64). Some fluorescent staining occurs in the normal cornea due to natural physiological desquamation of the epithelium (65), and for demonstrating corneal irritation by fluorescein, restricting the staining time to 15 seconds has been found to minimise confusion between normal corneal staining and that occurring from ocular irritation (66).

Loss or diminution of corneal sensitivity is a serious effect in eye irritation. Under normal conditions corneal sensitivity declines with age (67) and in different species seems to be roughly correlated with the acetylcholine content of the cornea (40). The corneal reflex may be elicited by gently touching the cornea with a nylon thread. The method has been quantitated by measuring the force of thread deformation needed to produce the reflex (67). The reflex can be abolished by local anaesthetics, the use of which has been suggested in the Draize test to minimise discomfort. Tests have been made on five irritant substances, with or without the prior use of butacaine sulphate, and differences in irritancy scores noted in only 4 of 29 comparisons. In each instance where a difference occurred, the corneal opacity scores were lower in the unanaesthetised eye. No clear-cut pattern of differences occurred between anaesthetised and unanaesthetised eye responses, so it was suggested that the use of butacaine sulphate should be considered in eye tests (68). On the other hand, local anaesthetics can be toxic to corneal epithelium and their surface-active properties may modify corneal permeability. They have been said to depress glycolysis and respiration of corneal epithelium, increase permeability to drugs and chemicals, and thus rendering the cornea more susceptible to injury (69). Delay in recovery from ocular damage has been noted where local anaesthetics were used prior to the test instillation of detergent materials, and in this respect the use of local anaesthetics for reducing discomfort was seen as counterproductive as a result of the subsequent augmentation of irritative effects which followed their use (32). These equivocal findings are perhaps not surprising, as local anaesthetics of very similar chemical constitution can differ in their effects on the cornea. The diethylaminoethyl esters of p-amino-m-butoxy and p-amino-m-propoxy benzoic acids were applied to the corneas of rabbits and their effects examined by ultramicroscopy. The propoxy caused considerably more marked and persistent corneal effects than did the butoxy member, although neither caused corneal damage of sufficient degree to be macroscopically visible (70). In any case, the use of local anaesthetics is treatment of the symptom rather than the cause, and it is better to design-out pain as far as possible by improved experimental procedure, or by blocking the pain mediation itself. Prostaglandin-potentiated histamine causes the typical florid irritant reaction in the rabbit eye, especially swelling and reddening of the conjunctivae, and also increases the sensitivity of the eye. It is also said to diminish corneal epithelial adhesion. Antihistamines, by blocking these potentiated histamine-mediated effects, might be more effective than local anaesthetics in reducing pain, as well as being non-toxic. It has already been seen how antihistamines can lower the temperature of inflamed conjunctivae, thereby reducing congestion. Is it possible that antihistamine cover, by reducing the conjunctival overreaction, could also reduce the incidence of corneal neovascularisation to which the rabbit eye is predisposed and thus render the rabbit eye response more akin to that seen in primates or man?

Correct management of eyes in ocular irritation studies is stressed; both with regard to the subjects' welfare and also on technical grounds. If an irritated eye is not kept clean and freely drained, infection or symblepharosis may occur, making irritation scores valueless.

Scoring and Data Handling

The conventional gathering and treatment of data in Draize-type eye testing methods has necessitated, first, a grading schedule for degrees of various aspects of eye irritation (redness, swelling of conjunctivae, etc.) to give numerical scores, then arithmetical treatment employing simple weighting factors, and summing, to give a total composite score which is taken to indicate the degree of irritant potential of the test compound on an irritancy scale with a maximum value of 110. The difficulty of satisfactorily scoring results according to a mandatory protocol, let alone the handling of the data and its subsequent interpretation, is shown by the wealth of published material on the subject. Ballantyne & Swanston (71) criticised the numerical Draize score as non-informative and non-meaningful, and published an expanded grading schedule derived from Draize, but showing the effects of eye irritation separately, namely, keratitis, iritis, discharge, swelling, etc., rather than combining all the irritant effects into a single numerical score value. Variation of scoring has been identified as occurring both between and within individual laboratories, especially through personal interpretation of printed guidelines and reading of tissue reactions (72), and the suggestion has been made that periodic methodology courses for newcomers to the field would be advantageous. Possible sources of variation are age, sex and strain of test animals, together with subjective and personal error between individual observers, insufficient numbers of animals in test groups and even the early release of eyelids following instillation. To counterbalance some of these sources of error, photographic recording, ophthalmoscopy and histology have been suggested as useful adjuncts to the central Draize technique (73). Kay & Calandra (74) suggested replacement of the final numerical score by interpreting the individual scores with an 8 point descriptive eye irritation rating table running from 0 (non-irritating) to 8 (maximally-irritating). They stressed that it is difficult, if not impossible, to devise a numerical system for either scoring or classifying eye irritants which is wholly accurate, and that the classification system they had suggested was not to be regarded as a substitute for the experience, training and judgement of a competent scientist. It has been pointed out that the area of the cornea involved should not be included in any scoring system, because this assumes uniform exposure to the test substance and under the conditions of the standard Draize technique there is no reason to suppose that this is so (52). Beckley (51) proposed a scoring method based on slit-lamp biomicroscopy examination and fluorescein staining reactions of the cornea and found that monkey results, when graded according to the suggested system, reflected effects in humans more satisfactorily. Griffiths et al. (55) used Draize grading and classified irritancy by application of the NAS Evaluative Criteria for Ocular Irritancy (56), defining irritancy on the basis of reversibility of response in terms of the median number of days for effects to clear, rather than the maximum derived from the most severe responder in the group, where the use of maximum rather than median assumes, without justification, that the worst case in a rabbit response can equate with a potentially worst case in humans.

DISCUSSION

General Considerations

The eye, in common with any other major organ in the body, is a co-ordinated system of interdependent functions, with homeostatic capabilities of compensation, renewal and repair. Irritation of the eye may affect a particular function or structure, or set off a chain of effects secondary to the original insult. Eyelids, conjunctivae, cornea, structures within the anterior chamber, or regulation of the internal pressure of the eye itself may all be affected. Eye irritancy testing is designed to take account of these factors in evaluating eye irritation potential, whence it is necessary to know:

a. What kind of damage may be caused (type).
b. How severe it might be (degree).
c. Its time of onset and the duration of the course of its development and the resolution of any lesions or inflammation (onset/duration).

d. Whether the tissues ever completely return to normal (reversibility).

Information may also be required on the effects of emergency measures in the event of eye contamination, such as water or saline irrigation, and the eye may be used as a model to evaluate the efficacy of ophthalmic medicaments such as antibiotics, decongestants, etc. Finally, if possible, it is useful to gain a rough approximation of the threshold dose at which significant irritation occurs.

From these requirements of a test for ocular irritancy potential and a review of current methodology, it is apparent that present alternatives cannot completely replace in vivo testing, as they are unable to take account of all the potential manifestations of irritancy outlined above or to function as models for evaluation of therapeutic measures. The investigators of in vitro methods for eye testing have been careful to stress that their tests are not models for ocular inflammation, cannot take account of all the factors in ocular irritancy and, like any new approach, will require considerable validation with known facts and in vivo experience. The desirability of a careful scientific approach is indicated by the speculation that to satisfy the testing requirements for irritancy on different parts of the eye, a bank of perhaps 10 in vitro tests might be needed to replace the Draize test (75). If the goal of replacement of in vivo by in vitro testing is ever to be achieved, it is likely to be best served by the gradualist approach of reduction with interim refinement of present in vivo methods.

The various alternative approaches used as screening or ancillary tests offer an opportunity for reduction in the scale and severity of in vivo eye testing by screening out caustic compounds and for reducing the testing burden in, for example, examining long series of compounds of similar class or constitution. At present, the rational aim should be to reduce in vivo irritancy testing wherever possible, but where it is required to ensure a reduction in the severity of the test and an increase in the scientific value of the results obtained. Several alternative approaches to this end can be considered in the light of the mechanisms, responses and data requirements previously discussed.

The first question should be, "Does testing need to be done at all?", and in some regulatory schemes the obligations to test for eye effects is waived if primary irritancy on the skin has been demonstrated. Caution, however, is needed because with effects other than demonstrable primary skin irritancy correlation between skin and eye irritation becomes very unpredictable. Even where primary irritancy has been shown, correlation is not absolute. In any case, when attempting to predict eye irritancy from experimental skin irritation data, this should be done on the basis of similar test conditions, i.e. similar concentrations for both membranes. As an illustration, some household detergents can, under certain somewhat artificial conditions, be made to produce quite marked skin irritations. Physicochemical properties have some relevance to the differences between skin and eye responses. A logical approach to eye irritancy evaluation would initially consider existing information and physicochemical data, prior to *in vitro* or *in vivo* investigations.

Testing *In Vitro*

Physicochemical Factors

Of the three major factors referred to in the context of eye damaging potential, two, i.e. penetration of the cornea and intimacy of contact, are concerned with bioavailability of the test substance to ocular tissues and depend upon physicochemical properties and characteristics. Relevant data include solubility and partition characteristics, pH, degree of ionisation and stability in the aqueous medium of the eye, and possible modification of these properties by the presence of solvents or wetting agents. The possibility may exist of preferential retention of the test substance in a solvent system of similar characteristic, such as a lipid compound in an oily vehicle, a situation which could affect bioavailability. A scheme for predicting the irritancy of aqueous solutions on mucous membranes by scoring for irritancy on the basis of pH and osmolality has been proposed by Bucher *et al.* (53).

Biochemical Approaches

The third factor in ocular irritation, namely, reactivity with tissues, might usefully be assessed by studies on protein denaturing ability, tissue binding by cationics, and affinity of anions for proteins. The binding of thiol groups essential for tissue integrity and leading to inhibition of thiol-dependent enzymes might merit study. Pyruvate oxidase and yeast hexokinase inhibition has been found to be associated with vesicant or lachrymatory potential, especially where such compounds contain reactive halogen groups. However, since the publication of the initial work on thiol enzymes and irritancy, much debate has appeared on this subject which has recently been usefully reviewed by Morton Grant (12). Heat precipitation of collagen/glycosaminoglycan solutions serving as a model for corneal proteins has been suggested as a test for corneal opacifacients. In this context, ox corneas, available as abbatoir material, represent a true model for corneal proteins in the natural state of tissue organisation.

Cell Culture and Isolated Organ Systems

Much of the work with cytological tests has been carried out on surfactant materials, and more validation with other types of compounds will be informative. Cytotoxicity, rather than histamine or serotonin release from mast cells, might be a more practical end-point for commercial testing (76), and the methodology is likely to offer more opportunities for development, e.g. specialised cell lines, such as corneal cells, "tailored" to requirements. Correlations of cytotoxicity with known *in vivo* irritancy potentials have been obtained with various series of surfactant materials; however, anomalous results, such as inverse correlations, indicate that further validation is needed and highlight the importance of data on mechanism of irritant action in evaluating such test systems.

The enucleated eye model has the advantage of screening out severe irritants on the eye, but in a non-sentient manner, leaving only those of milder or doubtful irritancy to be tested *in vivo*. Correlations with published effects appear satisfactory so far. However, compounds exist where the onset of irritation is delayed for several hours and progress thereafter, and this technique might not be applicable in such cases. Nor can the technique take account of conjunctival effects, healing, or effects within the anterior chamber, etc. Nevertheless, it could be of use in determining the corneal irritant thresholds of some compounds. If ox eyes from abbatoirs could be used for the same purpose, this would avoid the sacrifice of laboratory animals necessary to obtain the eyes. However, difficulties of control of supply, organ viability and freshness, and dissection procedure with abbatoir material would need careful consideration, and unless resolved could be sufficient to render such use impractical. The chorioallantoic membrane of the chick embryo is similarly a hybrid *in vivo/in vitro* technique and represents in effect an *in vivo* form of cell culture. The technique is at a speculative stage at present.

Testing *In Vivo*

The Present

Although it appears that *in vitro* methods are not yet able to replace *in vivo* testing, this does not imply that the present *in vivo* technology is above criticism on scientific and humane grounds.

The instillation of an excessive quantity or volume, such as 0.1ml, which exceeds the capacity of the eye sac, makes any actual exposure volume or statement of dose irrelevant, even with bland solutions. This is especially so where irritation occurs, leading to watering, blinking or squeezing of the eye, whence a significant portion of the instillate immediately spills onto the face of the animal, making grading of lachrymatory discharge pointless and possibly causing spurious blepharitis from external contamination of the eyelids.

In scientific terms, over-large volumes have no more relevance than the megadose LD50 in acute toxicity. The irrationality of instilling a large volume into a rabbit eye is further illustrated by the fact that the normal volume of fluid residing in the human eye is 0.01ml or less, and the addition of 0.01ml of extraneous fluid makes the eye appear quite watery (77). In practice, it is difficult for large volumes of fluid to enter and remain in the eye, and subjective estimates of fluid entering a human eye tend to be greatly exaggerated.

The Draize grading for area of cornea affected is of little value, being based upon the assumption of even exposure to the test substance when there is no justification for such as assumption. Use of an official photographic colour guide for grading of effects is not without drawbacks, since the redness of the untreated conjunctivae may vary in different animals from a pale pink (grade 0) to a definite red (grade 1-2). Is then the eye to be graded according to the protocol or against its untreated control? Moreover, the weighting given to the corneal and iris effects are a recognition that the conjunctival scores in the rabbit may be inflated by overreaction and, in effect, represents a compensation for defective experimental design.

Herein lie the seeds of the variability which has beset the Draize test over the years and has bedevilled interpretation, leading to a proliferation of published gradings, scorings and arithmetical treatments designed to overcome it.

The Future

As some in vivo testing will still be required for the present, proper use of the foregoing in vitro approaches should help to ensure that highly irritant materials are not tested in the eye and to ensure that for test materials in general doses are calculated so as to prevent any testing at a severe level. For a test designed to reduce variability and thus the necessity for repeat tests, a group of 6 animals appears to be the minimum number consistent with acceptable precision, but little benefit is to be gained from increasing the number above this. This would represent a reduction from the potential 18 animals required by present Draize-type schemes.

Resting the animals for 3 days (a weekend) allows a convenient period for the resolution of travel or recaging disturbance. Prior to the test, examination of the eye following a 15-second treatment with fluorescein will demonstrate minor corneal abrasions, etc. A dose of test substance of 0.01ml or 0.01g, is suggested, but the concentration in the case of solutions, or the actual weight or volume where solids or undiluted liquids are concerned, may be reduced in order to limit the judged degree of irritation to acceptable proportions. The eye should be kept well-managed and clean, if necessary by irrigation with sterile saline, but not with water. Freedom from infection should be ensured, as its occurrence will invalidate the test, and the predisposition of an inflamed or injured eye to infection is another good reason for avoiding marked degrees of irritation. The standard Draize-type scoring for irritant effects is simple to use, but the grading for corneal area is of doubtful value, as has been discussed. When a coloured photographic guide of effects is used, this should be in conjunction with comparison between treated and untreated eyes to bring out the benefit of an own control, unless a contralateral effect is expected (though this is unusual).

Use of local anaesthetics to reduce discomfort is of doubtful benefit because they may modify the corneal characteristics and the irritant response. Reducing the histamine flare response and the accompanying sensitivity to pain might be a better fundamental way of diminishing the overreaction of the rabbit eye to irritants. This would require validation of the effect of antihistamine on the eye response to test material.

Visual observation may be supported by slit-lamp biomicroscopy, and if desired, corneal thickness determinations, while vital staining procedures on the cornea can demonstrate epithelial damage or other membrane lesions. Other measurements such as intraocular pressure are best considered as discretionary techniques. Observation should continue until resolution is complete or residual effects seem likely to persist. Griffiths _et al._ (55) have suggested the use of the NAS Evaluative Criteria for Ocular Irritancy for interpretation of data and the classification of the 4 degrees of irritation listed in terms of the number of days to clear, using the group median rather than maximum value. The Criteria represent a fuller description of irritancy than many of the more arithmetic schemes based purely on numerical scores, and there is considerable benefit in good narrative raw data supporting the irritancy gradings where necessary. This interpretative scheme is not necessarily suggested as the one to be used to the exclusion of any other, but is quoted as a good example of a practical approach.

The ultimate "alternative" to animals is, of course, man. Some consumer products testing has been carried out on human volunteers in the past, but any scheme for such testing would require serious consideration of ethics and the problems of ensuring an adequate level of skilled supervision, such as that provided by ophthalmologists. The ethical problems involved in using man as a test subject for any other type of substance or preparation such as industrial chemicals, agrochemicals, etc., are likely to be insurmountable.

SUMMARY

1. A review of ocular irritancy testing demonstrates that mechanisms of chemical irritation in the eye and consequent responses to such irritation are not necessarily simple processes, but more often involve interactions of several factors, which themselves may be modified if the test substance consists of a mixture or formulation rather than a single substance.

2. In spite of potentially variable mechanisms, a reliable assessment of potential chemical hazard to the eye is necessary, because of the great psychological and physical significance of visual damage, impairment or loss in man. It is therefore not surprising that, to date, no *in vitro* methods have yet emerged that in certainty and scope have been judged to be equal to, or able to supersede the *in vivo* model for final safety clearance or hazard evaluation. Even a close approximation, such as the isolated eye preparation, is not seen as fully-substituting for the *in vivo* situation. Nevertheless, the fail-safe eye tests demanded hitherto have tended to be counterproductive, because the aim of eliciting the most potentially severe response, when allied to the variability inherent in their design, has made the results difficult to interpret, and virtually guaranteed the exclusion on safety grounds of materials which in practice would present only a minor hazard. Variations among the regulatory authorities and codes of practice, in terms of procedures and scoring systems, have not helped, nor has the tendency to overemphasise the quantitative aspect of what is essentially qualitative data.

3. Although total replacement of *in vivo* methods by *in vitro* testing for ocular irritancy is not yet possible, reduction in *in vivo* testing is desirable on the grounds of humanity, and the refinement of live animal testing is also necessary on scientific grounds. Whether the aim of complete replacement of *in vivo* irritancy testing by *in vitro* techniques can be achieved remains for the moment a matter for conjecture and ultimately will depend in large measure on the confidence the regulatory authorities feel able to place in making safety evaluations, recommendations, or clearances on the basis of data obtained from alternative techniques. Meanwhile, reduction of *in vivo* eye irritancy testing to a practical irreducible minimum by the use of physicochemical data and scientifically validated *in vitro* alternatives remains the most practical objective for the present.

RECOMMENDATIONS

1. A reduction in the scale of live animal ocular irritancy

testing and the avoidance of severe reactions in the eye should be sought by:

a. the gathering and application of all available physico-chemical data on the test compound relevant to ocular inflammation, as a first step to predicting eye injury potential and eliminating highly irritant compounds;
b. skin testing preceding eye tests, so that the data can be used, if not to absolutely predict eye effects, at least to assist in guiding the approach to the subsequent eye tests;
c. the use, where appropriate, of isolated eyes as irritancy models, obtained either from laboratory animals or, preferably, from animals already killed for other purposes (e.g. abattoir material).

2. In those situations where whole animal testing is still deemed necessary, testing procedures should be refined, to produce both a more humane and scientifically valid test and reduce the need for repeat tests. Under the present procedure, up to 18 animals may be required, owing to the possibility of repeat groups of animals, but it should be possible to obtain a result from no more than 6 animals. The following refinements of _in vivo_ testing are suggested:

a. a 10-fold reduction in the standard dose to 0.01ml or 0.01g;
b. direct application to the eye rather than to the conjunctival sac;
c. avoidance of irritant overreactions;
d. the use of a more descriptive rather than a purely numerical classification of irritant potential;
e. in the rabbit eye, prostaglandin-potentiated histamine causes marked conjunctival inflammation and local tenderness. The feasibility of using antihistamine during testing to reduce both discomfort to the animal and the spurious overreaction of the conjunctiva should be investigated.
f. The use of local anaesthetics in eye testing should not be encouraged, as their influence on the eye test is unclear and such use may eventually be counterproductive by prolonging irritant effects.

3. The considerable investment now being made in the search for alternatives to _in vivo_ testing, including eye irritancy, is likely to bring further advances in the ability of _in vitro_ tests to assist in routine safety testing or the investigation of mechanisms. Research should therefore be encouraged on biochemical tests for binding or denaturation of proteins, on the inactivation of enzyme systems concerned in tissue homeostasis,

Table I Some Characteristics of Present and Proposed Tests for Eye Irritant Potential

Test System	Predictiveness	Validation	Model for Eye Irritation	Remarks
Physicochemical	* –	** ++	No	* Good for pH; possible guide to other effects. ** Retrospective data available.
Biochemical (corneal protein pptn)	±	–	No	Mainly for astringents/caustics ionic effects on protein
Biochemical (-SH enzyme inhibition)	±	±	No	No recent work. Original research mainly involved sensory irritants.
Mast cell serotonin release	±	±	No	Limited at present to specific classes of compounds.
Cytotoxicity	(+)	+	No	Potentially versatile - corneal cell cultures etc. Concern over unexpectedly variable irritancy correlations.
Isolated eye	+	+	No	Not an animal alternative, but promising as a non-sentient animal model.
Standard Draize (maximised irritation)	++(primate) + (rabbit)	++	Yes	Inherent variability. Test conditions suspect - large dose-volume, intensity of chemical insult.
Modified Draize (mild irritation/standards)	+±(rabbit)	++	Yes	More humane, better control and data yield by testing under mild conditions with standards.
Suggested Draize	++(rabbit)	+	Yes	More humane, and more realistic dose-volumes which are reported to improve correlation with irritancy in humans.
MAN	+++		Yes	

on the development and validation of techniques employing isolated eyes, primary cell and organ cultures of eye-derived tissues, and general cell culture lines and strains.

REFERENCES

1. Draize, J.H., Woodward, G. & Calvery, H.O. (1944). Methods for the study of irritation and toxicity of substances applied topically to the skin and mucous membranes. Journal of Pharmacology and Experimental Therapeutics 82, 377-390.
2. Draize, J.H. (1959). Dermal toxicity. In "Appraisal of the Safety of Chemicals in Foods, Drugs and Cosmetics", pp. 46-59. Association of Food and Drug Officials of the USA.
3. Food and Drugs Administration, USA (1963). Test for eye irritation. Federal Register. June 12, Sec. 191.12.
4. Duke-Elder, S. (1954). "Textbook of Ophthalmology". St. Louis: Mosby.
5. Seabaugh, U.M., Osterberg, R.E. & Hocheisal, C.A. (1976). A comparative study of rabbit ocular reactions to various exposure times to chemicals. Abstract of the Fifteenth Annual Meeting of the Society of Toxicology.
6. Davies, R.E., Kynoch, S.R. & Liggett, M.P. (1976). Eye irritation tests - an assessment of the maximum delay time for remedial irritation. Journal of the Society of Cosmetic Chemists. 27, 301.
7. Maurice, D.M. (1955). Influence on corneal permeability of bathing with solutions of differing reaction and tonicity. British Journal of Ophthalmology 39, 463-473.
8. Swan, K.C. & White, N.G. (1942). Corneal permeability 1. Factors affecting penetration of drugs into the cornea. American Journal of Ophthalmology 25, 1043-1058.
9. Friedman, T.S. & Patton, T.F. (1976). Differences in ocular penetration of pilocarpine in rabbits of different ages. Journal of Pharmacological Science 65, 1095-1096.
10. Anon - Leading Article (1969). Ammonia in the eyes. British Medical Journal 3, 430.
11. Hughes, W.F. (1946). Alkali burns of the eye. Archives of Ophthalmology 35, 423-449.
12. Morton Grant, W. (1974). "Toxicology of the Eye", 2nd. edn. pp. 10-14. Springfield: Thomas.
13. Freidenwald, J.S., Hughes, W.F. & Hermann, H. (1946). Acid burns of the eye. Archives of Ophthalmology 35, 98-108.
14. York, M., Lawrence, R.S. & Gibson, G.B. (1982). An *in vitro* test for the assessment of eye irritancy in consumer products - preliminary findings. International Journal of Cosmetic Science 4, 223-234.
15. Morton Grant, W. & Kern, H.L. (1956). Cations and the cornea. American Journal of Ophthalmology 42, 167-181.
16. Mackworth, J.F. (1948). Inhibition of thiol enzymes by

lachrymators. Biochemical Journal 42, 82.
17. Stocken, L.A. & Thompson, P. (1946). British Anti Lewisite. 2. Dithiol compounds as antidotes for arsenic. Biochemical Journal 40, 535-547.
18. Peters, R.A. (1955). Biochemistry of some toxic agents. 1. Present state of knowledge of bichemical lesions induced by trivalent arsenical poisoning. Bulletin of Johns Hopkins Hospital 97, 1-20.
19. Dixon, M. & Needham, D.M. (1946). Biochemical research on chemical warfare agents. Nature, London 158, 432-438.
20. Eakins, K.E. & Bhattercherjee, P. (1977). Histamine, prostaglandins and ocular inflammation. Experimental Eye Research 24, 299-305.
21. Hermann, H. (1948). Effect of antihistamines on loss of adhesiveness of corneal epithelium after injection of histamine. Bulletin of Johns Hopkins Hospital 82, 208.
22. Patterson, C. & Pfister, R.R. (1975). Prostaglandin-like activity in the aqueous humour following alkali burns. Investigative Ophthalmology 14, 177-183.
23. Jampol, L.M., Neufeld, A.H. & Sears, M.L. (1975). Pathways for the response of the eye to injury. Investigative Ophthalmology 14, 184.
24. Maul, E. & Sears, M.L. (1976). Objective evaluation of experimental ocular irritation. Investigative Ophthalmology 15, 308-312.
25. Salem, H., Dunn, B.J. & Loux, J.J. (1975). Conjunctival temperature: a measure of ocular decongestant and anti-inflammatory activity. Annals of Ophthalmology 7, 819-824.
26. Mann, I., Pirie, A. & Pullinger, B.D. (1948). An experimental and chemical study of the reaction of the anterior segment of the eye to chemical injury, with special reference to chemical warfare agents. British Journal of Ophthalmology, monograph suppl. 13, 15-54.
27. Thomas, C.I. (1955). "The Cornea". 168 pp. Springfield: Thomas.
28. Maurice, D.M. (1966). The stimulus to neovascularisation in the cornea. Experimental Eye Research 5, 168-184.
29. Renard, G., Hirsch, M. & Pauliquin, Y. (1978). Corneal changes due to alkali burns. Transactions of the Ophthalmological Society of the UK 98, 379-382.
30. McCormack, J. (1982). In vitro irritancy. FRAME Technical News 6, 4.
31. Bettley, F.R. (1968). The toxicity of soaps and detergents. British Journal of Dermatology 80, 635.
32. Bell, M., Holmes, P.M., Nisbet, T.M., Uttley, M. & Van Abbé, N.J. (1979). Evaluating the potential eye irritancy of shampoos. International Journal of Cosmetic Science 1, 123-131.
33. Scaife, M. (1982). An investigation of the detergent action on cells in vitro and possible correlations with in vivo

data. International Journal of Cosmetic Science 4, 179-193.

34. Rotman, B. & Papermaster, B.W. (1966). Membrane properties of lining mammalian cells as studied by enzymatic hydrolysis of fluorogenic esters. Proceedings of the National Academy of Sciences of the USA 55, 134-141.
35. Simons, P.J. (1980). An alternative to the Draize test. In "The Use of Alternatives in Drug Research" (ed. A.N. Rowan & C.J. Stratmann), pp. 147-151. London: Macmillan.
36. Leighton, J. (1982). New focus on replacing animals in the lab. Science, New York 215, 35-38.
37. Burton, A.B.G., York, M. & Lawrence, R.S. (1981). The in vitro assessment of severe irritants. Food Drug Cosmetic Toxicology 19, 471-480.
38. Kastner, W. & Frosch, P.J. (1981). Skin irritation of various anionic surfactants in the Duhring-Chamber test on volunteers in comparison with in vitro and animal test methods. Fette Seifen Anstrichmittel 83, 33-46.
39. Prottey, C. & Ferguson, T. (1975). Factors which determine the skin irritation potential of soaps and detergents. Journal of the Society of Cosmetic Chemists 26, 29-46.
40. Hellauer, H.F. (1950). Sensibilitat und acetylcholingehalt der hornhaut verschiedenier tiere und des menschen. Zeitschrift Für Vergleichende Physiologie 32, 303-310.
41. Ballantyne, B. & Swanston, D.W. (1973). The irritant potential of dilute solutions of ortho-chlorobenzylidene malononitrile (CS) on the eye and tongue. Acta Pharmacologia et Toxicologia 32, 266-277.
42. Ballantyne, B. & Swanston, D.W. (1974). The irritant effects of dilute solutions of dibenzoxazepine (CR) on the eye and tongue. Acta Pharmacologia et Toxicologia 35, 412-423.
43. Gaunt, F. & Harper, K.H. (1964). The potential irritancy to the rabbit eye of certain commercially available shampoos. Journal of the Society of Cosmetic Chemists 15, 209-230.
44. Buehler, E.V. & Newmann, E.A. (1964). A comparison of eye irritation in monkeys and rabbits. Toxicology & Applied Pharmacology 6, 701-710.
45. Marzulli, F.N. & Simon, M.E. (1971). Eye irritation from topically applied drugs and cosmetics: pre-clinical studies. American Journal of Optometry 48, 61-79.
46. Panessa, B.J. & Zadunaisky, J.A. (1981). Pigment granules. A calcium reservoir in the vertebrate eye. Experimental Eye Research 32, 593-604.
47. Potts, A.M. (1964). The reaction of uveal pigment in vitro with polycyclic compounds. Investigative Ophthalmology 3, 405-416.
48. Marzulli, F.N. (1965). New data on eye and skin test. Toxicology & Applied Pharmacology 7, 78-85.
49. Carpenter, C.P. & Smyth, H.F. (1946). Chemical burns of the rabbit cornea. American Journal of Ophthalmology 29, 1363-1374.

50. Beckley, J.H. (1965). Comparative eye testing: man vs. animal. Toxicology & Applied Pharmacology 7, 93-101.
51. Beckley, J.H., Russell, T.J. & Rubin, L.F. (1969). Use of irritants. Toxicology & Applied Pharmacology 15, 1-9.52.
52. Battista, S.P. & McSweeney, S. (1965). Approaches to a quantitative method for testing eye irritation. Journal of the Society of Cosmetic Chemists 16, 119-137.
53. Bucher, K., Bucher, K.E. & Walz, D. (1981). The topically irritant substance: essentials - bio-tests - predictions. Agents and Actions 11, 515-519.
54. Ballantyne, B. & Swanston, D.W. (1976). The ophthalmic toxicology of dichloromethane. Toxicology 6, 173-187.
55. Griffiths, J.F., Nixon, G.A., Bruce, R.B., Reer, P.J. & Bannan, E.A. (1980). Dose-response studies with chemical irritants in the albino rabbit eye as a basis for selecting optimum testing conditions for predicting hazard to the eye. Toxicology & Applied Pharmacology 55, 501-513.
56. Committee for the Revision of NAS Publication 1138 (1977). "Principles and Procedures for Evaluating the Toxicity of Household Substances", pp. 41-54. Washington DC: National Academy of Sciences.
57. Williams, S.J., Graepel, G.J. & Kennedy, G.L. (1982). Evaluation of ocular irritancy potential: intralaboratory variability and effect of dosage-volume. Toxicology Letters 12, 235-241.
58. Burton, A.B.G. (1972). A method for the objective assessment of eye irritation. Food Drug Cosmetic Toxicology 10, 209-219.
59. Conquet, R., Durand, G., Lailler, J. & Plazonnet, B. (1977). Evaluation of ocular irritation in the rabbit: objective versus subjective assessment. Toxicology & Applied Pharmacology 39, 129-139.
60. Ballantyne, B., Gazzard, M.F. & Swanston, D.W. (1972). Effect of solvents and irritants on intraocular tension in the rat. Journal of Physiology 226, 12-14p.
61. Ballantyne, B., Gazzard, M.F. & Swanston, D.W. (1977). Applanation tonometry in ophthalmic toxicology. In "Current Approaches in Toxicology" (ed. B. Ballantyne), pp. 158-192. Bristol: Wright.
62. Callaway, S., Gazzard, M.F., Price-Thomas, D. & Swanston, D.W. (1973). The calibration and evaluation of a hand-held tonometer as a means of measuring the intraocular pressure in the conscious rabbit. Experimental Eye Research 15, 383-393.
63. Walton, R.M. & Heywood, R. (1978). Applanation tonometry in the assessment of eye irritation. Journal of the Society of Cosmetic Chemists 29, 365-368.
64. Norn, M.S. (1972). The mucous thread in conjunctival fornix. Acta Ophthalmologica, supplementum 113, 39-46.
65. Kikkawa, Y. (1972). Normal corneal staining with flour-

escein. Experimental Eye Research 14, 13-20.

66. Hickey, T.E., Beck, G.L. & Botta, J.A. (1973). Optimum fluorescein staining time in ocular irritation studies. Toxicology & Applied Pharmacology 26, 571-574.
67. Boberg-Ans, J. (1955). Experience in clinical examination of corneal sensitivity. British Journal of Ophthalmology 39, 705-726.
68. Ulsamer, A.G., Wright, P.L. & Osterberg, R.E. (1977). A comparison of the effects of model irritants on anaesthetised and non-anaesthetised rabbits eyes. Toxicology & Applied Pharmacology 41, 191-192.
69. Cremer-Bartells, G. (1977). Effect of drugs on corneal stroma. In "Drugs and Ocular Tissues" (ed. S. Dikstein), pp. 102-127. Basel: Karger.
70. Harnisch, J.P., Hoffman, F. & Dumitrescu, L. (1975). Side-effects of local anaesthetics on the corneal epithelium of the rabbit eye. Albrecht Von Graefes Archiv fur Klinische und Experimentel Ophthalmologie 197, 71-81.
71. Ballantyne, B. & Swanston, D.W. (1977). The scope and limitations of acute eye irritation tests. In "Current Approaches in Toxicology" (ed. B. Ballantyne), pp. 139-157. Bristol: Wright.
72. Weil, C.S. & Scala, R.A. (1971). Study of intra- and inter-laboratory variability in the results of rabbit eye and skin irritation tests. Toxicology & Applied Pharmacology 19, 276-360.
73. Weltman, A.S., Sparber, S.V. & Jurtshuk, T. (1965). Compartive evaluation and influence of various factors in eye irritation scores. Toxicology & Applied Pharmacology 7, 308-319.
74. Kay, J.H. & Calandra, J.C. (1962). Interpretation of eye irritation tests. Journal of the Society of Cosmetic Chemists 13, 281-289.
75. Stark, D. (1982). New focus on replacing animals in the lab. Science, New York 215, 35-38.
76. Sargeant, L.S. (1980). The Draize test and alternatives. Atla Abstracts 2, 105-107.
77. Ehlers, N. (1977). Pharmacology of the conjunctival sac. In "Drugs and Ocular Tissues" (ed. S. Dikstein), pp. 23-56. Basel: Karger.

In Vitro Studies on Ocular Irritancy

M. C. SCAIFE

The objectives of my postgraduate research were to develop and investigate the suitability and adequacy of in vitro methods for determining the order of irritant responses in compounds (especially synthetic surfactants) in the eye.

Two in vitro cytotoxicity techniques, namely the measurement of cell membrane integrity (using fluorescein diacetate and ethidium bromide) and quantitation of the release of a cell membrane-bound enzyme (alkaline phosphatase) gave consistent findings (1). These findings, well supported in the literature, indicated that an increase in the lipophilic characteristics of a series of amphiphiles resulted in increased cytotoxicity (shown for sodium and triethanolamine alkyl trimethylammonium bromides and Tweens 20, 40, 60 and 80 (2)). Moreover, an increase in the hydrophilic nature of the head group of a particular detergent, e.g. by increasing the degree of ethoxylation of sodium lauryl sulphate, resulted in greater cytotoxicity (3). The concentration required to evince a cytotoxic effect (50% cell damage) was below the concentration at which the detergent monomers aggregate (the critical micelle concentration).

The single instillation eye studies performed by a collaborating establishment were made on these same materials at a concentration far in excess of the aqueous solubility of these materials at 37°C. One should therefore note that the physical forms of the detergents were not equivalent in vivo and in vitro. For the anionic detergents, an inverse correlation was found for the in vitro/in vivo comparison - i.e. an increase in lipophilicity increased the in vitro cytotoxicity, but decreased in vivo irritancy. For the cationic detergents, the order of irritant responses seen in the conjunctivae and iris were similar to that found in vivo (i.e. an increase in lipophilicity increased the cytotoxicity and irritancy), although in the eye the differences were not statistically different (4). Ideally, the detergents should have been examined in vivo when in the monomer state, but that would have necessitated multi-dose eye studies.

Limited studies were undertaken using shampoos where all the constituents were completely soluble; the in vivo/in vitro correlations were found to be in accord and I recommended that further studies be made on a larger range of shampoos (1). Indeed, similar studies undertaken independently at another establishment have shown good in vivo/in vitro correlations; these data will be presented shortly by the researcher in question. Without pre-empting his findings, there are strong indications that a cytotoxicity procedure may give a good indication of whether a material may have an irritancy potential in the eye, provided that the substances tested are soluble and do not contain undissolved materials that have an aqueous solubility albeit limited.

In an attempt to try and explain the apparently anomalous correlation with the anionic detergents, I studied the ability of these substances to induce corneal opacity, reflecting a swollen state of the damaged cornea (1). Physical disruption of the cornea may result in the inability of the ionic pump mechanism within the cornea to maintain the deturgescence of the cornea; the consequence is corneal swelling. Measurements were taken of the electrical impedance changes across the isolated rabbit cornea in the presence and absence of various anionic detergents. The conclusion drawn from the results, using anionic detergents, was that the shorter chain length alkyl sulphates caused faster swelling than the longer chain compounds. These findings correspond to the order of irritancy of these detergents in the in vivo rabbit eye.

These results are of importance in attempting to explain the apparent anomaly with anionic detergents in the previous in vitro tests, namely, that an increase in cytotoxicity occurred as the lipophilicity increased. If the longer chain length detergents do not penetrate the cornea (as suggested by the rate of corneal swelling) as fast as the smaller detergents, then the cytotoxicity findings would be reversed in the eye test results.

In conclusion, the findings suggest that a simple cytotoxicity procedure is capable of mirroring the in vivo situation only when the major difference between studies on complex tissues such as the eye and cells in culture is obviated, namely, that the penetration barrier in the in vivo situation is removed (one presumes that shampoos by their very nature have maximal detergent solubilising and penetration characteristics). However, other factors should be considered such as the interactive effects of materials in enzymes, their adsorption characteristics and their ability to liberate inflammatory mediators. As lucidly pointed out in Mr Swanston's paper, classes of substances may have entirely different modes of action in the eye - e.g. arsenical vesicants, caustics and acids, and shampoos. It is perhaps too naïve to aim for one test that would be suitable for all classes of materials.

REFERENCES

1. Scaife, M.C. (1981). An investigation of possible in vitro methods for studying eye irritancy potential. CNAA: Ph.D. Thesis (Leicester Polytechnic).
2. Imokawa, G. & Mishima, Y. (1979). Cumulative effect of surfactants on cutaneous horny layers of lysosome labilizing action. Contact Dermatology 5, 151-162.
3. Gibson, W.T. (1980). Lysis of rabbit polymorphonuclear leucocyte granules by surfactants of differing structure and irritancy. Food Drug Cosmetic Toxicology 18, 511-515.
4. Scaife, M.C. (1982). An investigation of detergent action on cells in vitro and possible correlations with in vivo data. International Journal of Cosmetic Science 4, 179-193.

An Isolated Rabbit Eye Technique

MICHAEL YORK

The FRAME Toxicity Committee Report gives a balanced view of in vivo eye testing and the variety of in vitro methods which might be used as alternatives to the test.

It is clear from the report that at this time there is no in vitro procedure which will satisfactorily or reliably replace all of the features of an in vivo eye test. There remains, therefore, the need to carry out limited in vivo eye testing. Such testing should be carried out under the best possible conditions and should yield the maximum information possible, while minimising the trauma to the experimental animals.

I fully support the use of procedures which minimise trauma to the animals, provided this does not prejudice the result, since in the long run this could lead to further in vivo testing. Perhaps one of the most important changes in the approach to in vivo eye testing recently has been the reduction of the amount instilled to 10µl. This not only reduces trauma for the animals, but also represents a realistic amount of material which might enter the human eye, and I fully support its use.

The use of antihistamine to reduce the degree of post-treatment conjunctival inflammation is of questionable value, since it is likely to involve the use of more animals to carry out properly controlled experiments.

Such live animal experiments should not be carried out unless there is no other way of gaining the required information, and as responsible toxicologists we should look towards a form of in vitro procedure which will reduce animal usage. The approach in our laboratory is to use the enucleated rabbit eye procedure (1,2). We believe that by proper use of the system we can obtain a significant amount of information on the eye irritancy potential of various products or ingredients, and that it has a number of advantages over other possible in vitro systems:

a. The system will identify materials which have the potential to be extremely irritant to the in vivo eye. Such materials cause direct clearly visible damage to the in vitro cornea following a very short period of contact.
b. The system investigates the effects of the products/chemicals in the form in which they might enter the human eye. The system does not need to rely on dilution of that material to identify that it is particularly toxic to cells.
c. As materials are applied directly on to the cornea, the system can be used for a very wide range of irritants, from corrosive materials such as sodium hydroxide to totally non-irritant materials such as glycerol. The test's versatility across this wide range of irritants is of considerable advantage, and it is doubtful whether other in vitro systems would be able to cope adequately with products or ingredients which differ widely in their irritation potentials. For example, in a cell culture system, sodium hydroxide would need to be present at a misleadingly high concentration to cause an effect, and therefore it might appear to be less of a hazard than it really is.

One criticism of the whole eye in vitro technique is that it is not too difficult to predict severe eye irritants anyway. This is true and it has always been one of our objectives that, to be of major practical use, the in vitro system should differentiate between test materials which are not severely irritant in vivo. We have had some success in this area and have found that by adjusting treatment conditions we can rank a number of products based on different concentrations of anionic or non-ionic surfactants in an order of irritancy which is consistent with their in vivo irritancy. These findings have been very encouraging and have led us to investigate the effects of different types of products. It has become evident from these studies that different types of materials affect the in vitro cornea in different ways. Substantivity to corneal cells and penetration into the cornea are extremely important factors. As we continue working on the system it is clear that we will need to gain a better understanding of these factors.

REFERENCES

1. Burton, A.B.G., York, M. & Lawrence, R.S. (1981). The *in vitro* assessment of severe eye irritants. Food and Cosmetic Toxicology 19, 471-480.
2. York, M., Lawrence, R.S. & Gibson, G.B. (1982). An *in vitro* test for the assessment of eye irritancy in consumer products - preliminary findings. International Journal of Cosmetic Science 4, 223-234.

Dosage-volume, Sample Size and Predictability

S. J. WILLIAMS

The goal of these studies was to investigate modifications of current standard methods of ocular irritancy testing which could reduce the numbers of animals used in such tests and decrease the likelihood of causing severe damage with minimal compromise of data quality. In the first set of studies (Table I), a series of seven previously tested materials (0.1ml dose-volume) with graded irritancy ratings were tested in rabbit eyes, using a dose-volume of 0.01ml applied directly to the cornea of 6 rabbits for each material. One material also was tested using 0.1ml in 36 rabbits. Eyes were evaluated up to 21 days post-exposure using standard techniques. When the corneal and conjunctival scores from animals dosed with 0.01 or 0.1ml of one material are compared, a clear dose-effect relationship is discernible (Fig. 1). When the materials are ranked according to maximum score or duration of effect, the order is the same as that obtained in previous studies using the higher dose, but the effects are mollified (Fig. 2). From the 36 rabbits dosed with 0.1ml, some indication of the effect of sample size on test reproducibility was obtained. Thus, for a material with an average Draize score of 42 at 1 day, the probability of being within 10 units of the mean using a sample size of 6, 3 or 2 rabbits is 99, 94, or 87%, respectively (Table II). The use of primary skin irritation test results as predictive of ocular irritancy potential also was examined (Table III). A literature survey (1968-1982) was conducted to find all DuPont materials which were severe primary skin irritants and had been tested also for ocular irritancy. Of the sixty materials which met both

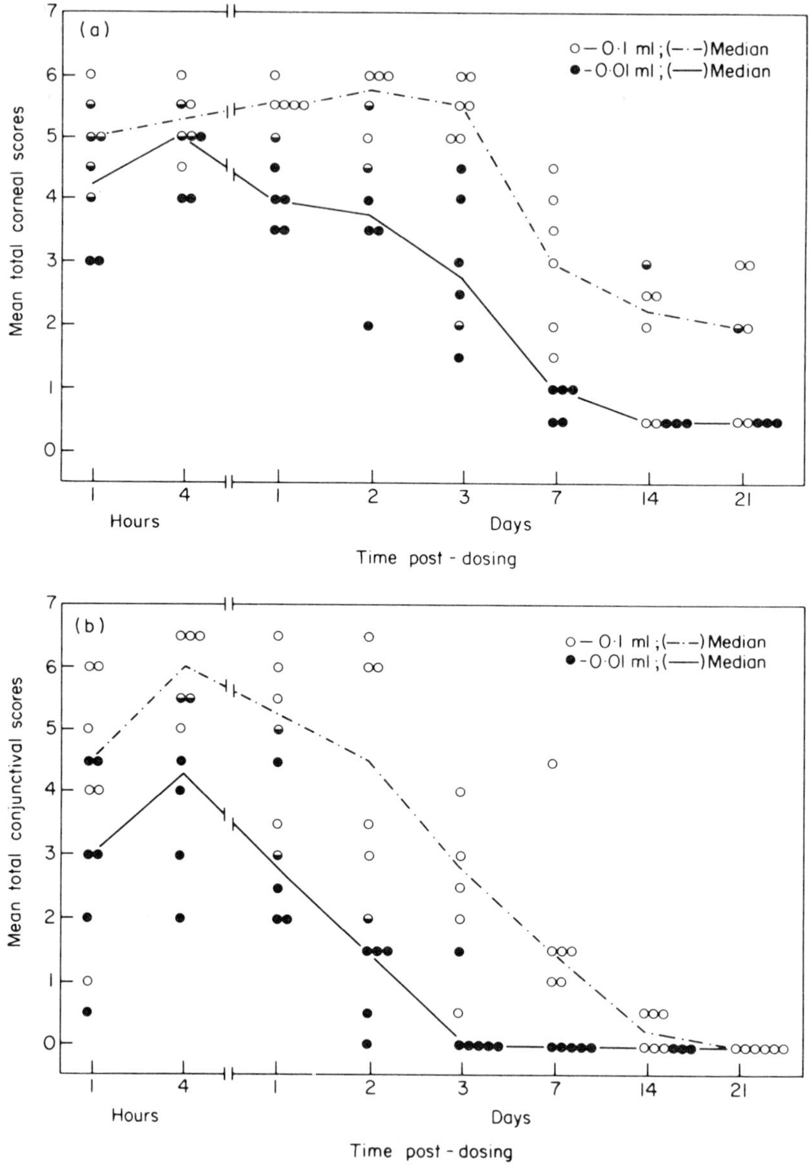

Figure 1 Dose effect relationship of 1-decanol, titanium (4+) salt applied to right eyes of rabbits at a dose of 0.1ml or 0.01ml. Each point represents the mean of the total scores obtained by the two readers. Each line represents the median value of the mean scores obtained from the six rabbits at each dose (—0.01ml;—.—0.1ml). (A) Total corneal scores; (B) total conjunctival scores.

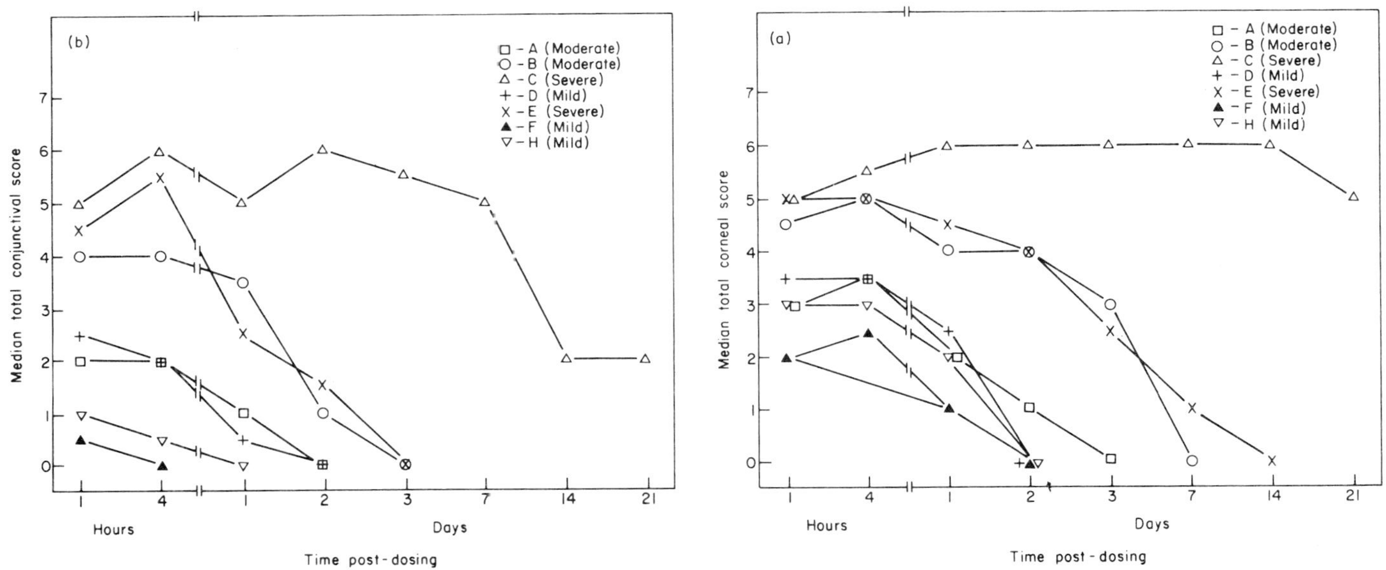

Figure 2 Median scores obtained for a series of liquid irritants tested for ocular irritancy potential using a test volume of 0.01ml. Each point represents the median total score obtained for the cornea (A) or the conjunctiva (B). The irritancy classifications of the test materials as determined previously using a dose-volume of 0.01ml are shown in the figure keys.

of these criteria (Table IV), 39 were severe eye irritants (severe effect at any time or any degree of damage ≥21 days), 15 were non-irritants to minimal-irritants (no effect or mild injury in any tissue ≤3 days) and 6 were moderate irritants (mild to moderate injury which resolves in 5 to 14 days). Therefore, severe primary skin irritation was predictive of a similar degree of ocular response for only 65% of the materials tested.

Table I

Test Materials Used in the Evaluation of Eye Irritancy Potential

Irritancy Classification at Dose of 0.1ml	Test Material (Formulation)	Letter Code
Mild	Poly(difluoromethylene), alpha-fluoro-omega-[2-(sulfoxy)ethyl]-, ammonium salt (15% in H_2O)	D
Mild	Hexa(methoxymethyl)melamine, partially transetherified with a quaternary ammonium polyethylene glycol derivative, formulated with an antioxidant and a wetting agent (99% pure)	F
Mild	Pentaerythritol tetra (C_8-C_{10} acids) (67% in surfactants)	H
Moderate	Formamide, N,N-dimethyl- (100%)	A
Moderate	1-Decanol, titanium (4+) salt (100%)	B,G
Severe	Quaternary ammonium compounds, bis[alpha-hydropoly (oxy-1,2-ethanediyl)-omega-yl]-(2-hydroxethyl)(tallow alkyl)-, hydroxy-acetates (66% in H_2O)	C
Severe	1-Hexanol, 2-ethyl-, titanium (4+) salt (95% pure)	E

CONCLUSIONS

1. Reducing the test volume from 0.1ml to 0.01ml for a series of known, graded irritants does not alter the irritancy rank (correlation coefficients 0.78-0.80).

2. The number of animals used for determination of ocular irritation should be determined according to the desired accuracy of results.

3. Results obtained from primary skin irritation tests probably do not provide a reliable index of ocular irritation potential.

Table II

Probability of an Obtained Mean Draize Score Being Within "X" Units of a True Mean Score for Moderate Material

	Probability (%)					
	Sample Size					
	2		3		6	
Draize Units from Mean	4 hr[1]	1 day[2]	4 hr[1]	1 day[2]	4 hr[1]	1 day[2]
2.5	29.8	25.9	36.1	31.5	49.3	43.4
5.0	55.6	49.2	68.2	58.2	81.5	74.8
7.5	74.9	67.9	84.0	77.6	95.3	91.5
10.0	87.4	81.4	93.9	89.5	99.2	97.8

[1] Mean score of 36 rabbits is 43.6 + 9.2
[2] Mean score of 36 rabbits is 42.8 + 10.7

Table III

Ocular Responses to Materials Determined to be Either Severe Primary Irritants or Corrosive on the Skin

Material Tested	Tissue Response: Skin	Tissue Response: Eye	Class
1	Corrosive (DOT)	Severe permanent corneal opacity with vascularisation	1
2	Necrotic erythema with severe oedema	Corrosive; permanent corneal opacity	1
3	Severe erythema and oedema	FHSA (+) - severe corneal opacity with eversion of the eyelids	1
4	Severe erythema with moderate oedema	FHSA (+) - moderate corneal opacity at 72 hrs.	1
5	Necrotic erythema with severe oedema	Severe, generalised, penetrating corneal opacity	1
6	Necrotic erythema with moderate oedema	Severe, irreversibly corrosive	1
7	Severe to necrotic erythema with mild oedema	Mild, corneal opacity reversible in 3 days, eye normal at 14 days	2
8	Necrotic erythema with moderate to severe oedema	FHSA-non-irritant	3
9	Corrosive (DOT)	Generalised, permanent penetrating opacity	1
10	Severe to mild necrosis with mild oedema	Severe, permanent corneal opacity	1
11	Necrotic erythema with moderate oedema	Severe, permanent corneal opacity	1

Table IV

Ocular Responses to Materials Determined to be Either Severe Primary Irritants or Corrosive on the Skin

	Ocular Irritancy Classification (Definition)	Number of Occurrences (Out of 60)
1	Severe (severe injury in any ocular tissue at any time or any degree of damage persisting ≥21 days)	39
2	Mild or Non-irritant (no effect or mild injury in any ocular tissue which resolves in ≤3 days)	15
3	Moderate (mild to moderate injury in any ocular tissue which resolves in 5-14 days)	6

General Discussion

N. J. VAN ABBÉ

Rapporteur

The Chairman, Mr VAN ABBÉ, said that, until such time as the prediction of eye irritancy was able to rely entirely on in vitro methods, it was highly desirable to ensure as far as possible that any in vivo testing was carried out in such a way as to minimise any pain or discomfort experienced by the animals used. The principle should be universally endorsed that predictive eye irritancy tests should never be conducted in living animals under conditions whereby it could reasonably be predicted that severe responses were likely to occur. In many laboratories, this was already acknowledged and tests were restricted to the study of dilutions which did not produce more than mild effects in the eye. Testing of this kind discriminated more effectively between different levels of irritancy than testing under more severe conditions. It was to be hoped that all laboratories would in future make every effort to avoid testing under conditions likely to cause significant pain or distress.

The Chairman added that the need for eye irritancy testing could not be judged from skin irritancy data unless concentration of the test material was taken into account. Typical concentrations used for skin testing might well elicit positive responses on the skin, but this did not necessarily show whether dilutions likely to come into contact with the eyes would be tolerated or not. For example, many surfactants are skin irritants as normally tested but, at lower concentrations, some are fairly severe eye irritants whereas others only produce mild effects in the eyes; it is quite important to be able to make a distinction. However, this did not mean that materials which were powerful skin irritants even at low concentrations would require separate eye irritancy testing. Dr Ruth CLAYTON drew attention to the fact that most ocular toxicity studies were intended to predict acute hazards, whereas long-term effects could also be extremely important, especially in relation to delayed changes in the eye and retina. Topical corticosteroids administered as eye-drops could be associated with delayed cataract development. She was specially worried about enhanced susceptibility in juveniles. Studies using radiotracer labelled detergents showed penetration and binding throughout the ocular tissues, along with relatively slow subsequent release. Mr SWANSTON felt that measurement of intra-ocular tension could be relevant, so long as the cornea was intact; he also suggested that slit-lamp biomicroscopy might be helpful. However, Dr CLAYTON did not feel that such approaches would suffice to detect the risk of delayed changes.

Dr Mary DAWSON referred to problems mentioned by Dr Scaife with in vitro cytotoxicity studies concerned with particulate substances. She noted that anything insoluble, even if relatively inert, was liable to appear toxic in cell culture studies. Cultured conjunctival cells had proved satisfactory in the study of topical anaesthetics. Tests of formulations were important, rather than just the testing of individual constituents in terms of ocular toxicity.

Addendum on Dermal and Ocular Toxicity

N. J. VAN ABBÉ

After the conclusion of the Meeting, the Chairman (Mr N.J. Van Abbé) made the following suggestions to FRAME:

> "The concept of rating samples in topical toxicity tests by simultaneous comparison with a reference control under mild exposure conditions has several advantages. However, these do not seem to be widely appreciated and I should like to put my point of view for your consideration.
>
> "My suggestion is that whenever it is feasible to design a study on appropriate lines, it is desirable to (a) select dose-levels, concentrations and other exposure conditions such that responses are positive but only mild, and (b) undertake simultaneous comparison with a reference control already known to be tolerated satisfactorily when used for the same intended purpose. This applies mainly to studies on acute skin and eye irritancy and to work on either human volunteers or laboratory animals.

"No investigation should be expected to give optimal discrimination at the extremes of its dose-response but, on the contrary, reliability and sensitivity are likely to be maximised in intermediate conditions, especially somewhere along a straight region of the curve. For example, in a "classical" Draize rabbit eye test, it is impossible to make any distinction between two samples each of which produces a severe response, although these samples may differ considerably in their effects in human eyes under normal exposure conditions.

"Simultaneous comparisons under mild conditions imply that testing should rarely if ever have distressing effects, whether the subjects are human or animal, so I feel that FRAME should seriously consider advocating such a principle. Additional benefits are, in my view, that the approach overcomes the more unreliable features of arbitrary scoring and of time-dependent variability of test subjects.

"It is important to note that published test methods seldom offer guidance on how to reach pass/fail decisions, although these are the ultimate requirements in industry. However, simultaneous comparison with a suitable reference control helps to solve the problem, and even to minimise uncertainty with regard to interspecies extrapolation, if it is ruled that the "test" must not be any more toxic then the "control" under the chosen experimental conditions. This needs to be enforced quite strictly; if the "test" is more toxic (however small the tolerance permitted), there is no way of interpreting significance of the excess toxicity in terms of risk during normal use."

Short-term Tests for Genotoxicity

B. J. DEAN and
PETER HODGES

INTRODUCTION

In recent years, there has been growing scientific, regulatory and public awareness of the potential carcinogenic and mutagenic hazards involved in the introduction of many thousands of new chemicals (drugs, pesticides and industrial chemicals) into the environment. Allied to this has been an equally growing awareness of the limitations, both scientific and logistical, of currently used animal methods for investigating these hazards. These factors have led to the development of a wide variety of short-term/*in vitro* (although the two terms are not necessarily synonymous) tests for potential genotoxicity. Generally, these tests have been based on some sort of mutational event. Genotoxicity is an indication of the ability of a chemical to interact with DNA and such interaction may result in mutagenicity or carcinogenicity, or both. Further tests specifically identify carcinogenic potential (e.g. cell transformation assays) or mutagenic potential (e.g. heritable translocation assays). Until the introduction of short-term assays, potential carcinogens and mutagens could only be identified by studies involving large numbers of animals. The possible further development of such techniques into other areas, such as the prediction of teratogenicity, remains to be fully explored.

Interest in the range of short-term tests available for determination of genotoxic potential has been reflected in the number of recent reviews from a variety of sources (1-7). A major international collaborative experimental programme has been carried out (8), and other, more limited, collaborative studies (9-11) have also been undertaken and workshops have been held (10,12-14). In addition, the US Environmental Protection Agency (EPA) through its Gene-Tox programme is carrying out a major in-depth review of the literature on the various tests, and the first results of this work have been published (15-26). A survey of the results of testing by UK pharmaceutical companies is also being undertaken by the ABPI (27), the results of which, when published, should aid the assessment of the value of the various tests. The International Commission for Protection Against Environmental Mutagens and Carcinogens (ICPEMC) was established in 1977, with as one of its functions "to apply scientific expertise to the interpretation and validation of short-term screening tests to detect genotoxic activities of chemicals" (28).

In the context of the FRAME Toxicity Committee's work, the effort expended and the progress made in the area of short-term tests for genotoxicity are of major importance, since a number of potentially useful test systems have been developed. This document is an overview of the field of genetic toxicology, which concentrates on those systems that seem to show greatest potential for use as test systems for environmental agents. It also seeks to provide indications of where further lines of research might usefully be explored.

This paper is divided into sections describing tests for overall genotoxic activity, including gene and chromosomal mutations, tests specifically designed to study heritable genetic damage, i.e. to the germ cells, and tests more relevant to carcinogenic chemicals, followed by an outline of the deployment of these assays, and, finally, the current state of the art and the direction of future research in genetic toxicology are discussed.

For a detailed review of mutagenicity testing procedures, the reader is referred to the DHSS Guidelines for the Testing of Chemicals for Mutagenicity (5), and for a review of short-term tests in the prediction of carcinogenicity to Dean (3).

TESTS FOR GENOTOXIC ACTIVITY

Microbial Systems

Bacterial Systems

Bacteria have a very simple arrangement of genetic material in a single circular molecule of DNA. The DNA is thus readily accessible to any mutagen that can penetrate the cell. The now classic example of this type of assay is the *Salmonella*/microsome ("Ames") test (29,30). This uses a set of tester strains of *Salmonella typhimurium* with mutations conferring a nutritional requirement for histidine. The bacteria have been specially developed to have cell walls that are permeable to "foreign" chemicals and to lack enzymes that are responsible for DNA repair. Some strains also possess plasmids making them even more sensitive to mutagens (31). However, many compounds require metabolic activation before they can exert a genotoxic action, and the bacteria as such do not have such metabolic capacity. The incorporation of an enzyme preparation of rat or mouse liver (the S9 mix) provides some approximation to the metabolic activation in the whole mammal.

The *Salmonella*/microsome assay is probably the most widely used and tested of all mutagenicity assays. Many hundreds of chemicals have been tested, with a high degree of correlation between mutagenicity findings and results of animal bioassays (32). Factors influencing the correlation between the results of short-term tests and animal studies were reviewed by Rinkus & Legator (33).

"False" negative results would be expected to arise from agents that express their carcinogenic effect directly through a non-mutational process or indirectly through a physiological or hormonal effect on the test animal, e.g. chloroform or diethylstilboestrol (DES). It is not to be expected that compounds operating by such epigenetic mechanisms would be detected by mutation-based tests, though they may be detected in other test systems. DES, for example, is reported to induce sister chromatid exchanges in human skin fibroblast cultures (34). "False" results of either type may result from inadequacies in the metabolism system to adequately activate or deactivate the test substance. The reactions required for activation or deactivation vary widely and may include oxidation, reduction, hydrolysis, and conjugation. The enzymes necessary for all these reactions may not be active in the liver microsomal preparation conventionally used in the *Salmonella*/microsome test. Special systems may be required, for example, for hydrolysis of glycosides, such as cycasin, by faecal extracts (35) or activation of nitro-compounds by cell-free extracts of anaerobic bacteria (36).

"False" positive responses may result from the "exposed" nature of the DNA in bacterial cells (37) or the deficiencies in DNA repair which have been deliberately built into the *Salmonella*/microsome tester strains. Thus, the bacteria may demonstrate a genotoxic potential that is not manifested in *in vivo* mammalian systems.

The test identifies compounds that interact with DNA and thus identifies potential mammalian carcinogens and mutagens. However, no quantitative correlation appears to exist between the mutagenic and carcinogenic potencies. Therefore, the results of this and other such short-term tests cannot predict carcinogenic potency and cannot be used for human risk assessment in quantitative terms.

Microbial assays may be adapted to examine body fluids, notably plasma and urine, for the presence of mutagenic materials (38). In this respect the test might be carried out in conjunction with orthodox toxicity trials. This technique has also been used for epidemiological studies on workers exposed to potentially harmful chemicals (39,40) or hazardous environmental agents, such as cigarette smoke (41).

Histidine-requiring auxotrophs of *S. typhimurium* are also used in the fluctuation assay, a liquid culture technique that seems particularly effective in the detection of weak carcinogens (42).

Other bacterial systems have been developed based on auxotrophic strains of *Escherichia coli* and *Bacillus subtilis.* However, the data base for such systems remains relatively small, and a Gene-Tox panel review of the available literature on the *E. coli* system concluded that it did not contribute results that would not be obtained by careful application of the *Salmonella*/microsome test (16).

All the systems outlined above are reverse-mutation assays, i.e. they depend on the reversal of a pre-existing mutation leading to nutritional independence. A theoretical argument can be made that this introduces a selectivity into the mutagens which may be detected by particular strains, due to a need for interaction between the mutagen and a specific point on the DNA molecule. This objection could be overcome by the use of forward-mutation-based test systems. Such systems have been developed in *S. typhimurium* (43) and *B. subtilis* (44), but evidence available to date does not appear to indicate any significant advantage over the *Salmonella*/microsome reverse-mutation test.

Other bacterial assays based on growth inhibition in repair-deficient strains have been developed for *E. coli*, *B. subtilis*, and *S. typhimurium*. However, technical and other problems lead to the conclusion that these tests are probably of less general value than the *Salmonella*/microsome test.

Systems Utilising Eukaryotic Microorganisms

Eukaryotic microorganisms, such as the yeasts (*Saccharomyces* and *Schizosaccharomyces*) and moulds (*Aspergillus* and *Neurospora*) occupy a position between the simple prokaryotic bacteria and the higher eukaryotic mammalian cells. Superficially at least, the eukaryotic microorganisms appear to have a number of potential advantages as a basis for a mutagenicity test system. The DNA is structurally similar and organised into chromosomes in a manner analogous to mammalian cells. They have the theoretical advantage that both haploid and diploid forms can be used in genetic tests.

The haploid fungus *Neurospora crassa*, can be used as a two-component heterokaryon to provide what is, in effect, a diploid test organism. Heterokaryons are constructed from biochemically different haploids and, in this way, test systems can be designed to detect chemically-induced mutations over the whole genome (45). *Neurospora* systems offer a sophisticated research tool for studying DNA lesions induced by genotoxic chemicals and/or monitoring the genetic consequences of such lesions at the gene and chromosome levels.

Saccharomyces cerevisiae is a unicellular, uninuclear yeast which occurs in haploid and diploid forms during its life-cycle and is widely used in genetic toxicology. Tests are available for detecting both reverse and forward mutations, mitotic crossing over, and mitotic gene conversion. Logarithmic phase cultures have some mixed-function oxidase activity, but it is common practice to complement this by the incorporation of a rodent liver microsomal fraction when testing chemicals for genotoxic activity. *S. cerevisiae* is a regular component of test batteries using mitotic gene conversion as the genetic end-point and positive results are generally regarded as an indication of primary DNA damage. The assay is particularly useful as it responds to chemicals that produce a number of different types of mutation in bacteria, and occasionally detects genotoxic activity where bacterial assays are negative. Mitotic gene conversion leads to accurate transfer of small segments of DNA containing some 100 to 200 nucleotides between homologous chromosomes. This may lead to the formation of new alleles. For example, in the diploid yeast JDI, which is heteroallelic at the histidine and tryptophan loci, and which requires both amino acids for growth, mitotic gene conversion at either of these loci restores the ability of the cell to synthesise histidine and tryptophan, respectively. A recent finding of potential importance is the discovery that many tumour promoters, including phorbal esters and oleic acid, induce aneuploidy in an appropriate strain (D6) of *S. cerevisiae* (46). This is particularly interesting in the context of recent theories that associate tumour promotion with mitotic segregation events (47).

Tests for Gene Mutation Using Mammalian Cells in Culture

Tests for gene mutations in mammalian cells in culture provide a useful component of short-term test batteries. Although cell culture assays have not been validated to the same extent as bacterial systems, at least two systems are widely used and are listed by legislative authorities (2,5). The first involves the use of the Chinese hamster V79 or CHO cells and two genetic markers, i.e. resistance to the lethal base-analogues, 8-azaguanine or 6-thioguanine, and resistance to the steroid ouabain. Base-analogue resistance is determined by the activity of hypoxanthine-guanine phosphoribosyl transferase (HGPRT) which catalyses the incorporation of pre-formed bases into DNA. Normal cells fail to survive in culture medium containing 8-azaguanine or 6-thioguanine; mutation of the HGPRT locus results in loss of enzyme activity and such mutants can proliferate in the presence of the base-analogues. Ouabain-resistance is associated with a mutation inhibiting activity of membrane ATPase which controls membrane cation transport (48). The second system utilises a mouse lymphoma-derived cell line (L5178Y/TK$^{+/-}$), which is heterozygous at the thymidine kinase locus. The assay detects mutation from TK$^{+/-}$ to TK$^{-/-}$, using lethal analogues of thymine monophosphate such as 5-bromodeoxyuridine or trifluorothymidine as selective agents (49).

The cells used in both these systems lack adequate foreign compound metabolising capability and, for screening purposes, this deficiency is corrected by incorporating either a rat liver microsomal fraction or by co-cultivation with a feeder layer of metabolically competent cells, e.g. hamster embryo cells (50). Increasing interest is being shown in using cells that have intrinsic metabolising activity for gene mutation studies. The use of rat liver epithelial-type cells for detecting mutation induction by pre-carcinogens is an example of this approach (51).

Cytogenetic Assays

Cytogenetic assays are used to determine structural or numerical chromosomal changes which may be visualised by the light microscope, as distinct from the gene mutations described previously. Techniques exist for the detection of chromosome aberrations, for the detection of exchanges of chromosomal material between sister chromatids (sister chromatid exchange [SCE]), and for the detection of fragments resulting from chromosome breakage (micronucleus assay). The detection of chromosomal abnormalities may be carried out using *in vivo* (whole mammal) or *in vitro* techniques.

In Vitro Chromosome Techniques

Cell culture techniques are very convenient and rapid systems for screening chemicals for chromosome breaking activity (51), and human lymphocytes (53) and rodent-fibroblasts (e.g. V79 cells) have been widely used for this purpose. Most cell types require additional metabolic activity in the form of a microsomal enzyme preparation, and such a procedure using lymphocytes has proved useful in testing for genotoxicity. For example, the system successfully identified a number of carbamate carcinogens that had not been detected in microbial systems (54). An alternative technique utilises a rat liver-derived cell line that retains sufficient metabolic activity to detect the induction of chromosome damage by many carcinogenic and mutagenic chemicals (55).

Interchange of replicating DNA between chromatids at apparently homologous loci as a result of DNA breakage and reunion, produces sister chromatid exchanges (SCE) which can be demonstrated in metaphase chromosomes. The frequency of SCEs is increased by exposure to DNA-damaging chemicals, and the procedure has proved capable of detecting genotoxic compounds in both human lymphocytes and fibroblasts in culture (56).

In Vivo Chromosome Techniques

The most widely used *in vivo* technique is to examine bone marrow metaphase chromosomes from treated rodents following exposure to the test compound, although other tissues have also been used. A variation employs *in vivo* exposure to the test compound followed by *in vitro* cultures of peripheral lymphocytes. This latter technique is especially interesting in that it has been used as a basis for surveying human populations exposed to potentially mutagenic substances (53,57). Although not completely satisfactory, this technique and the urine/microbial assay system provide the only practicable screening tests for human genetic damage *in vivo*.

The classical technique for studying the induction of chromosome damage *in vivo* utilises bone marrow cells from rodents which are processed for metaphase chromosome analysis. The micronucleus test is a modification of this approach, in which residual chromosome fragments in polychromatic erythrocytes are recorded as indicative of chromosome breakage (58,59). The micronucleus test compares favourably with metaphase analysis in terms of sensitivity to many mutagenic chemicals and is regarded as a quicker and simpler technique. However, types of chromosome aberration other than simple breakage, e.g. exchanges and translocation, can be detected only by the metaphase technique. Conflicting results have been reported on the validity of the micronucleus assay as a screening test for carcinogens (60,61), and it may be that assays in which bone marrow cells are the sole target are inadequate to detect the genotoxicity of chemicals that require tissue-specific activation.

Techniques are also available for studying SCE induction in bone marrow cells (62,63). The data base on SCE studies remains quite small, and the mechanism of induction of SCEs and the interpretation of their significance remain unclear. However, the data available do suggest that SCE induction does have a role to play in screening for mutagenic effects at the chromosomal level.

Tests Using Insects

The most widely studied insect for genetic purposes is the fruit fly, *Drosophila melanogaster* (64,65). In addition to its well-characterised genetics, it has the advantage of possessing enzymes capable of carrying out many of the reactions performed by mammalian mixed-function oxidases. A variety of genetic end-points can be detected, but the most widely studied is the sex-linked recessive lethal (SLRL) assay. This assay is based on treatment of f_0 males, followed by detection of a damaged X-chromosome in the f_2 males after mating of f_1 females with untreated males. A growing body of data on testing of chemicals in Drosophila indicate that its potential for identification of mutagens is quite high. The isolation of new strains that are more sensitive to chemical mutagens could improve the spectrum of mutagens that can be detected using Drosophila.

Mammalian Coat Spot Test for Somatic Gene Mutation

The mammalian coat spot test is a modification of the Specific Locus test, but detects mutations in somatic cells rather than in germ cells. The method utilises a tester strain of mice homozygous for a series of recessive mutations affecting coat colour (66,67). A cross between the wild-type mouse and the tester strain results in progeny that are heterozygous for the marker mutations. The female is treated at 8-11 days of pregnancy, when precursors of pigment cells are proliferating. Mutation of the wild-type allele results in an embryonic melanocyte with a mutant phenotype that is expressed as contrasting colour spots in the fur of the fully-developed progeny. The test is sensitive to relatively low doses of mutagenic chemicals, though the chemicals must be capable of passing the placental barrier.

TESTS FOR TRANSMISSIBLE MUTATION

Detection of Mammalian Gene Mutation In Vivo

The major assay for the detection of mammalian gene mutation in germ cells is the Specific Locus test (68,70). The principle of the method lies in the fact that if homozygous wild-type mice are mated with mice homozygous for recessive traits at seven genetic loci, the offspring will be heterozygous at those loci and hence will appear phenotypically as wild-type. If these wild-type parents are treated with a mutagen, a mutation may be induced at one of the seven loci, in which case the offspring will be homozygous for the recessive trait and will express the mutation. In practice, at least 10,000 offspring are raised and examined for mutations at the seven loci. The expected spontaneous mutation rate is 1 in 16,000 animals. Consequently, an enormous number of animals may be required to establish a statistically-significant positive response. Clearly this test is a large, complex, time-consuming and expensive experiment, which would have no place as a screening test, but may sometimes be useful for clarification of effects seen in non-mammalian systems (71).

Detection of Germ Cell Chromosome Damage

The Dominant Lethal Assay

Dominant lethal mutations in mammalian reproduction result in the failure of a fertilised egg to implant (pre-implantation loss) or the failure of an implanted egg to develop (post-implantation loss). In practice, male rodents are treated with a compound, and then mated with groups of untreated females each week for several weeks to sample sperm from all stages of the spermatogenic cycle. Females are sacrificed at day 12 or 13 after mating and examined for evidence of dominant lethality (72). Although the dominant lethal effect is believed to result from gross chromosomal damage, its precise genetic aetiology cannot be determined since the fetuses are not viable. The test has also been criticised for its lack of sensitivity. In conclusion, the dominant lethal assay does not seem to constitute a suitable screening test for mutagenic potential. It may, however, have a significant role in the clarification or augmentation of results obtained from other systems.

Heritable Translocations

Heritable translocations are a direct consequence of chromosome breakage in male or female germ cells (73). They can be detected cytologically by examination of chromosomes in dividing spermatocytes or oocytes or by mating treated parents and examining f_1 progeny for reduced fertility. F_1 males with reduced fertility can be studied cytologically to confirm the presence of heritable translocations. The test has the advantage over the dominant lethal assay of allowing observation of live progeny and of the genetic event leading to fertility loss. The test remains, however, a large-scale experiment that could in no way be considered a screening test. The data-base at present is correspondingly small.

Sperm-head Abnormalities

Sperm-head abnormalities in mice have been shown to arise from treatment with radiation or with chemical mutagens (74). Although a genetic basis for the sperm-head abnormalities has not been firmly established, there is some evidence to indicate that there is at least some genetic control over sperm-head shape. The test is quite simple and requires relatively few animals. However, the chemical spectrum of activity in this test is not yet fully elucidated, though this may emerge more fully from the Gene-Tox programme. An added attraction of this test is that it may be extended to population monitoring, as, for example, in a survey of cigarette smokers (75).

TESTS FOR POTENTIAL CARCINOGENICITY - NEOPLASTIC TRANSFORMATION

The tests for gentotoxicity detect overall genotoxicity of chemicals and can be interpreted in terms of potential carcinogenicity or mutagenicity. An assay that is specifically relevant to carcinogenesis involves the transformation of normal diploid or pseudodiploid cells to a neoplastic state. The ultimate test of neoplastic transformation is the ability of a relatively small inoculum of the cells to proliferate and form a tumour in a suitable animal host. This tumourigenic property is closely associated with certain morphological and growth characteristics that are used to identify transformation in *in vitro* assays. Most available procedures are based on rodent fibroblasts (e.g. mouse C3H 10TI/2, Syrian hamster BHK, hamster embryo cells) though, as some 85% of human cancer is of epithelial origin, the development of assays using epithelial-type cells may be a significant advance (76,78).

Criteria for Transformation

Cultures of normal fibroblasts produce colonies with a characteristic "sheaves of corn" formation, which eventually form a monolayer of cells over the growing surface. When the growing surface is completely covered, cell division ceases, though the cells remain viable in a state described as post-confluence inhibition. Fibroblasts that have undergone transformation form colonies in which the cells show a random "criss-cross" pattern, often three or four cells deep, and confluent cultures are multilayered. This change from ordered to random growth is a widely used criterion of transformation. Another characteristic of transformed cells is their ability to form colonies in semi-solid media such as agar or methocel. Under these conditions, normal cells undergo three or four cell divisions before growth ceases. Transformation removes the need for anchorage to a solid surface, enabling transformed cells to proliferate and form spherical colonies.

Other factors that have been used to characterise transformation include a relatively infinite lifespan in culture, less stringent cultural conditions, increased protease production, reduced cyclic AMP, altered membrane characteristics, and increased fibrinolytic activity.

Transformed epithelial cells rarely differ morphologically from the norm, either individually or in their growth pattern. In some cases there is evidence of increased saturation density and multi-layered growth, but the most reliable *in vitro* criterion of transformation is growth in a semi-solid medium.

The observed properties of transformed cells are acquired sequentially during a period of proliferation after treatment with a transforming chemical. The cell surface changes that influence multi-layered growth and loss of anchorage dependence appear late in the process. Certain cell lines such as baby hamster kidney (BHK21) can form colonies in soft agar immediately after a single exposure to a carcinogen and are considered to be partly transformed in the "normal" culture. Primary human cells (79) require extensive subculture through many cell divisions before transformed clones can be detected.

Assays for Chemically-induced Transformation

Three distinct types of transformation assay are in current use, though validation of each of them is an ongoing exercise. They include Syrian hamster embryo cells (80), mouse fibroblasts C3H 10T1/2 (81) and BALBc 3T3 (82), and the baby hamster kidney BHK21 system (83).

An assay using primary and secondary hamster embryo cells was introduced by Berwald & Sachs (84), further developed by Di Paulo's group (85), and refined as a screening assay by Pienta et al. (78). Hamster embryo cells are seeded at low density on a feeder layer of irradiated secondary hamster cells. After exposure to the test chemical, transformed colonies are identified on the basis of cell and colony morphology. A feeder layer of cells supports a high cloning efficiency in the sparsely-seeded target cells and also provides additional metabolising activity for certain pre-carcinogens. Since embryonic tissues produce a heterogeneous population of cells in culture, the identification of transformed colonies is a subjective procedure and requires a clear definition of transformation criteria. Pienta et al. (80) have carefully standardised the technique and, by introducing cryopreservation and defining criteria for transformation, inter-study reproducibility is very good. These workers have demonstrated a high correlation between rodent carcinogenicity and transformation of hamster embryo cells.

Fibroblasts derived from mouse tissues have also provided valuable systems for investigating neoplastic transformation. The C3H 10T1/2 is representative of this cell type (81). Clones are selected for properties such as sensitivity to post-confluence inhibition of cell division, low spontaneous transformation rate, sensitivity to chemically-induced transformation, and the stability of these properties over prolonged culture. Transformed foci appear as multi-layered groups of cells against a thin, monolayer background.

The third system utilises the growth characteristics of BHK cells in soft agar culture as a measure of transformation (83). The near-transformed state of BHK cells before treatment confers a high degree of sensitivity to the activity of carcinogens. However, great care must be taken in the selection of suitable clones with low spontaneous transformation and in the rigid standardisation of procedures to eliminate the possibility of false results. A standardised and reproducible procedure is capable of discriminating between carcinogens and non-carcinogens with 90% accuracy (86).

The three types of transformation assay described each have advantages and failings. Mouse fibroblasts and BHK cells require additional metabolising activity in the form of rat liver microsomal enzymes. The hamster embryo technique depends on a highly subjective identification of transformed colonies in a heterogeneous cell population. This assay and the BHK assay rarely travel well, i.e. it is often difficult to establish a reproducible procedure in a new laboratory. The BHK system occasionally breaks down and requires regular recloning to obtain cultures with acceptable characteristics.

Two alternative approaches are being pursued in various laboratories, i.e. transformation of primary human cells and assays using rat epithelial cells. Successful transformation of primary human fibroblasts has been described only rarely, though Kakunaga (79) describes characteristic morphological and cultural changes in cells derived from a skin biopsy after treatment of the culture with either 4-nitroquinoline-N-oxide or methyl nitrosoguanine. However, 3-methylcholanthrene failed to induce transformation and the cells appeared to lack the appropriate oxidative enzymes.

Probably the most promising recent studies on in vitro transformation utilise epithelial-type cells derived from rat liver. Epithelial-type cells can be isolated from liver tissue by a variety of techniques (87), and, although a major part of cytochrome P-450 activity is lost fairly rapidly in the primary culture (76), sufficient metabolic capability is retained in long-term cultures to allow the conversion of most pre-carcinogens into reactive forms (88,89). Unlike fibroblast systems, transformed epithelial-type cells do not show the morphological changes associated with transformation, i.e. random and multi-layered growth. Some morphological features such as irregular cell outlines (88) and increased nuclear:cytoplasmic ratio (78) have been described in transformed cells, but these do not appear to be reliable criteria. The most consistent growth characteristic of transformation in epithelial-type cells is proliferation in soft agar (78,90). One drawback to the system is that complete transformation of epithelial-type cells by carcinogens takes a number of weeks before it is expressed as growth in soft agar. Although this may not be a serious disadvantage, efforts are being made to find earlier markers of transformation. A biochemical marker that seems promising is the presence of glutamyl-transpeptidase in chemically-transformed cells and also in cells from hepatocarcinomas (87).

Where transformation assays have been adapted for use as short-term screening procedures, they are generally reliable indicators of putative carcinogenicity. However, the relevance of the findings is dependent, in part, on the competence of the metabolising enzymes and results should be interpreted with this in mind. Neoplastic transformation in cultured cells cannot be equated directly with in vivo neoplasia.

DEPLOYMENT OF SHORT-TERM TESTS FOR GENOTOXICITY

In the International Collaborative Study (8), some thirty assay systems were evaluated for their ability to differentiate between carcinogenic and non-carcinogenic chemicals. As a result of this and similar studies, strategies have emerged for testing chemicals for genotoxicity which are being deployed in many testing laboratories and which are recommended by many regulatory authorities.

The most basic screen consists of a microbial/microsome assay and an in vitro or in vivo test for chromosome damage. The complexity of the basic tests is governed by the nature and potential usage of the chemical. For example, in the early stages of the development of a drug or of an industrial chemical for which widespread human exposure is unlikely, these two assays may provide sufficient information for judging potential genotoxicity. In later stages of drug development or where wider human contact with a chemical is envisaged, the basic screen may be extended to include a mammalian cell assay for gene mutation or neoplastic transformation and may demand an in vivo test of some type, e.g. cytogenetics. An alternative strategy for selection of the basic test battery may be determined by the total tonnage of a chemical manufactured.

Results of the basic screen represent a decision point on the fate of a development chemical or on the handling of an existing product. A second phase of testing may then be implemented to determine the potential carcinogenic or mutagenic risk in qualitative terms. This may include more-complex in vitro assays, in vivo studies for heritable effects, or metabolism/DNA-interaction experiments. The objective is to assemble sufficient data on the genotoxicity, metabolism and in vivo behaviour of a chemical to allow a judgement of its potential genotoxicity under the conditions of use of the chemical. The next stage of the exercise is to attempt to assess the risk of genotoxicity to man in quantitative terms. This subject is still in its infancy and, although several approaches have been proposed, a wider data-base is required before they can be applied in practice.

Tests for Carcinogens

How can these tests best be deployed in order to maximise the chance of detection of a suspect carcinogen? The "tier-system" (91) proposes the use of a single test (e.g. a Salmonella/microsome test) at the first stage, with further stages of progressively-increasing complexity only if a positive response is obtained at the first stage. However, since the correlation between genotoxicity and carcinogenicity is not 100%, it is readily apparent that the effectiveness of such a system is dependent on the effectiveness of the first test. No one test is totally effective in detecting all carcinogens, and even a potent carcinogen such as hexamethylphosphoramide would be missed using the Ames test as the first stage test (92). The alternative system, which has been promulgated in a number of proposed regulatory guidelines, is the "battery" approach in which a number of tests are conducted more or less in parallel, so that a package of data is generated. In this way deficiencies in one test may be compensated for by strengths elsewhere. This view received some support from the International Collaborative Trial (8), from which the general conclusion was drawn that when "two tests using different end-points are considered as a battery, the accuracy increases in comparison with the performance of a single test". There were, however, examples where the use of two tests conferred no advantage. Nevertheless, the use of a battery of tests with a variety of end-points usually gives a very good chance of detecting a genotoxic chemical.

Using the most comprehensive battery of assays currently available, there will still remain a proportion of "false" positive and "false" negative results. These may occur for a number of reasons, the most important being the enormous difference between the metabolic capabilities of in vitro systems and the complex physiological factors that influence the in vivo fate of a chemical. Carcinogenesis is considered to be a multi-stage process, two distinct stages, initiation and promotion, being the most clearly defined. Most of the screening assays are based on interaction of the chemical with DNA and, even assuming that this is a critical event in the carcinogenic process (i.e. the initiation stage), there are classes of carcinogen that have not been shown to interact with DNA. Thus, the mutation-based assays are unlikely to detect these classes of carcinogens or to identify tumour promoters. However, transformation assays are being refined to detect promoters such as phorbol esters (93-95).

Detection of Mutagenic Activity

Epidemiological studies have verified the potential for induction of cancers in humans by a number of agents such as vinyl chloride and beta-naphthylamine, thus verifying the predictive nature of the animal experiments. Such agents are also detected by the tests for genotoxicity, so we may reasonably extrapolate from such tests to man. In the case of mutagenic hazards to man, epidemiologic data are difficult to obtain and interpret. There are data to suggest that genetic disease constitutes a significant proportion of the human disease burden (for review, see (96)), although data are lacking as to what part of this genetic disease burden may be due to chemical mutagenesis. The posture usually adopted is that any compound showing genotoxic activity in a battery of tests may, under suitable circumstances, interact with the genetic material in man to give rise to heritable damage. However, the tests available are not yet capable of allowing risk analysis, and conclusions can only be reached on the broadest basis, by considering the results of mutagenicity tests alongside other toxicity, metabolism and kinetics data.

Tests for Other Effects

There have been suggestions made that screening for genotoxic effects might also give an indication of possible teratogenic activity. Instinctively, this does not seem an unreasonable suggestion. However, the possibilities do not seem to have been systematically explored, although there are isolated reports in the literature of a possible correlation between teratogenic activity and some genetic effect in vitro. For example, Holden et al. (97) elaborated on earlier work of Delatour & Richard (98) in showing that a number of teratogenic benzimidazoles induced significant increases in mitotic index, apparently as a result of spindle disruption. The correlation between teratogenicity and induction of mitotic arrest was not 100% in either direction, due to variations that might be ascribable to metabolic or pharmacokinetic effects. Diphenylhydantoin is also a known teratogen in mice (99), which has been shown to be a mitotic inhibitor (100), although the relevance of animal teratology and cytogenetic findings to man has been questioned (101). The relationship between teratogenic and genotoxic effects in these studies is tenuous at best. Nevertheless, there is sufficient evidence to suggest that further work to clarify the situation would be worthwhile.

DISCUSSION

The animal bioassay for carcinogenic potential has evolved over many years as a large, highly complex and extremely expensive scientific experiment, involving large numbers of animals (usually rodents, but sometimes others), to which a test substance is administered, frequently at high doses, for a large part of their lifespan. At the end of such an experiment, one is still left with major questions in relation to the extrapolation of the results to man. Many questions have been raised about the animal bioassay for carcinogens, but it remains true that almost all known human carcinogens (arsenic and benzene are notable exceptions) may be detected in animal bioassays.

Major criticisms levelled at animal bioassays are their relative insensitivity and inability to detect weak carcinogens, and, in the context of their huge size, cost and duration, their inability to begin to deal with the large numbers of chemicals to which people are exposed in the workplace, in the home and in the environment generally. It is largely in response to these points that mutation-based tests for carcinogens have been developed.

Of all the areas of toxicology, it is probably in testing for genotoxicity that the application of the philosophy of replacement of animals has been most successful. The development of *in vitro* test systems for mutagenicity testing has resulted in a marked reduction in the utilisation of animal tests such as the dominant lethal assay, host-mediated assays and, to a lesser extent, *in vivo* cytogenetics. A major contributary factor has been the development and utilisation of metabolic activation systems.

In testing materials for carcinogenicity, it is questionable whether the development of *in vitro* techniques has yet resulted in any significant reduction in the actual numbers of animals used. However, what has undoubtedly happened is that these techniques, when used as a preliminary screen, have allowed the early elimination of compounds showing positive genotoxic activity. The animal resources devoted to orthodox carcinogenicity trials are thus better employed. In addition, the *in vitro* techniques have probably prevented an expansionary phase in toxicology, since for many industrial chemicals they can provide adequate data to satisfy legislative requirements without the need for additional animal data.

The application and limitation of rodent bioassays are discussed elsewhere in these Proceedings. One major limitation illustrates one area in which the application of *in vitro* or short-term *in vivo* assays may contribute towards a more balanced interpretation of animal studies. Probably the major problem in carcinogenicity testing is the extrapolation of bioassay results to human hazard, and this is almost entirely due to a lack of understanding of the mechanisms of neoplasia and of the significance of species differences in these mechanisms. With increasing knowledge of the mechanisms leading to the development of tumours in animals and, in particular, identification of the critical events involved, then short-term procedures designed to detect these critical events will almost certainly be developed. Such procedures may be aimed at identifying the DNA-interactions necessary for initiation, the relationship between tumour-initiation and gene mutation in mammalian cells, etc. Although it is not possible to reproduce all aspects of mammalian biotransformation of chemicals in an *in vitro* system, techniques can be envisaged in which, for example, the initial events of neoplasia are induced in the intact animal and the subsequent changes leading to overt neoplasia monitored or identified in primary tissue culture. This would allow the introduction of promoters or other modifiers of the process into the cell cultures. This type of approach is being investigated in a number of laboratories and offers the prospect of identifying carcinogenic chemicals in tens, rather than hundreds of animals, and in periods of weeks rather than years.

Other areas of research that appear to offer genuine prospects for progress include refinements of transformation assays to include epithelial cells with intrinsic metabolising activity, wider validation of mammalian cell culture techniques for detecting mutagens, again with cells that do not require additional metabolising systems, and a better approach to in vivo cytogenetics (i.e. using tissues in addition to bone marrow).

SUMMARY AND CONCLUSIONS

The last ten years has seen the introduction of a series of short-term in vitro and in vivo tests that have been used with varying degrees of success to detect chemicals that are potentially genotoxic to man. The number and diversity of the tests in current use illustrate the shortcomings of many of them, and with continuing research it is inevitable that the present generation of short-term assays will be superseded by new tests with better predictive value.

Current practice is to use a battery of assays representing different genetic end-points, e.g. point mutations, chromosome aberrations, and incorporating some form of metabolic activation system. The results of such batteries cannot be accepted as firm evidence of the presence or lack of a human genotoxic hazard, but have a number of valuable applications. They can be used to screen new chemicals at an early stage of development to identify those with possible carcinogenic or mutagenic activity. By testing series of analogues, it is feasible to select non-genotoxic compounds as candidates for further development. Both these applications can produce increased cost-effectiveness in the development of new drugs, food additives and agricultural chemicals. The results of short-term assays on industrial intermediates can be used to establish safe handling procedures in the design of new chemical processes. A further application lies in the testing of existing chemicals to aid the assessment of priorities for animal bioassays. The intelligent use of short-term genotoxicity assays is now an integral part of general toxicity testing. However, the interpretation of these tests in terms of human hazard is not well established and should be approached with caution. Realistic risk analysis is not possible with the present generation of short-term tests.

Further development of short-term tests for the identification of carcinogenic chemicals will be determined to a great extent by progress in the elucidation of the mechanisms of neoplasia. The major task is to identify the critical events that occur during the transformation of a normal cell to an overt neoplastic state, with the objective of developing techniques based on the mechanisms of neoplasia rather than the numerical correlation between the results of short-term tests and animal bioassays.

The whole area of genotoxicity testing is a rapidly changing scene and the existing array of test systems will certainly be refined and changed, possibly dramatically. Further developments will undoubtedly improve the predictive value of *in vitro* tests for carcinogenic and mutagenic hazards to man and will possibly extend to cover other toxicological end-points. Every additional refinement added to the *in vitro* test systems will result in the better use of animal resources. Whether scientifically-valid *in vitro* test systems that will render the orthodox carcinogenicity bioassays redundant can ever be developed must remain a matter for conjecture. At the moment such a situation seems unlikely, and, in any event, even *in vitro* tests are to a greater or lesser extent dependent on utilisation of animals, for example in the provision of metabolic activation systems and mammalian cell cultures.

With the above comments on future developments in short-term tests in mind, a number of recommendations and research objectives have been identified, the main emphasis being on the development of mammalian cell assays to supersede the existing bacterial tests.

1. Development of *in vivo/in vitro* (e.g. primary culture) techniques to investigate the critical cellular, genetic and molecular events associated with neoplastic transformation.

2. Isolation and characterisation of more-appropriate mammalian cell lines, particularly of an epithelial-type, that retain representative intrinsic metabolising activity.

3. Development of sensitive, inexpensive short-term procedures for detecting chemically-induced heritable (germ cell) mutations, e.g. based on DNA adduct formation, etc.

4. Development of *in vitro* mammalian cell assays for detection of chemically-induced aneuploidy.

5. Introduction of *in vivo* chromosome assays of greater sensitivity and relevance than the existing bone-marrow cell procedures.

6. Wider use and refinement of techniques for detecting non-genotoxic carcinogens and promoters.

GLOSSARY OF TERMS (taken from DHSS (5) and other sources)

ANEUPLOID(Y). Cells or individuals with one or more chromosomes of the euploid (see DIPLOID) set of chromosomes absent from or additional to this set. In the case of addition to a basically diploid set of two (or more) homologues, the extra chromosome causes trisomy (tetrasomy, polysomy) of that chromosome. If one chromosome of a pair is missing, the result is monosomy of that particular chromosome (absence of the pair is called nullisomy).

DIPLOID(Y). In general, the body cells of higher organisms are diploid, i.e. they have two homologous sets of chromosomes, one derived from the father and one from the mother. Homologues are similar in size and genetic make-up. The exception is the XY pair in the male, in which the homologues are unequal in size. The general term "ploidy" refers to the number of chromosome sets per cell. The term "euploid(y)" is often used to describe cells (or individuals) with one complete chromosome set, or with whole multiples of the basic chromosome number characteristic of the species.

EUKARYOTES. Eukaryote organisms, in contrast to prokaryotes, are those higher plants and animals whose cells have a nucleus in which the DNA is organised into characteristic sets of chromosomes. Cell division occurs by the process of mitosis or, in the case of gamete formation, by meiosis, when germ cells undergo reduction division.

HAPLOID(Y). The cells of an individual, including the primordial germ cells, possess two sets of chromosomes, one from each parent, and are therefore diploid. In gametogenesis, the germ cells undergo meiotic division, whereby the double set of chromosomes is reduced to one set (the haploid state) in the gametes.

HETEROKARYON. A fungus cell containing nuclei derived from genetically different hyphae.

HETEROZYGOTE. In diploid eukaryotes, each cell (gametes excepted) has two complete sets of chromosomes, one from each parent. The pairs of equivalent chromosomes are called homologous, and are taken to be structurally the same. At precisely equivalent locations (loci) on the DNA molecules of the homologues, alleles (allelic forms) of a gene occur, which serve the same function. Often these pairs of alleles are not identical. If so, one allele might express itself dominantly, at the expense of the other, which acts recessively. However, this is not necessarily so. When the alleles are not identical, the individual is described as heterozygous for the particular gene at the given locus. If the alleles are identical, the individual is described as homozygous (i.e. is a homozygote).

MEIOSIS. The term used to describe that special sequence of cell divisions, and the concomitant behaviour of the diploid set of chromosomes, which leads to the formation of haploid gametes. During meiosis there are two cell divisions which follow each other, but only one round of replication of the chromosomal DNA. This precedes the first meiotic division and is similar to the replication that occurs before mitosis. Subsequently, during the meiotic prophase (see MITOSIS), homologous chromosomes associate as pairs, and crossing-over occurs between homologous chromatids, namely at the four-strand stage; thus there is recombination of linked genes (which results from an exact exchange of genetic material between homologous chromatids). At the first meiotic division, which follows, the previously paired homologues separate from each other, each chromosome consisting of two (sister) chromatids. Where recombination has occurred, the two chromatids (although originally genetically identical) differ genetically. The second meiotic division then follows. This is similar to a mitotic division but differs from it in that the dividing cell has only a haploid set of chromosomes. At this division the chromatids of each chromosome separate from each other. Between them the two divisions give rise to four products of meiosis, all haploid, and all potentially genetically different from each other. In the male, these four haploid products mature into sperm. In the female, only one of them matures into the oocyte; the others form polar bodies.

METAPHASE. A stage in cell division, either meiotic or mitotic, when the nuclear membrane has disappeared, and the chromosomes, in their most condensed form, are arrayed across the equatorial region of the cell, on the fibrous spindle. The function of the spindle is to separate from each other the sister chromatids of each chromosome, at mitotic metaphase or at second meiotic division (or the homologous chromosomes at first meiotic division). If the formation and function of the spindle fibres are inhibited at metaphase, the two chromatids remain attached to each other, and condensed, and this is especially favourable for microscopic study. The substance most commonly employed for deliberately blocking chromatid separation at metaphase is colchicine.

MITOSIS. The process of cell division, whereby the sister chromatids of each replicated chromosome separate from each other and migrate to opposite poles of the dividing cell. The sister chromatids are exact copies of each other and their segregation ensures the transmission of genetic information from mother cells to daughter cells. Mitosis is divided into a number of phases, of which metaphase is of special practical importance. Metaphase is preceded by prophase, and is followed by anaphase, during which the spindle draws one set of chromatids to each pole, where they form the chromosomes within the nuclei of the two daughter cells (telophase).

NEOPLASTIC. An uncontrolled, undifferentiated multiplication of cells, as applied to cancerous growth.

NON-DISJUNCTION. The failure of paired chromosomes to separate at the anaphase stage of cell division.

PLASMIDS. Small elements of DNA found in bacteria, which are separate from the single, circular, bacterial chromosome. They determine properties such as resistance to drugs and bacterial conjugation, and can transfer from one cell to another during bacterial division and independently of the bacterial chromosome.

PROKARYOTES. The simplest of living organisms, namely viruses, bacteria, and some blue-green algae, in which the genetic material is arranged into one chromosomal complex consisting of a single, circular, molecule of DNA (or RNA in some viruses). There is no nuclear organisation, and mitosis and meiosis do not occur, although nucleotide polymerisation (chromonema) replication takes place, and division and multiplication follow.

TRANSLOCATION. Refers to a change in the position of a section of a standard chromosome following its breakage and reunion. A translocation may occur within a chromosome, between one chromosome and its homologue, or between different, non-homologous chromosomes.

REFERENCES

1. Butterworth, B. & Golberg, L. (eds.) (1979). "Strategies for Short-term Tests for Mutagens and Carcinogens". 127 pp. West Palm Beach, Florida: CRC Press.
2. Committee for Proprietary Medicinal Products. (1979). "Notes for Guidance on the Testing of Medicinal Products for their Mutagenic Potential (III) (630/78-Env Rev)". 18 pp. Brussels: CPMP.
3. Dean, B.J. (1980). Short-term tests in the prediction of carcinogenicity. In "Scientific Foundations of Oncology" (ed. T. Symington & R.L. Carter), pp. 31-48. London: Heinemann.
4. DHEW. (1979). "Approaches to Determining the Mutagenic Properties of Chemicals". 84 pp. Bethseda, Md.: DHEW.
5. Committee on Mutagenicity of Chemicals in Food Consumer Products and the Environment. (1981). "Guidelines for the Testing of Chemicals for Mutagenicity", 95 pp. London: DHSS.
6. Hollstein, M., McCann, J., Angelosanto, F.A. & Nichols, W.W. (1979). Short-term tests for carcinogens and mutagens.

Mutation Research 65, 133-226.

7. IARC. (1980). "Long-term and Short-term Screening Assays for Carcinogens: a Critical Appraisal". 426 pp. Lyon: IARC.
8. De Serres, F. & Ashby, J. (eds.) (1981). "Evaluation of Short-term Tests for Carcinogens", Progress in Mutation Research, vol. I, 827 pp. Amsterdam: Elsevier/North-Holland.
9. Leonard, B.J. (1978). Report on the ABPI working party on mutagenicity. Mutation Research 53, 219-220.
10. Seiler, J.P., Mattern, I.E., Green, M.H.L. & Anderson, D. (1980). Meeting report: second European workshop on bacterial *in vitro* mutagenicity test systems. Environmental Mutagenesis 2, 97-100.
11. Grafe, A., Mattern, I.E. & Green, M. (1981). A European collaborative study of the Ames assay 1. Results and general interpretation. Mutation Research 85, 391-410.
12. Von Borstel, R.C., Hastings, P.J. & Shahin, M.M. (1977). Report on the workshop on mutagenesis and predictive carcinogenesis. Edmonton, May 1-6, 1977. Mutation Research 46, 409-411.
13. Mattern, I.E. & Greim, H. (1978). Report of a workshop on bacterial *in vitro* mutagenicity test systems. Mutation Research 53, 369-378.
14. Brusick, D. (1980). Meeting report on the second EMS workshop. Environmental Mutagenesis 2, 431-432.
15. Green, S. & Auletta, A. (1980). Editorial introduction to "The Gene-Tox Programme": an Evaluation in GENEtic TOXicology. Mutation Research 76, 165-168.
16. Brusick, D., Simmon, V.F., Rosenkranz, H.S., Ray, V.A. & Stafford, R.S. (1980). An evaluation of the *Escherichia coli* WP2 and WP2uvrA reverse mutation assay. Mutation Research 76, 169-190.
17. Generoso, W.M., Bishop, J.B., Gosslee, D.G., Newell, G.W., Sheu, C.J. & von Halle, E. (1980). Heritable translocation test in mice. Mutation Research 76, 191-215.
18. Hsie, A.W., Casciano, D.A., Couch, D.B., Krahn, D.F., O'Neill, J.P. & Whitfield, B.L. (1981). The use of Chinese hamster ovary cells to quantify specific locus mutation and to determine mutagenicity of chemicals. Mutation Research 86, 193-214.
19. Latt, S.A., Allen, J., Bloom, S.E., Carrano, A., Falke, E., Kram, D., Schneider, E., Schreck, R., Tice, R., Whitfield, B. & Wolff, S. (1981). Sister chromatid exchanges. Mutation Research 87, 17-62.
20. Bradley, M.O., Bhuygan, B., Francis, M.C., Langenbach, R., Peterson, A. & Huberman, E. (1981). Mutagenesis by chemical agents in V79 Chinese hamster cells: a review of the literature. Mutation Research 87, 81-142.
21. Preston, R.J., Au, W., Bender, M.A., Brewen, J.G., Carrano, A.V., Heddle, J.A., McFee, A.F., Wolff, S. & Wassam, J.S. (1981). Mammalian *in vivo* and *in vitro* cytogenetics assays.

Mutation Research 87, 143-188.
22. Leifer, Z., Kada, T., Mandel, M., Zeiger, E., Stafford, R. & Rosenkranz, H.S. (1981). An evaluation of tests using DNA repair-deficient bacteria for predicting genotoxicity and carcinogenicity. Mutation Research 87, 211-297.
23. Kafer, E., Scott, B.R., Dorn, G.L. & Stafford, R. (1982). Aspergillus nidulans: systems and results of tests for chemical induction of mitotic segregation and mutation. I. Diploid and duplication assay systems. Mutation Research 98, 1-48.
24. Scott, B.R., Dorn, G.L., Kafer, E. & Stafford, R. (1982). Aspergillus nidulans: systems and results of tests for induction of mitotic segregation and mutation. II. Haploid assay systems and overall response of all systems. Mutation Research 98, 49-94.
25. Larsen, K.H., Brash, D., Cleaver, J.E., Hart, R.W., Maher, V.M., Painter, R.B. & Sega. G.A. (1982). DNA repair assays as tests for environmental mutagens. Mutation Research 98, 287-318.
26. Legator, M.S., Bueding, E., Batzinper, R., Connor, T.H., Eisenstadt, E., Farrow, M.G., Fiscor, G., Hsie, A., Seed, J. & Stafford, R.S. (1982). An evaluation of the host-mediated assay and body fluid analysis. Mutation Research 98, 319-374.
27. Anon. (1981). Good response by UK companies to ABPI's questionnaire on testing aids. Scrip 559, 3.
28. ICPEMC. (1980). International Commission for Protection against Environmental Mutagens and Carcinogens. News No. 3. Mutation Research 76, 217-226.
29. Ames, B.N., Lee, F. & Durston, W. (1973). An improved bacterial test system for the detection and classification of mutagens and carcinogens. Proceedings of the National Academy of Sciences, USA 70, 782-786.
30. McCann, J., Choi, E., Yamasaki, E. & Ames, B.N. (1975). Detection of carcinogens as mutagens in the Salmonella/microsome test: assay of 300 chemicals. Proceedings of the National Academy of Sciences, USA 72, 5135-5139.
31. McCann, J., Spingarn, N.E., Kobori, J. & Ames, B.N. (1975). Detection of carcinogens as mutagens: bacterial tester strains with R-factor plasmids. Proceedings of the National Academy of Sciences, USA 72, 979-983.
32. McCann, J. & Ames, B.N. (1977). The Salmonella/microsome mutagenicity test: predictive value for animal carcinogenicity. In "Origins of Human Cancer" (ed. H.H. Hiatt, J.D. Watson & J.A. Winsten), pp. 1431-1450. New York: Cold Spring Harbor.
33. Rinkus, S.J. & Legator, M.S. (1979). Chemical characterisation of 465 known or suspected carcinogens and their correlation with mutagenic activity in the Salmonella typhimurium system. Cancer Research 39, 3289-3318.

34. Rudiger, H.W., Haenisch, F., Metzler, M., Oesch, F. & Glatt, H.R. (1979). Metabolites of diethylstilboestrol induce sister chromatid exchange in human cultured fibroblasts, Nature, London 281, 392-394.
35. Tamura, G., Gold, C., Fervo-Luzzi, A. & Ames, B.N. (1980). Fecalase: a model for activation of dietary glycosides to mutagens by intestinal flora. Proceedings of the National Academy of Sciences, USA 77, 4961-4965.
36. McCoy, E.C., Speck, W.T. & Rosenkranz, J.S. (1977). Activation of a procarcinogen to a mutagen by cell-free extracts of anaerobic bacteria. Mutation Research 46, 261-264.
37. Greim, H., Goggelmann, W., Summer, K.H. & Wolff, T. (1980). Mutagenicity testing with the Salmonella/microsome test. Archives of Toxicology 46, 31-40.
38. Ficsor, G., Bordas, S., Wade, S.M., Muthiani, E., Wertz, G.F. & Zimmer, D.M. (1977). Mammalian host and fluid-mediated mutagenicity assays of captan and streptozotocin in Salmonella typhimurium. Mutation Research 48, 1-16.
39. Falck, K., Grohn, P., Sorsa, M., Vainio, M., Heinonen, E. & Holsti, L.R. (1979). Mutagenicity of urine of nurses handling cytostatic drugs. Lancet i, 1250-1251.
40. Falck, K., Sorsa, M., Vainio, H. & Kilpikari, I. (1980). Mutagenicity in urine of workers in rubber industry. Mutation Research 79, 45-52.
41. Yamasaki, E. & Ames, B.N. (1977). Concentration of mutagens from urine by absorption with the non-polar resin XAD 2: cigarette smokers have mutagenic urine. Proceedings of the National Academy of Sciences, USA 74, 3555-3559.
42. Green, M.H.L., Rogers, A.M., Muriel, W.J., Ward, A.C. & McCalla, D.R. (1977). Use of a simplified fluctuation test to detect and characterise mutagenesis by nitrofurans. Mutation Research 44, 139-143.
43. Stopek, T.R., Liber, H.L., Kvolewski, J.J. & Thilly, W.G. (1978). Relative sensitivities of forward and reverse mutation assays in Salmonella typhimurium. Proceedings of the National Academy of Sciences, USA 75, 4465-4469.
44. MacGregor, J.T. & Sacks, L.E. (1976). The sporulation system of Bacillus subtilis as the basis of a multigene mutagen system. Mutation Research 36, 271-286.
45. De Serres, F.J. & Malling, H.V. (1971). Measurement of recessive lethal damage over the entire genome and two specific loci in the ad-3 region of Neurospora crassa with a two component heterokaryon. In "Chemical Mutagens, Principles and Methods for their Detection" (ed. A. Hollaender), vol. II, pp. 311-342. New York: Plenum Press.
46. Parry, J.M., Parry, E.M. & Barrett, J.C. (1981). Tumour promoters induce mitotic aneuploidy in yeast. Nature, London 294, 263-265.
47. Radman, M. & Kinsella, A.R. (1980). Chromosomal events in carcinogenic initiation and promotion: implications for

carcinogenicity testing and cancer prevention strategies. In "Molecular and Cellular Aspects of Carcinogen Screening Tests" (ed. R. Montesano, H. Bartsch & L. Tomatis), sc. publn. 27, pp. 75-90. Lyon: IARC.

48. Baker, R.M., Brunette, D.M., Mankovitz, R., Thompson, L.H., Whitmore, G.F., Siminovitch, L. & Till, J.E. (1974). Ouabin-resistant mutants of mouse and hamster cells in culture. Cell 1, 9-21.
49. Clive, D., Johnson, K.O., Spector, J.F.S., Batson, A.G. & Brown, M.M.M. (1979). Validation and characterisation of the L5178Y/TK$^{+/-}$ mouse lymphoma mutagen assay system. Mutation Research 59, 61-108.
50. Huberman, E. & Sachs, L. (1976). Mutability of different genetic loci in mammalian cells by metabolically activated carcinogenic polycyclic hydrocarbons. Proceedings of the National Academy of Sciences, USA 73, 188-192.
51. Dean, B.J. (1979). Cytogenetic aspects of mutagenicity testing. In "Mutagenesis in Sub-mammalian Systems: Status and Significance" (ed. G.E. Paget), pp. 135-145. Lancaster: MTP Press.
52. Tong, C. & Williams, G.M. (1980). Definition of conditions for the detection of genotoxic chemicals in the adult rat-liver epithelial cell/hypoxanthine-guanine phosphoribosyl transferase (ARL/HGPRT) mutagenesis assay. Mutation Research 74, 1-9.
53. Evans, H.J. & O'Riordan, M.L. (1977). Human peripheral blood lymphocytes for the analysis of chromosome aberration in mutagen tests. In "Handbook of Mutagenicity Test Procedures" (ed. B.J. Kilbey, M. Legator, W. Nichols & C. Ramel), pp. 261-274. Amsterdam: Elsevier/North-Holland.
54. Ishidate, M. & Odashima, S. (1977). Chromosome tests with 134 compounds on Chinese hamster cells in vitro - a screening test for chemical carcinogens. Mutation Research 48, 337-354.
55. Dean, B.J. & Hodson-Walker, G. (1979). An in vitro chromosome assay using cultured rat liver cells. Mutation Research 64, 329-337.
56. Latt, S.A., Allen, J.W., Rogers, W.E. & Juergens, L.A. (1977). In vitro and in vivo analysis of sister chromatid exchange formation. In "Handbook of Mutagenicity Test Procedures" (ed. B.J. Kilbey, M. Legator, W. Nichols & C. Ramel), pp. 275-291. Amsterdam: Elsevier/North-Holland.
57. Miller, R.C., Hill, R.B., Nichols, W.W. & Meadows, A.T. (1979). Acute and long-term cytogenetic effects of childhood cancer chemotherapy and radiotherapy. Cancer Research 38, 3241-3246.
58. Schmid, W. (1976). The micronucleus test for cytogenic analysis. In "Chemical Mutagens: Principles and Methods for their Detection" (ed. A. Hollander), vol. IV, pp. 31-53. New York: Plenum Press.

59. Salamone, M., Heddle, J., Stuart, E. & Katz, M. (1980). Towards an improved micronucleus test. Mutation Research 74, 347-356.
60. Wild, D. (1976). Effects of indirect mutagens and carcinogens in micronucleus test in mouse bone marrow. Mutation Research 38, 105.
61. Trzos, R.J., Petzold, G.L., Brunden, M.N. & Swenberg, J.A. (1978). The evaluation of sixteen carcinogens in the rat using the micronucleus test. Mutation Research 58, 79-86.
62. Vogel, W. & Bauknecht, T. (1976). Differential chromatid staining by in vivo treatment as a mutagenicity test system. Nature, London 260, 448-449.
63. Stetka, D.G. & Wolff, S. (1979). Sister chromatid exchange as an assay in genetic damage induced by mutagens-carcinogens. 1. In vivo test for compounds requiring metabolic activation. Mutation Research 41, 333-342.
64. Vogel, E. & Ramel, C. (1980). Mutagenesis assays with Drosophila. In "Long-term and Short-term Screening Assays for Carcinogens: a Critical Appraisal", pp. 157-183. Lyon: IARC.
65. Vogel, E. & Sobels, F. (1976). The function of Drosophila in genetic toxicology testing In "Chemical Mutagens: Principles and Methods for their Detection" (ed. A. Hollander), vol. IV, pp. 93-142. New York: Plenum Press.
66. Fahrig, R. (1977). The mammalian spot test with mice. Archives of Toxicology 38, 87-98.
67. Russel, L.B. (1978). Somatic cells as indicators of germinal mutations in the mouse. Environmental Health Perspectives 24, 113-116.
68. Russell, W.L. (1951). X-ray induced mutations in mice. Cold Spring Harbor Symposia on Quantitative Biology 16, 327-336.
69. Russell, W.L. (1978). Specific locus test of the possible mutagenic effect of polycyclic hydrocarbons in the mouse. Mutation Research 53, 256.
70. Searle, A.G. (1975). The specific locus test in the mouse. Mutation Research 31, 277-290.
71. Bishop, J.B. & Kodell, R.L. (1980). The heritable translocation assay: its relationship to assessment of genetic risk for future generations. Teratogenesis, Carcinogenesis and Mutagenesis 1, 305-332.
72. Bateman, A.J. (1977). The dominant lethal assay, in the male mouse. In "Handbook of Mutagenicity Test Procedures" (ed. B.J. Kirkby, M. Legator, W. Nichols & C. Ramel), pp. 325-334. Amsterdam: Elsevier/North-Holland.
73. Generoso, W.M., Cain, K.T., Huff, S.W. & Gosslee, D.G. (1978). Heritable translocation test in mice. In "Chemical Mutagens: Principles and Methods for their Detection" (ed. A. Hollander & F. de Serres), vol. V, pp. 55-77. New York: Plenum Press.
74. Wyrobek, A.J. & Bruce, W.R. (1975). Chemical induction of sperm abnormalities in mice. Proceedings of the National

Academy of Science, USA 72, 4425-4429.

75. Evans, H.J., Fletcher, J., Torrance, M. & Hargreave, T.B. (1981). Sperm abnormalities and cigarette smoking. Lancet i, 627-629.
76. Williams, G.M. (1976). The use of liver epithelial cells for the study of chemical carcinogens. American Journal of Pathology 85, 739-753.
77. Montesano, R., Bannilov, G., Drevon, C., Kuroki, T., Saint-Vincent, L. & Tomatis, L. (1980). Neoplastic transformation of rat liver cells in culture. Annals of the New York Academy of Sciences 349, 323-331.
78. Montesano, R., Drevon, C., Kuroki, T., Saint-Vincent, L., Handleman, S., Sanford, K.K., Defoe, D. & Weinstein, I.B. (1977). Test for malignant transformation of rat liver cells in culture: cytology, growth in soft agar, and production of plasminogen activation. Journal of the National Cancer Institute 59, 1651-1658.
79. Kakunaga, T. (1978). Neoplastic transformation of human diploid fibroblast cells by chemical carcinogens. Proceedings of the National Academy of Sciences, USA 75, 1334-1338.
80. Pienta, R.J., Poiley, J.A. & Lebherz, W.B. (1977). Morphological transformation of early passage golden Syrian hamster embryo cells derived from cryo-preserved primary cultures as a reliable in vitro bioassay for identifying diverse carcinogens. International Journal of Cancer 19, 642-655.
81. Reznikoff, C.A., Bertram, J.S., Brankow, D.W. & Heidelberger C. (1973). Quantitative and qualitative studies of chemical transformation of cloned C3H mouse embryo cells sensitive to post-confluence inhibition of cell division. Cancer Research 73, 3239-3249.
82. Ishii, Y., Elliot, J.A., Mishra, N.K. & Lieberman, M.W. (1977). Quantitative studies of transformation by chemical carcinogens and ultraviolet irradiation using a subclone of BHK21 clone 13 Syrian hamster cells. Cancer Research 37, 2023-2029.
83. Styles, J.A. (1977). A method for detecting carcinogenic organic chemicals using mammalian cells in culture. British Journal of Cancer 36, 558-563.
84. Berwald, Y. & Sachs, L. (1975). In vitro transformation of normal cells to tumour cells by carcinogenic hydrocarbons. Journal of the National Cancer Institute 36, 641-661.
85. Di Paulo, J.A., Nelson, R.L. & Donovan, P.J. (1972). In vitro transformation of Syrian hamster embryo cells by diverse chemical carcinogens. Nature, London 235, 278-280.
86. Purchase, I.F.H., Longstaff, E., Ashby, J., Styles, J.A. Anderson, D., Lefevre, P.A. & Westwood, F.R. (1978). An evaluation of 6 short-term tests for detecting organic chemical carcinogens. British Journal of Cancer 37, 873-959.
87. Borek, C. (1980). Differentiation, metabolic activation and

malignant transformation in cultured rat liver cells exposed to chemical carcinogens. In "Mammalian Cell Transformation by Chemical Carcinogens" (ed. N. Mishra, V. Dunkell & M. Mehlman), pp. 297-318. New Jersey: Senate Press.

88. Williams, G.M., Elliot, J.M. & Weisburger, J.H. (1973). Carcinoma after malignant conversion in vitro of epithelial-like cells from rat liver following exposure to chemical carcinogens. Cancer Research 33, 606-612.

89. Tong, C. & Williams, G.M. (1978). Induction of purine analog-resistant mutants in adult rat liver epithelial lines by metabolic activation-dependent and -independent carcinogens. Mutation Research 58, 339-352.

90. San, R.H.C., Shimada, T., Maslansky, C.J., Kreiser, D.M., Laspia, M.F., Rice, J.M. & Williams, G.M. (1979). Growth characteristics and enzyme activities in a survey of transformation markers in adult liver epithelial-like cell cultures. Cancer Research 39, 4441-4448.

91. Bridges, B.A. (1973). Some general principles of mutagenicity screening and a possible framework for testing procedures. Environmental Health Perspectives 6, 221-227.

92. Longstaff, E., Clive, D. & Pienta, R. (1979). Recommendations for practical strategies for short-term testing for mutagens/carcinogens. In "Strategies for Short-term Testing for Mutagens and Carcinogens" (ed. B. Butterworth & L. Golberg), pp. 90-92. West Palm Beach, Florida: CRC Press.

93. Sivak, A. (1977). Comparison of the biological activity of tumour promoter phorbal myristate acetate and a metabolite phorbolol myristate acetate in the cell culture. Cancer Letters 2, 285-290.

94. Sivak, A., Rudenko, L. & Simmons, I. (1978). Carcinogen-induced neoplastic transformation in BALB/c3T3 cells. Proceedings of the American Association for Cancer Research 19, 36.

95. Colburn, N.H., Koehler, B.A. & Nelson, K.J. (1980). A cell culture assay for tumour-promoter-dependent progression toward neoplastic phenotype: detection of tumour promoters and promotion inhibitors. Teratogenesis, Carcinogenesis and Mutagenesis 1, 87-96.

96. Carter, C.O. (1977). The relative contribution of mutant genes and chromosome abnormalities to genetic ill health in man. In "Progress in Genetic Toxicology" (ed. D. Scott, B.A. Bridges & F. Sobels), pp. 1-14. Amsterdam: Elsevier/North-Holland.

97. Holden, H.E., Crider, P.A. & Wahrenburg, M.G. (1980). Mitotic arrest by benzimidazole analogues in human lymphocyte cultures. Environmental Mutagenesis 2, 67-73.

98. Delatour, P. & Richard, Y. (1976). Proprietes embryotoxiques et antimitotiques en serie benzimidazole. Therapie 31, 505-515.

99. Gibson, J.E. & Becker, B.A. (1968). Teratogenic effects of diphenylhydantoin in Swiss-Webster and A-J Mice. Proceedings of the Society for Experimental Biology and Medicine 128, 905-909.
100. MacKinney, A.A., Vyas, R. & Powers, K. (1978). Morphologic effect of hydantoin drugs on mitosis and microtubules of cultured human lymphocytes. Journal of Pharmacology and Experimental Therapeutics 204, 195-202.
101. Alving, J., Jensen, M.K. & Meyer, H. (1977). Chromosome studies of bone marrow cells and peripheral blood lymphocytes from diphenylhydantoin-treated patients. Mutation Research 48, 361-366.

Cytogenetic Monitoring of Human Populations

D. J. KIRKLAND

INTRODUCTION

There is a popular movement, at present, to use humans as an adjunct to toxicity testing, where possible. However, as it will be impossible to eliminate all potentially mutagenic and carcinogenic substances from our environment, it is just as important to monitor human populations exposed to such substances, in order to estimate the carcinogenic or mutagenic hazard associated with such exposure, and to assess the safety of various manufacturing procedures and the equipment employed.

As many carcinogens and mutagens induce chromosome breakage, the measurement of chromosome damage in the circulating lymphocytes of exposed individuals is a means of monitoring the health risks associated with exposure to chemicals, radiation and biological agents, without having to wait many years for the statistics of mortality and disease which are the usual implements of traditional epidemiology.

Exposure to a variety of drugs, solvents, metals, organic chemicals, radiation, tobacco smoke and alcohol have been shown to present a health hazard in terms of elevated levels of cytogenetic damage in exposed individuals. It has even been possible to achieve dosimetry with such population monitoring: the more extensive the exposure, the greater the frequency of chromosome

Group	No. of subjects	Age (mean ± S.D.)	No. of cells analysed	Gaps		BREAKS						NUMERICAL ABERRATIONS					
						No. of cells with one or more breaks		No. of breaks		Dicentrics, rearrange-ments		Hyper-diploid		Polyploid		Endore-duplicated	
				Total	Per cell	Total	Mean	Total	Per cell	Total	Per cell	Total	Mean	Total	Mean	Total	Mean
Male controls	9	29.2 ±7.7	900	54	0.060	28	3.10	34	0.038	4	0.004	4	0.44	1	0.11	0	0
Male tinters	18	28.1 ±10.6	1800	116	0.064	56	3.10	64	0.036	6	0.003	3	0.17	0	0	2	0.11
Female controls	12	27.3 ±7.4	1200	63	0.053	23	1.90	32	0.027	6	0.005	4	0.33	1	0.08	1	0.08
Female tinters	23	22.9	2300	151	0.066	48	2.09	52	0.023	2	0.0009	4	0.17	1	0.04	2	0.90

<u>Table I</u> <u>Chromosome Aberrations in Peripheral Lymphocytes of Controls and Tinters, Excluding Subjects with History of X-ray Exposure and/or Recent Virus Infection.</u>

Group	No. of subjects	Age (mean ± S.D.)	No. of cells analysed	Gaps		BREAKS: No. of cells with one or more breaks		BREAKS: No. of breaks		Dicentrics, rearrange-ments		NUMERICAL ABERRATIONS: Hyper-diploid		NUMERICAL ABERRATIONS: Polyploid		NUMERICAL ABERRATIONS: Endore-duplicated	
				Total	Per cell	Total	Mean	Total	Per cell	Total	Per cell	Total	Mean	Total	Mean	Total	Mean
Males, own hair not dyed	17	31.8[a] ± 10.1	1700	124*	0.073*	63[b]	3.71[c]	75*	0.044*	9	0.0053[b]	6	0.35	1	0.06	0	0
Males, own hair dyed	10	22.7 ± 5.1	1000	46	0.046	21	2.10	23	0.023	1	0.0010	1	0.10	0	0	2	0.20
Females, own hair not dyed	19	24.1 ± 6.9	1900	107	0.056	29	1.53	35	0.018	4	0.0021	4	0.21	0	0	2	0.11
Females, own hair dyed	16	25.1 ± 6.2	1600	110	0.069	42[b]	2.63[b]	49[b]	0.031[c]	4	0.0025	4	0.25	2	0.13	0	0

a $t = 2.66$, $p < 0.02$ (25 degrees of freedom)
* $p < 0.01$
b $p < 0.05$
c $p < 0.02$

Table II Chromosome Aberrations in Peripheral Lymphocytes of Subjects Dyeing or not Dyeing Their Own Hair, Excluding Subjects with History of X-ray Exposure and/or Recent Virus Infection

Subject	Sex	Age	Type of dye*	PRE-DYE SAMPLE			6-H POST-DYE SAMPLE			7-DAY POST-DYE SAMPLE		
				No. of cells scored	Mean SCE/ cell	S.D.	No. of cells scored	Mean SCE/ cell	S.D.	No. of cells scored	Mean SCE/ cell	S.D.
A	F	41	P	100	10.28	4.27	100	11.57	4.15	100	11.41	3.88
B	F	66	SP	50	9.30	4.04	100	10.67	4.04	99	10.46	3.61
C	F	32	P	100	10.53	3.46	68	9.21	3.81	50	10.68	4.04
D	F	70	P	39	14.92	7.65	45	11.48	4.69	11	11.64	3.50
E	F	53	P	87	9.97	4.15	61	9.71	3.14	54	11.67	4.79
F	F	45	P	100	12.06	4.03	0	-	-	100	12.05	4.57
G	F	54	P	25	13.64	5.37	74	11.82	5.26	88	12.44	4.62
H	M	22	SP	64	8.38	3.61	51	8.86	3.73	85	8.69	3.49
J	F	40	P	85	11.62	4.50	74	11.39	3.81	57	10.54	3.95
K	F	47	P	100	10.57	3.68	61	10.19	3.31	29	8.62	4.05
L	F	44	P	95	11.42	4.38	40	10.68	3.96	24	9.54	3.92
M	F	50	SP	69	9.39	3.89	100	9.79	3.09	88	10.15	3.67
N	F	32	SP	34	12.38	4.22	88	13.19	4.87	13	10.23	4.95
P	F	50	P	68	9.60	3.52	72	10.33	4.33	57	11.16	4.36
Totals				1016	10.77	4.34	934	10.77	4.01	855	10.82	4.11

Table III Sister-chromatid Exchanges in the Peripheral Lymphocytes of 14 Subjects Before and After Hair-dyeing. The Data are Pooled from Duplicate Cultures Made From Each Blood Sample

damage for people exposed to vinyl chloride (1), tobacco smoke (2), and alcohol (3), for example. However, there are a number of pitfalls to be aware of in the organisation of such studies, and I shall use our experiences at the Institute of Cancer Research in assessing exposure of humans to hair dyes to illustrate these problems (4,5).

IDENTIFICATION OF CORRECT POPULATION AND CORRECT ROUTE OF EXPOSURE

As a number of laboratories had shown that hair dyes cause chromosome damage in cells *in vitro*, cytogenetic monitoring of people exposed to hair dyes was a logical step. We chose to look at professional hair tinters as we believed these would show the most severe occupational exposure. It can be seen from Table I that tinters did not have elevated levels of chromosome damage when compared with controls of the same sex who were carefully matched for age, smoking and drinking habits, etc.

When these people were all re-grouped according to hair dye usage (Table II), it was discovered that females who dyed their own hair had significantly more chromosome damage in their peripheral lymphocytes than women, closely matched for age, etc., who did not dye their own hair. Men with dyed and undyed hair could not be matched for age, and older men with undyed hair had more chromosome damage than younger men with dyed hair. We suggested several explanations for these results (4), one of which was that exposure of the scalp rather than the hands, in women at least, was leading to more significant absorption of hair dyes, with resultant biological effects.

This study showed us the importance of accurate matching of groups and identification of appropriate route of exposure.

UNIFORMITY OF AGENT

In a follow-up study, we therefore looked at exposure to hair dyes via the scalp only, and eliminated the need for matched groups by measuring sister chromatid exchanges (SCE) in individuals before and after using hair dyes, i.e. all individuals served as their own controls.

As can be seen from Table III, some individuals showed increases and some showed decreases in SCE after hair dye use. As a group there was no overall change. The fact that individuals chose their own hair dyes - some permanent, some semi-permanent and many different shades - was a problem, because it was not possible to identify whether increases and decreases in SCE were related to particular types of dye or ingredient.

This study highlighted for us the need, where possible, to

have only a single agent or uniform mixture under test for all exposed individuals.

CONCLUSION

Cytogenetic monitoring of exposed human populations can be a useful method in genetic toxicology, but in order to be able to confidently assess a health hazard in such studies, it is critical to match exposed and control groups extremely accurately, to be examining a single agent or uniform mixture wherever possible, and to clearly identify the most appropriate route as well as extent of exposure.

REFERENCES

1. Purchase, I.F.H., Richardson, C.R., Anderson, D., Paddle, G.M. & Adams, W.G.F. (1978). Chromosomal analysis in vinyl chloride exposed workers. Mutation Research 57, 325-334.
2. Evans, H.J. (1981) Cigarette smoke induced DNA damage in man. In "Progress in Mutation Research" (ed. A. Kappas), vol. II, pp. 111-128. Armstrong: Elsevier/North-Holland, Biomedical Press.
3. Obe, G. (1981). Mutagenicity and carcinogenicity of alcohol. In "Progress in Mutation Research" (ed. A. Kappas), vol II, pp. 19-24. Amsterdam: Elsevier/North-Holland.
4. Kirkland, D.J., Lawler, S.D. & Venitt, S. (1978). Chromosomal damage and hair dyes. Lancet ii, 124-128.
5. Kirkland, D.J., Honeycombe, J.R., Lawler, S.D., Venitt, S. & Crofton-Sleigh, C. (1981). Sister chromatid exchanges before and after hair dyeing. Mutation Research 90, 279-286.

Some Comments on Genotoxicity Testing

ERIC LONGSTAFF

I would like to congratulate the speakers on an excellent paper with which, in the main, I entirely agree. Like them, I am anxious that the number of animals used in chronic toxicity testing is reduced, not only for economic, but also for humanitarian reasons. I dislike using animals in experiments, but at this time I cannot see any scientific alternative if we are to continue to develop as an industrialised society, while simultaneously insisting on high levels of safety and hazard-free consumer products.

For the purposes of this discussion, I believe it is important to clearly separate out the principles of *in vitro* predictive screening for potential carcinogens from the idea that we can use mutagenicity tests to identify potential human mutagens: they may be identical tests, but the interpretation is quite different. In predicting carcinogenic activity, we are attempting to identify those chemicals which would cause cancer if subjected to long-term animal studies. We do this on the assumption that cancer is induced by interaction of the chemical, or its metabolites, with DNA, resulting in mutant cells which in some way form the precursors of tumours. Short-term tests, in the main, measure the possibility of a chemical interacting with DNA, and the validation studies that have been done to date use animal data to retrospectively assess the predictive value of such tests. In the early validation studies (1), the tests were selected which were known to react positively to a few potent carcinogens, such as mycotoxins, polycyclic aromatics, and alkylating agents and, inevitably, these tests had a high predictive value when sometimes even arbitrary tests with empirical end-points (cell transformation, etc.) were tested against a small selected population of carcinogens. However, more recent validation studies (2) deliberately used a wider range of carcinogens, e.g. hexamethylphosphoramide, safrole, chloroform, diethylstilboestrol, etc., to assess the limitations of the tests. These studies revealed gross deficiencies in the ability of *in vitro* tests to identify such carcinogens and there is currently another international study (3) attempting to find which tests may identify carcinogens missed by bacterial assays such as the Ames test.

A problem with these studies, which causes me some considerable concern, is that they are currently being "validated" with chemicals which I do not always feel have been adequately shown to be carcinogenic, or at least with chemicals which have been shown to be carcinogenic by methods which need not interest the industrial toxicologist. The sort of compound I mean is, for example, diethylhexylphthalate (DEHP) which has to be termed carcinogenic but this property is only manifest in rats at very high dose-levels (4) and almost certainly results from prolonged perturbation of the animal's physiology rather than from any phenomenon that can realistically be extrapolated to the level of DEHP to which man is exposed. Likewise, I believe it is wrong to use benzene as an example of a carcinogen not detected by *in vitro* tests. I know the International Agency for Research on Cancer classify it as a human carcinogen (5), but the animal experiments to date fail to provide convincing evidence that benzene is a carcinogen. Benzene does, however, cause chromosome damage *in vivo*, but this should not be taken as evidence that such tests are predictive for carcinogenicity, or worse, that it provides further proof that benzene is an animal carcinogen. It follows, therefore, that we need to reconsider what we should expect of short-term *in vitro* tests. I suggest that Ames negatives with DEHP and benzene are the "right" results and the "correct" predictions, and not, as is suggested by some investigators, false negatives. To me the danger is that if we do not clearly define our expectations of short-term tests they may be erroneously and prematurely discredited, and that, I suggest, would be a tragedy.

These validation studies are, of course, *retrospective* studies. That is to say, they employ known animal carcinogens to find the predictive value of *in vitro* tests. Before the true value of such predictive tests can be assessed they will have to demonstrate they can reliably predict the carcinogenicity of "unknown" chemicals; i.e. *prospective* validation studies. In one such study conducted at ICI, an attempt was made to verify the predictions of short-term tests with a series of fluorocarbons (6). To our disappointment, we found one fluorocarbon was very strongly carcinogenic to rats which was not detectable by bacterial or cell transformation tests as potentially carcinogenic (FC133a), and another material, which was Ames test positive, was not carcinogenic at all under the conditions of the test (FC22). However, one such material that we anticipated would be carcinogenic was found to be so (FC31), but in general it can be said that for this group of chemicals, the short-term tests used were totally inadequate for predicting their potential carcinogenicity. Nevertheless, there are examples, e.g. tris(2,3,dibromopropyl)phosphate, which were first detected as potentially carcinogenic by such tests, so they must have a useful screening role to play. It must be obvious, however, that total reliance, i.e. replacement of animal studies by short-term *in vitro* tests, is at this time not practical and it would be foolhardy to suggest it were possible on the current evidence.

Clearly then, *in vitro* short-term tests have limitations which prevent them being adopted as the only predictive tests for carcinogens, and a limitation of the tests worth exploring further is misinterpretation. Take, for example, the case of industrial-grade trichloroethylene (TCE). If it were to be included in a screening exercise, a bacterial *in vitro* assay of the material would almost certainly return a positive dose-related response. The authors of the study would then claim TCE was mutagenic and further claim their test predicted the carcinogenicity of TCE. Superficially, this would seem to be the correct prediction for TCE, since everyone knows this material causes cancer in mouse liver (7). However, the true explanation of all this is more complicated than at first appears.

Industrial-grade TCE contains a trace of stabiliser which is highly mutagenic and totally accounts for the mutagenic activity seen with TCE (pure TCE is not mutagenic). The very low level of stabiliser present is most unlikely to pose any toxicological threat to man, but even so, it could be argued that the predictive tests were right about the carcinogenicity of TCE, even if it were for the wrong reasons. However, when we come to examine the reported carcinogenicity of TCE in the mouse, we find that it is pure TCE which is carcinogenic, and that the mouse metabolism at very high doses of TCE is unique and creates an indirect effect on liver DNA which does not occur in other species (8). It is debatable, therefore, whether TCE should be classified as a carcinogen at all, since it seems the effect is simply an artefact of long-term animal study techniques. If this argument were acceptable, it can be seen that the original interpretation of the Ames test positive is quite erroneous with respect to the potential carcinogenicity of TCE and that great care is needed when attempting to extrapolate genotoxic situations from *in vitro* to *in vivo*. A further serious limitation of short-term tests is that they provide no basis on which to predict carcinogenic potency.

The original claims by proponents of short-term tests that potency *in vivo* could correlate with *in vitro* activity has not stood the test of time. A recent and surprising example of a lack of potency correlation is provided by the results from studies with ethylene oxide (EO). *In vitro* tests of all kinds predicted EO to be a highly potent genotoxin, but in animals the observed level of mutagenic activity was considerably reduced, and chronic animal studies using inhalation exposure indicated only a very weak carcinogenic response (9). Nevertheless, it could be argued that *in vitro* studies accurately predict the carcinogenic potency of EO when administered by subcutaneous injection or by gastric gavage. In both cases a significant carcinogenic response was observed. Which is the correct approach in terms of human risk assessment is not too clear, but I suspect the inhalation route of exposure for EO is the more realistic and the latter two studies are confounded by chronic irritancy factors.

As a biological phenomenon, mutagenicity *per se* can readily be detected by both *in vitro* and *in vivo* short-term tests, and it can be argued that chemicals capable of causing mutation in these tests may be capable of causing mutation in man. However, I know of no example of a chemical causing clinical disorders as a result of mutation in man. However, it is a worthwhile precaution to avoid mutagens in our environment, and this would seem to make good sense, except in the case of unique microbial mutagens. Difluoromethane, for example, seems to be uniquely mutagenic to bacteria (10), and as Flamm *et al.* pointed out in 1977 (11), it seems inappropriate to attempt to control or restrict human exposure to "bacterial only" mutagens. Chemicals causing dominant lethal and other effects in vivo, of course, represent a much more formidable and undesirable threat to human health, and exposure should be minimised as far as is reasonably practical.

To summarise:

1. Short-term in vitro tests are not yet suitable replacement techniques either for the identification of carcinogens or for the prediction of their potency.

2. In vitro short-term tests adequately detect mutagens, but these do not always show activity in man or higher organisms.

3. In spite of these short-comings, I am dedicated to the idea of replacement of animals in toxicology and I am actively looking for ways of reducing the number of animals used in carcinogenicity studies.

REFERENCES

1. Purchase, I.F.H., Longstaff, E., Ashby, J., Styles, J.A., Anderson, D., Lefevre, P.A. & Westwood, F.R. (1978). An evaluation of 6 short-term tests for detecting organic chemical carcinogens. British Journal of Cancer 37, 873-959.
2. De Serres, F. & Ashby, J. (eds.) (1981). "Progress in Mutation Research, vol. I. Evaluation of Short-term Tests for Carcinogens", 827 pp. Amsterdam: Elsevier/North-Holland.
3. International Programme on Chemical Safety (IPCS). (1982). "Collaborative Study of Short-term In Vitro Genotoxicity Assays". Geneva: Division of Environmental Health, WHO.
4. US National Toxicology Program. (1982). "NTP Technical Report on the Carcinogenesis Bioassay of Di(2-ethylhexyl) phthalate (CAS No.117-81-7) in F344 Rats and B6C3F1 Mice (Feed Study)", rpt. 217, 127 pp. Research Triangle Park, North Carolina: National Technical Information Service, US National Toxicology Program.
5. IARC. (1982). Monographs on the evaluation of the carcinogenic risk of chemicals to humans, vol. XXIX, pp. 94-148. Lyon: IARC.
6. Longstaff, E., Robinson, M., Bradbrook, C., Styles, J.A. & Purchase, I.F.H. (1982). Carcinogenicity of fluorocarbons: assessment by short-term in vitro tests and chronic exposure in rats. Toxicologist 2, 86.
7. US National Toxicology Program. (1982). "NTP technical report on the carcinogenesis bioassay of trichloroethylene (CAS No.79-01-6) in F344/N rats and B6C3F1 mice (Gavage Study)", rpt. 243, 231 pp. Research Triangle Park, North Carolina: National Technical Information Service, US National

Toxicology Program.
8. Elcombe, C.R., Pratt, I.S. & Green, T. (1982). The rate of trichloracetic acid (TCA) formation determines the species difference in hepatic peroxisome proliferation due to trichloroethylene (TRE). The Pharmacologist 24, 173.
9. European Chemical Industry Ecology and Toxicology Centre. (1982). "Toxicity of Ethylene Oxide and its Relevance to Man", tech. rpt. 5, 75 pp. Brussels: ECETOC.
10. Loprieno, N. & Abbondandolo, A. (1980). Comparative mutagenic evaluation of some industrial compounds. In "Short-term Test Systems for Detecting Carcinogens" (ed. K.H. Norpoth & R.C. Garner), pp. 333-356. Berlin: Springer-Verlag.
11. Flamm, W.G., D'Anguanno, W., Fishbein, L., Green, S., Malling, H.V., Mayer, V., Prival, M., Wolff, G. & Zeiger, E. (1977). "Approaches to Determining the Mutagenic Properties of Chemicals". 59 pp. Bethseda Md: DHEW.

In Vitro Assays

J. M. PARRY

The two processes of division characterisic of somatic and germ cells, namely mitosis and meiosis, must give rise to exact distributions of chromosomes or chromatids to daughter cells if the chromosome number and genetic integrity of a species is to be maintained as a constant. However, these division processes may be perturbed in some way, such that the resulting cells may become euploid or aneuploid. Euploidy describes chromosome numbers which are multiples of the haploid number, whereas aneuploidy describes chromosome numbers which are not multiples of the haploid number.

Aneuploid cells may result from non-disjunction, which is a failure of paired chromosomes or sister chromatids to pass to opposite poles of the spindle at the anaphase of meiosis or mitosis. Aneuploidy may also result from anaphase lagging, in which chromosomes or chromatids separate normally in the early stages of cell division but one chromosome or chromatid moves slowly to the spindle pole and is not included in the nucleus of either daughter cell.

Aneuploidy resulting from meiotic non-disjunction usually

gives such a gross imbalance of chromosomes as to be fatal. In man, many types of autosomal aneuploids have been found in spontaneously aborted embryos, but only the trisomic conditions of some of the smaller autosomes or the sex chromosomes are compatible with postnatal life unless in a mosaic form (1). Such surviving aneuploids represent a considerable individual and social burden. A number of autosomal trisomies are now well established in man, e.g. trisomy 21, 18 and 13, all three of which show an increased maternal age at birth. At least a fraction of the observed chromosome aneuploidy in the human population may result from the damaging effects of external agents, such as radiation, upon the apparatus of cell division (2).

There is also increasing evidence that chromosome aneuploidy represents an important step in the multi-stage process of carcinogenesis. For example, trisomy of chromosome 15 is the most common chromosome change in murine T-cell leukaemia, regardless of the origin of the condition, whether chemically, physically or virally induced (3). In man, the trisomies 21, 13, 18 and XXY, together with the monosomy XO, all show elevated levels of specific cancers, and chromosome studies of human and rodent uterine cervix have shown aneuploidy and mitotic abnormalities in the pre-neoplastic stages of invasive carcinoma of the cervix (4).

The synthetic oestrogen diethylstilboestrol (DES) has been extensively used by us as a model compound for the study and development of genetic and cytological systems capable of assaying the induction of chromosome aneuploidy. Exposure to this compound leads to an increased risk of vaginal carcinoma in prenatally exposed women (5). In such cases, pre-malignant vaginal lesions show aneuploid DNA contents (6). _In vitro_ exposure of cultured mammalian cells to DES results in induced morphological transformation and high levels of aneuploidy in the absence of induced point mutation (7).

In view of the potential human health hazard represented by the production of chromosome aneuploidy in both somatic and germ cells, it is of importance that we are able to detect and eliminate from our environment chemicals which may have the potential to induce these events. Such chemicals have been named "aneuggens" (8) to distinguish them from those capable of inducing point mutation, although there are now a number of examples of agents that have been shown to be capable of inducing both events.

In our laboratory at Swansea, my colleagues and I have undertaken the development of a series of _in vitro_ assays designed to identify chemicals that are capable of inducing chromosome aneuploidy and to characterise those agents that are capable of damaging the mechanical apparatus of cell division. These assays involve the use of both fungal and cultured mammalian cells and a series of biochemical, cytological and genetic end-points.

The detection of chromosome aneuploidy requires the use of eukaryotic cells with their characteristic chromosome structure and division cycle. At the simplest level, changes in chromosome number may be measured by the use of appropriately marked strains of fungi, in which abnormal chromosome constitutions may be recognised by phenotypic characteristics such as growth on selective media, colony colour and morphology. A number of specialised strains of the budding yeast Saccharomyces cerevisiae are now available which are capable of detecting the production of changes in chromosome number during either mitotic or meiotic cell division (8). Such strains may be exposed to test chemicals, and after plating upon appropriate selective media may be used to detect changes in chromosome number above the spontaneous level.

We have utilised yeast strains to assay a diverse range of environmental chemicals for their ability to induce changes in chromosome number. Such studies indicate that aneugenic activity may be detected amongst carcinogens, tumour promoters, and previously ascribed "non-genotoxic" carcinogens (8-10).

The accurate segregation of duplicated chromosomes during the cell division cycle in all eukaryotes depends upon the functioning of the microtubular proteins of the nuclear spindle. These spindle microtubules assemble during chromosome condensation in the prophase of division, are mechanically involved in chromosome separation during anaphase, and depolymerise during telophase. If the structure of the nuclear spindle is aberrant, abnormalities of chromosome segregation may occur. We have undertaken the evaluation of a number of preparative methods and staining techniques which may be used to study the action of environmental chemicals upon the morphology of the nuclear spindle and chromosomes in cultured mammalian cells.

Preparations of dividing mammalian cells fixed in the presence of appropriate (to the cell line) levels of Mg^{2+} and Ca^{2+} maintain their spindle proteins and cellular integrity. Such cells may then be treated with brilliant blue R and safranin which stain the spindle and chromosomes blue and red respectively (11).

Using the above staining procedure, we have demonstrated that exposure to DES results in dose-dependent disturbances to the cell division cycle. After low doses of DES, structural abnormalities of the spindle and chromosome dislocation were observed. After high doses of DES (>20μg/ml), the nuclear spindle was completely absent, presumably due to the failure of the microtubules to assemble during prophase (12). We have therefore demonstrated the validity of this technique for the elucidation of the biological action of some chemicals which may act as mitotic poisons and are potential inducers of chromosome aneuploidy, an important group at present missed by the current bacterial and clastogenic tests.

Microtubules have been shown to consist of a protein (tubulin) as a structural subunit which binds to the cell division inhibitor, colchicine (13). Procedures have been developed which allow the isolation of a highly-purified form of the colchicine-binding protein from mammalian brain (14,15), under conditions which allow the reassembly of microtubules *in vitro* (16). Under these conditions, the purified protein exhibits the full range of drug binding characteristics of the protein demonstrated *in vivo*.

The ability of tubulin to bind colchicine is one of the primary characteristics of this protein, and methods have been developed which demonstrate not only the binding of this drug, but other chemicals, which have been shown to possess anti-mitotic activity (17,18). These studies have shown that tubulin contains one binding site for colchicine which is thought to reside on the β-tubulin subunit (19).

Assays have been developed, based upon the premise that the binding of radiolabelled colchicine can be determined by the measurement of radiolabelled protein bound to DEAE-cellulose filters. The activity of a chemical that binds at the colchicine site, or at a site near enough to stearically inhibit the binding of the radiolabel, can therefore be calculated by measurement of the inhibition of radiolabel incorporation. This procedure, which is outlined below, is based upon the extraction of microtubule protein from brain homogenate derived from 2-3 week old Syrian hamsters, by an assembly-disassembly procedure originally described by Shelanski *et al.* (15). Immediately before the experiment, microtubules are allowed to polymerise in the presence of GTP, at 37°C, then centrifuged at 10,000 x g for 1 hour to ensure that only microtubules retaining their ability to assemble are used in the subsequent experiment.

^{3}H-colchicine Binding Assay

1. Reassembly of microtubules.

2. Inhibition Treatment

   a. Addition of chemical for 1 hour
   b. Addition of ^{3}H-colchicine for 2 hours
   c. Binding to DEAE-cellulose filters

3. Control Treatment

   a. Addition of ^{3}H-colchicine for 2 hours
   b. Addition of colchicine to 10^{-3}M
   c. Addition of chemical for 1 hour
   d. Binding to DEAE-cellulose filters

4. Measurement of radiolabelled protein bound to filter.

Experiments utilising the procedures outlined above have demonstrated that antimitotic agents are capable of binding to microtubule protein. Some typical results are illustrated in Fig. 1. The mitotic inhibitor podophyllotoxin, used in these experiments as a positive control (18), inhibits the binding of radiolabelled colchicine. Vincristine, an antimitotic agent which binds at a site distinct from both the colchicine and podophyllotoxin sites (20), has been shown not to inhibit the binding of the radiolabel and is used as a negative control. Using this assay, we have been able to demonstrate the inhibition of the colchicine-binding site by diethylstilboestrol and thus to confirm the interaction of this compound with the microtubules, as previously shown with the staining technique.

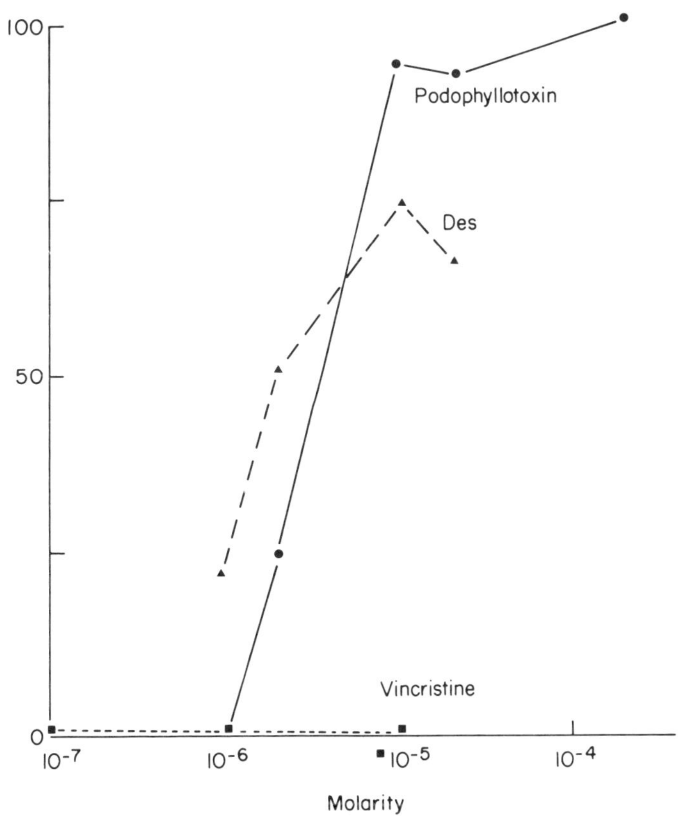

Figure 1 ^{3}H-colchicine Binding

(data provided by Dr D.C. Sharp)

The assessment of changes in chromosome number in mammalian cells by examination of metaphase preparations has a number of different technical requirements from that required to estimate clastogenic activity. First, cells must be allowed to reach their second metaphase following treatment in order to determine chromosome loss or gain occurring at the first anaphase. Secondly, the chances of chromosome loss during slide preparation must be avoided. In an attempt to minimise the latter, Chinese hamster primary fibroblasts derived from liver (CH1-L), kidney (CH1-K) and lung (CH1-P), have been utilised using a number of modified harvesting procedures. In these techniques, cultures were grown on microscope slides, given short hypotonic treatments and fixed in situ. These techniques allow the chromosomes to be retained within the cytoplasm and thus prevents accidental chromosome loss. Chinese hamster primary cells are particularly suitable for this study, since their chromosome number is relatively stable and there is relatively little overlapping of chromosomes on the metaphase plates.

The assay systems described in this paper provide a suitable package of tests for the in vitro assessment of aneugenic environmental chemicals which are capable of inducing changes in chromosome number with the biological consequences discussed in this paper.

ACKNOWLEDGEMENTS

The author wishes to acknowledge the contributions of his co-workers, Dr E.M. Parry, Dr N. Danford and Dr D.C. Sharp, to the development of the assays described in this paper.

REFERENCES

1. McDermott, A. (1975). "Cytogenetics of Man and Other Animals". 301 pp. London: Chapman & Hall.
2. Sankaranarayanan, K. (1979). The role of non-disjunction in aneuploidy in man. An overview. Mutation Research 61, 1-28.
3. Klein, G. (1979). Lymphoma development in mice and humans: diversity if initiation is followed by convergent cytogenetic evolution. Proceedings of the National Academy of Sciences, USA 76, 2442-2446.
4. Spriggs, A.I. (1974). Cytogenetics of cancer and precancerous states of the cervix uteri. In "Chromosomes and Cancer" (ed. J. German), pp. 423-450. New York: Wiley.
5. Herbst, A.L., Ulfelder, H. & Poskanzer, D.C. (1971). Adenocarcinoma of the vagina, association of maternal stilboestrol therapy with tumour appearances in young women. New England Journal of Medicine 284, 878-881.
6. Fu, Y.S., Regan, J.W., Richart, R.M. & Townsend, D.E. (1979).

Nuclear DNA and histologic studies of genital lesions in diethylstilboestrol exposed progeny. American Journal of Clinical Pathology 72, 503-514.

7. Tsutsui, T., Naizumi, H., McLachlane, J.A. & Barrett, J.C. Aneuploidy induction and cell transformation by diethylstilboestrol. Cancer Research (in press).
8. Parry, J.M., Sharp, D. & Parry, E.M. (1979). Detection of mitotic and meiotic aneuploidy in the yeast Saccharomyces cerevisiae. Environmental Health Perspectives 31, 97-111.
9. Parry, J.M., Parry, E.M. & Barrett, J.C. (1981). Tumour promoters induce mitotic aneuploidy in yeast. Nature, London 294, 263-265.
10. Parry, J.M. & Sharp, D. (1981). Induction of mitotic aneuploidy in the yeast strain D6 by 42 coded compounds. In "Progress in Mutation Research" (ed. E.J. Ashby & F.J. de Serres), vol. I, pp. 468-480. Amsterdam: Elsevier/North-Holland.
11. Wissinger, W.L., Estervig, D.N. & Wang, R.J. (1981). A differential staining technique for simultaneous visualisation of mitotic spindle and chromosomes in mammalian cells. Stain Technology 56, 221-226.
12. Parry, E.M., Danford, N. & Parry, J.M. (1982). Differential staining of chromosomes and spindle and its use as an assay for determining the effect of diethylstilboestrol on cultured mammalian cells. Mutation Research 105, 243-252.
13. Borisy, G.G. & Taylor, E.W. (1967). The mechanism of action of colchicine: binding of colchicine-^{3}H to cellular protein. Journal of Cell Biology 34, 525-533.
14. Weisenberg, R.C., Borisy, G.G. & Taylor, E.W. (1968). The colchicine-binding protein of mammalian brain and its relation to microtubules. Biochemistry 7, 4466-4479.
15. Shelanski, M.L. Gaskin, F. & Cantor, C.R. (1973). Microtubule assembly in the absence of added nucleotides. Proceedings of the National Academy of Sciences, USA 70, 765-768.
16. Weisenberg, R.C. (1972). Microtubule formation in vitro in solutions containing low calcium concentrations. Science, New York 177, 1104-1105.
17. Borisy, G.G. (1972). A rapid method for quantitative determination of microtubule protein using DEAE-cellulose filters. Analytical Biochemistry 50, 373-385.
18. Wilson, L. (1970). Properties of colchicine-binding protein from chick embryo brain. Interactions with vinca alkaloids and podophyllotoxin. Biochemistry 9, 4999-5007.
19. Cabral, F., Sobel, M.E. & Gottesman, M.M. (1980). CHO mutants resistant to colchicine, colcemid or griseofulvin have an altered β-tubulin. Cell 20, 29-36.
20. Bryan, J. (1972). Definition of three classes of binding sites in isolated microtubule crystals. Biochemistry 11, 2611-2616.

General Discussion

PETER HODGES

Rapporteur

A recent review of the mutagenicity and carcinogenicity of dyestuffs (Mutation Research 98, 101-248, 1982) indicated that less than 50% of mutagenicity tests were positive and, overall, around 60% of different tests for the same genetic end-point gave comparable results. In view of this disparity between laboratory results how is a potential human mutagen to be defined operationally? The solution would seem to be a more careful use of terms and careful choice of tests for extrapolation to man. Thus, it is preferable to avoid blanket definitions such as "a mutagen" in favour of more precise terms such as "a bacterial mutagen". Although results from bacterial mutation assays indicate the intrinsic mutagenic potential of a compound, i.e. the ability to interact with DNA in such a way as to result in a specific DNA lesion irrespective of test organism, they do not allow direct extrapolation to man. However *in vivo* tests, such as rodent bone marrow cytogenetics, are much more likely to be truly predictive.

We are at present unaware of the critical steps in neoplasia and the theoretical rationale for the correlation between short-term tests for mutagenicity and bioassays for carcinogenicity. However, work currently in progress leads to the expectation of a more detailed understanding of mechanisms of neoplasia and thus more directly relevant tests for carcinogens, probably in mammalian cells, rather than simple numerical correlations between results from short-term tests and carcinogenicity.

Allied to this must be a concentrated effort to define variables in tissue culture systems, such as the need to include serum. This would lead to a vast improvement in tissue culture techniques, allowing the maintenance of cell systems relevant to animals or man for periods sufficient to allow identification of critical interactions at the gene level.

Validation studies need to be carefully controlled to include compounds which are truly "carcinogenic". Thus, diethylhexylphthalate, included in the WHO/IPCS programme, shows a carcinogenic response in rodents only at doses so high as to cause chronic perturbation of the animal as a result of gross overdosing of a non-toxic chemical.

Epidemiology may be extremely valuable in monitoring human exposure. However, it is important to screen human populations only for those effects shown to occur *in vitro* (e.g. chromosome damage) and to recognise that dose-responses may be masked by other exposures.

DES-induced damage to spindle tubulin (as described by Dr Parry) is reversible, and washing out the DES gives recovery and restoration of tubulin synthesis. At high levels, complete "wipe-out" can occur with no tubulin synthesis, no spindle, and cells unable to continue in cell division. At lower levels, aberrations such as multipolar spindles indicate a common mechanism of action between chemically-induced and virally-induced tumours, in a similar manner to murine T-cell leukaemias which are almost always trisomies, irrespective of methods of induction.

Evaluation of Toxicity in Man

N. W. SHEPHARD

INTRODUCTION

Man is always the ultimate experimental animal. Our very survival and evolution has been dependent upon adaptation and on trial-and-error in the selection of food and environment. The evaluation of the safety of any substance is dependent upon our devising techniques and methodologies which enable us to determine hazards that are likely to occur in man and to avoid such happenings. Being realistic, our aim must be to reduce the incidence of undesirable effects to within acceptable limits, both in nature and in duration. The old maxim that a substance which produces no side-effects in man is probably inert, certainly applies to medicines and most probably to many environmentally applied chemicals.

The timescale for gross adaptation phenomena is too great for us to consider, but that man has the power to adapt in the short-term is demonstrated by many cellular activities, such as the proliferation of liver enzymes following ingestion of certain chemicals, e.g. barbiturates.

The purpose of this paper is to consider some aspects of methodology available to us, and currently used, in the assessment of toxicity of compounds in man, and to suggest means by which safety need not be impaired, but animal experimentation may be reduced. This might also serve as an introduction to the issue as to the extent to which man may be used as an experimental animal.

PRELIMINARY SCREENING

The aim of preliminary screening is to determine whether man should be exposed to a substance at all and, if exposed, what side-effects may be produced; what systems or "target" organs may be affected and what pharmacological effects are likely to develop. Do we know or can we hazard a reasonable guess as to the metabolic pathways? Is the substance likely to produce mutagenic or teratogenic effects, and does it produce or induce tumours?

The answer to these multiple questions is sometimes simple. The substance may be so toxic that in no way can one allow man to come into contact with it. Sometimes we can clearly say that toxicity is so marked that any potential benefit to humanity is too high a price to pay. It is the substances which carry no such stigma that we must consider most carefully.

In order to try and answer these questions, there have developed the very extensive toxicological animal research programmes we know today. There are very many variables and idealistic pathways which could be taken; for instance, the matching of animal metabolic pathways to those in man indicating which species of animal should be the one most carefully studied for long-term toxicity. However, this may not be the most appropriate species for predicting pharmacological activity in man. We all recognise that there are difficulties in predicting a chemical's behaviour in man from animal experience. It is equally true that a large number of happenings are predictable.

Some of the difficulties in predicting behaviour in man from animal studies have been reviewed by Fletcher (1). He reported that, as a very approximate estimate for any individual drug, up to 25% of the toxic effects observed in animal studies might be expected to occur as adverse reactions in man; it was also possible to say that the evidence suggested that some toxic effects in animals (particularly gastrointestinal effects) are much more likely to occur in man than others which are commonly seen in animals, but rarely in man (e.g. some CNS effects). Similarly, the negative correlation, although much less frequent, is certainly within our experience, a recent example being the agent which produced hypotension in dogs, but hypertension in man. When, and only when, all this preliminary data have been considered and deemed satisfactory, is the decision made that it is safe, or unsafe to expose man to the substance.

It has to be our opinion in the light of the knowledge available to us today that it would be quite wrong to eliminate all preliminary animal assessments - in spite of their shortcomings.

The very best animal data available to the physician assessing the hazards are derived from rationally devised and carefully conducted animal studies and not necessarily from a list of tests produced by some official body satisfying, in some instances, political rather than scientific requirements. At all times a specific programme has to be devised, and frequently amended, for each substance.

METHODOLOGY IN MAN

The methodology for the assessment of effects in man is divided into stages:

a. Controlled exposure to normal humans for the first time.
b. In the case of medicines, controlled exposure to ill humans.
c. Controlled extension of experience before general availability, including relevant, specialised testing for allergies, photosensitivity, etc.
d. A possible return to animal studies.
e. Post-marketing surveillance.
f. Epidemiological studies.

Controlled Exposure in Normal Humans

The various regimes used at present are all variations on a theme. The exposure commences with a single very low dose of the substance under tightly controlled conditions; this initial dose-level may approximate to 1/100th of that likely to be used and is determined by the results of the toxicity and pharmacologically active levels found in animals. There is a detailed assessment of the effects upon biochemistry, haematology and general physical observations, including ECG and ophthalmological tests, and any other tests suggested by the animal studies. This is then repeated with increasing doses. When the single dose stage is completed satisfactorily, then multiple exposure may be started: this will extend to, say, 3 days, and then to a week, and probably to 14 days or longer, depending upon the substance and the likely duration of use.

The principal areas of exposure are studied. For instance, with a spray that is to be used on fields, one must consider the amount ingested by inhalation and by exposure to the skin. As far as possible, these environmental conditions should be reproduced in the initial testing stages. In the case of some substances, we need to look at special toxicological aspects revealed in the animal testing, for example, cholinesterase activity in the red cells. At these early stages, the number of subjects is small and the gradually increasing doses are taken to a point where it can be demonstrated that there is no effect at the likely level of exposure and above or, in the case of environmental studies, until a factor of several times the maximal estimated exposure has been passed, or that the side-effects produced are acceptable. Also at this very early stage in the study of a new compound in man, it is essential that at each step as much new information as possible is obtained. Not only must toxicological parameters be looked for and tested, but an endeavour must be made to study the pharmacokinetics and the metabolic behaviour of the substance in man. This is not always easy because of analytical problems, but if at all possible, and without resorting to too many radiolabelling studies, this study should be undertaken.

So far, we have considered highly controlled experimental work in a selected small number of volunteers. For an environmental pollutant, be it a chemical, a fertiliser or a food additive, the controlled exposure of large numbers of individuals is not at all easy to arrange; but this is an area for future development.

Controlled Exposure to Ill Humans

Here, we have to determine two effects. First, the efficacy of the chemical as a therapeutic agent, which involves dose-response studies and clinical trials, and secondly, that it is safe to give to patients whose metabolism and absorption may well be altered because of disease conditions.

Controlled Monitoring of Experience, Before Marketing

Finally, there comes the monitoring and development of a substance before it is allowed to be generally released or prescribed. This demands the controlled monitoring of experience in larger numbers of volunteers or patients. So far in the assessment, a relatively small number of people have been used. When the numbers are increased, then some of the toxicological problems which were unsuspected, may arise.

There is a consistent underestimation of the toxicity of new agents and the reasons for this are four-fold:

a. The toxic reaction may be a rare event. It may be an idiosyncratic response, for example, prolonged apnoea after the use of succinyl choline-induced or primoquin-induced haemolytic anaemias and porphyrias produced by drugs. All of these are genetically-induced. Or, an aplastic anaemia may develop, such as that associated with chloramphenicol which has a very low incidence indeed, between 1 in 50,000 and 1 in 100,000 patients. In the controlled monitoring of experience at this early stage, it is unlikely that an effect which has an incidence of only 1 in 50,000 will be found.
b. Rare, toxic reactions may occur only after a longer exposure to the substance.

c. The toxic effect may be unique to man. Reactions between monoamine oxidase inhibitors and cheese, for instance, would never have been determined by animal experiments.
d. There may be an abnormal distribution of the substance in a certain proportion of people; for example, copper in some individuals suffering from Wilson's disease.

From past experience, fenclozic acid was tested extensively in animals before going into clinical trial and was introduced into man with confidence. There was then a quite unexpected onset of jaundice in a few patients. This led to the withdrawal of the drug and a vast research programme into why jaundice had occurred. There was no satisfactory animal model.

A dose of a compound given for one indication may not be tolerated in another. For instance, 6-azauridine is an anti-metabolite and is well tolerated up to a dose of 400mg per day in patients suffering from leukaemia. The drug was administered to patients suffering from rheumatoid arthritis and had to be withdrawn after 2-5 days because of a delayed hypersensitivity reaction, probably related in some way in these individuals to their rheumatoid arthritis.

The Swiss chemical companies have reported upon the numbers of patients who were studied before the development of a new drug was abandoned (2). In all therapeutic areas the mean number of patients was of the order of 181. For drugs acting upon the central nervous system the mean was 203, with a range from 4 to 2539; in cardiovascular drugs and diuretics, the mean was 238 and the range from 24 to 1920. Similar figures are not available for chemicals produced outside the pharmaceutical industry. This does suggest that if we are exceedingly careful in our preliminary studies of any substance in man, without necessarily exposing anyone to serious risk, an assessment can be made as to the hazard of the substance in man, possibly eliminating much animal work. The extension of experience prior to general availability is, of necessity, less well controlled than for the initial human studies, particularly outside medicine.

A Return to Animal Studies

It can be readily seen that if some untoward effect is produced or some unexplained phenomenon is discovered and yet the compound is still worth studying further, it may be necessary to return to animal testing after preliminary or quite extensive exposure in man. A relatively recent experience of this concerns a medicine, aminorex, which had been marketed for a number of years. It was suggested that a very small number of people who had taken the drug were developing pulmonary hypertension. It was therefore necessary to look at the problem in two ways. First, an epidemiological study was undertaken to assess as far as possible just what had happened to patients who had received this drug (3). Secondly, animal studies were set up in species which were known to be sensitive to crotolaria, a substance which produces primary pulmonary hypertension, in an endeavour to confirm a doubtful clinical finding (4). The drug was withdrawn from the market and a very interesting aspect of pulmonary toxicity emerged from these studies which can now be incorporated into toxicity evaluation.

Once a substance is made available for general use, the low incidence of an unexpected effect may emerge. It is clear that for some substances a detailed follow-up of effects should be made prospectively, i.e. a form of post-marketing surveillance, and in the future it may be shown to be necessary for prospective observations in one form or another to be part of the routine in the initial marketing period. Again in recent experience, the collection of data regarding the phenoxyacetic herbicides and the non-steroidal anti-inflammatory agent, benoxaprofen, needs careful assessment, not only to tell us what we might have failed to observe, or where new techniques of study are required, but also to show how the information reaching us is obtained and interpreted. Should deliberate means of obtaining such information be set up? Outside medicine we are still very dependent upon epidemiological studies.

CONCLUSION

We have a moral obligation to do all in our power to ensure the maximum degree of safety comparable with activity for all new chemical entities in contact with man. Our obligation extends to minimising the necessary trauma caused to animals. There is enormous potential for substitutes to animal experiments and we must do all we can to validate these methods. There is considerable potential for reducing animal screening by the sensible selection of appropriate animal models and tests. At the same time, we must constantly review man's role as an experimental animal.

REFERENCES

1. Fletcher, A.P. (1978). Drug safety tests and subsequent clinical experience. Journal of the Royal Society of Medicine 71, 693-696.
2. Bein, H.J., Eichenberger, E., Jung, G., Polzer, C., Stamm, W. & Taeschler, M. (1971). Comparison of experiments and clinical findings: and analysis of clinical trial preparations. Proceedings of the European Society for the Study of Drug Toxicity 12, 179.

3. Gurtner, H.P. (1971). Hypertensive pulmonary vascular disease: some remarks on its incidence and aetiology. Proceedings of the European Society for the Study of Drug Toxicity 12, 81.
4. Heath, D., Kay, J.M. & Smith, P. (1971). A quantitative pathological study of the heart and pulmonary arteries in rats and dogs after prolonged feeding with aminorex fumerate. Proceedings of the European Society for the Study of Drug Toxicity 12, 96.

Drug and Chemical Toxicity in Humans

P. N. BENNETT

This paper considers the study of drug and chemical toxicity in humans by methods that avoid or limit the use of animals. Two types of toxicity may be contrasted: first, that due to industrial chemicals for which even tracer-dose kinetics in humans often do not exist, and secondly, drugs which are taken by man in overdose. Both may present important and changing medical problems that demand the development of rational modes of treatment.

Man is exposed to toxic quantities of industrial chemicals by reason of accident, suicide or homicide. Collection of data from individual cases, though necessary, is a laborious way of building an understanding of the noxious effects of a chemical, especially if it is uncommon. The study of subtoxic doses of industrial chemicals administered to healthy volunteers would provide valuable information, but is seldom undertaken. An alternative approach involving computer modelling is presented. This proved useful in devising approaches to managing toxicity with the herbicide, paraquat.

The organs principally affected by paraquat are the kidney and the lung. Renal failure can be adequately managed by dialysis until recovery occurs, but the pulmonary lesion of paraquat is usually lethal. While the kidneys rapidly eliminate a small dose of paraquat, a curious feature of pulmonary tissue is the slow rate at which it accumulates the chemical (1). Analysis of the plasma concentration-time profile of a bolus of ^{14}C-labelled paraquat in dogs indicated that disposition could be described by a three-compartment open model with elimination from a central compartment (2). A computer simulation of the concentration of paraquat in each compartment appears in Fig. 1a, in which 1 represents the central compartment which includes the plasma and high blood flow organs, and 2 and 3 are rapidly and slowly equilibrating peripheral compartments, respectively. The model is compatible with certain established facts about the disposition of paraquat, since elimination occurs from the kidney which may be considered part of the central compartment, and the lung, which accumulates paraquat slowly, may be represented by compartment 3. Figure 1b describes concentrations of paraquat in the three compartments when the rate of elimination is reduced 19-fold, as would occur when renal failure develops. Now the concentration in the slowly equilibrating peripheral compartment 3 is increased 5-fold. The implication is that renal failure, in itself not necessarily life-threatening, prevents the elimination of paraquat and permits the development of the lethal lung lesion. This computer simulation of paraquat poisoning helped in the evolution of a rational approach to treating paraquat poisoning by drawing attention to the importance of early intervention with haemodialysis or haemoperfusion to reduce plasma paraquat concentration and to protect renal function.

Demands of regulatory authorities ensure that there is adequate information about pharmacological and therapeutic doses of a drug before it is released on the market. Assimilation of data on the effects of overdose presents a more difficult problem. In the United Kingdom most cases of drug overdose are managed in general medical wards and the extra requirements which a special study of overdoses would entail are placed secondary to routine needs of other patients. Thus, a valuable source of information is not being tapped. The answer lies in the establishment of more poisons treatment centres, for such units not only develop special therapeutic skills, but also provide the opportunity to study, in man, metabolism and excretion of drugs taken in toxic doses.

In the Clinical Pharmacology Unit at the Royal United Hospital in Bath, four high-dependency beds are devoted to the management of poisoning and drug overdose. About 400 patients are treated each year from a population of 380,000. Tranquillisers are most frequently taken (38%), followed by analgesics (28%) and anti-depressants (15%).

An example of the type of study that can readily be undertaken in such a unit appears in Table I, which shows the effect of the antidotes methionine and N-acetylcysteine (NAC) on the excretion of metabolites in the urine by a patient who took an overdose of paracetamol (3). In therapeutic doses, paracetamol is metabolised to glucuronide (PG) and sulphate (PS) conjugates, and also by oxidation to a highly reactive intermediate which is inactivated by glutathione and appears in the urine as

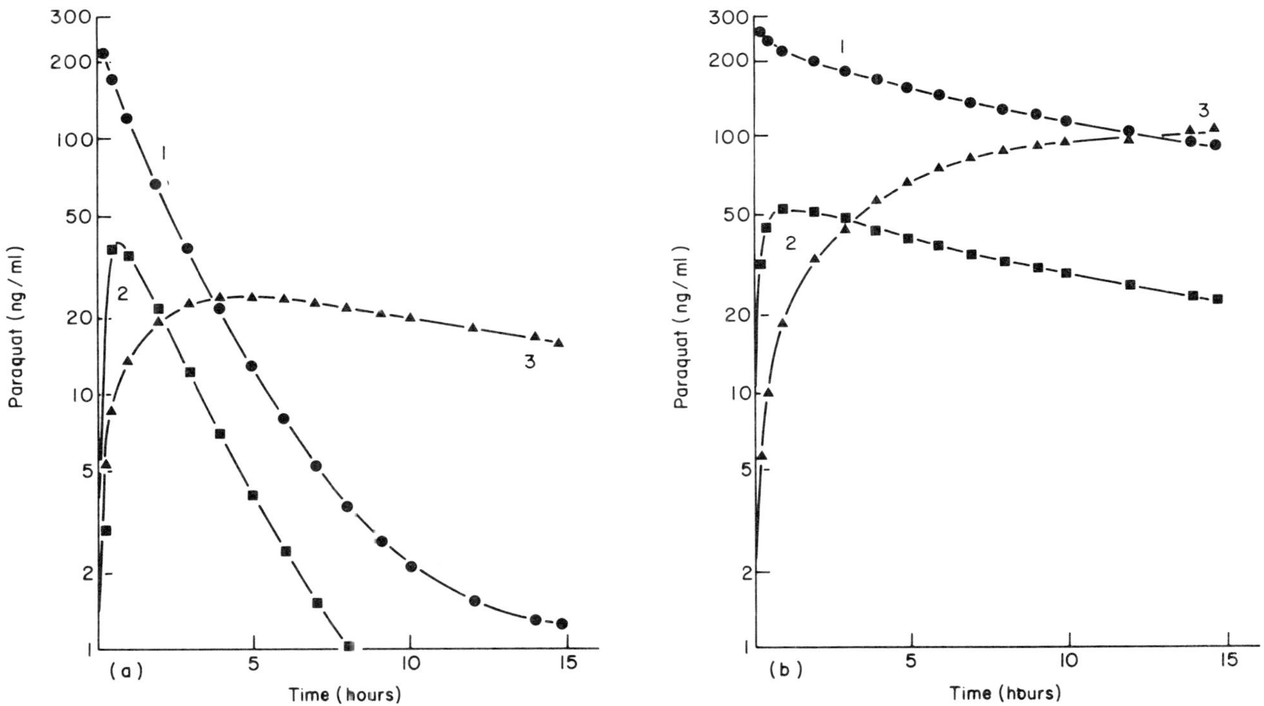

Figure 1 Computer simulation of paraquat kinetics in the dog following a bolus administered intravenously. 1 represents the central compartment which includes the kidney, the only route of elimination, and 2 and 3 are rapidly and slowly eliminating peripheral compartments respectively. The first-order rate constant for elimination from the central compartment in 1b is 19-fold less than that in 1a, simulating renal failure.

paracetamol cysteine (PC) and paracetamol metcapturic acid (PM). An overdose of paracetamol depletes hepatic glutathione and the active intermediate is then believed to combine covalently with cell macromolecules to cause liver necrosis (4). The increasing recovery of PC and PM shown in Table I are compatible with the hypothesis that NAC and methionine replenish hepatic glutathione and combine with an active intermediate of paracetamol.

Table I

Urinary Excretion of Paracetamol Metabolites in a Patient with Paracetamol Overdose (Female, 49 Years)

Time	Event	PG (mg*)	PS (mg*)	PC + PM (mg*)
16.00	Admission	4090	24.9	15.3
16.20	Methionine 2.5 g p.o.	-	-	-
17.00	NAC 9 g i.v.	-	-	-
17.15	NAC 3 g i.v.	-	-	-
19.15	-	3940	308	305
21.20	NAC 6 g i.v.	-	-	-
22.30	-	5752	1287	696
03.00	-	2312	711	198
05.30	-	1443	446	168
07.00	-	98	31	19.7
08.30	-	131	42	35.5

* Expressed as equivalent of paracetamol

See text for abbreviations

(Table I is taken from ref. 3 with permission from The Macmillan Press Ltd.)

However, an additional mechanism is suggested by the rise in PS, namely, that NAC and methionine provide free sulphate for conjugation and that the maintenance of the alternative route of sulphate conjugation is important in protecting the liver against the effects of paracetamol overdose. This information was provided by a straightforward study that involved only the making of timed urine collections and measurement of metabolites. But it was facilitated by being conducted in a ward that is designed for the treatment and study of drug overdose. Such facilities are all too uncommon in this country, yet annually we admit thousands of cases of drug overdose to our hospital beds. By reorganising our services to establish more poisons treatment centres, we would also be creating an opportunity to study drug toxicity in our own species.

REFERENCES

1. Rose, M.S., Smith, L.L. & Wyatt, I. (1974). Evidence for energy-dependent accumulation of paraquat in rat lung. Nature, London 252, 314-315.
2. Hawksworth, G.M., Bennett, P.N. & Davies, D.S. (1981). Kinetics of paraquat elimination in the dog. Toxicology & Applied Pharmacology 57, 139-145.
3. Bennett, P.N., Dixon, A.St.J., Notarianni, L.J. & Oldham, H.G. (1981). Paracetamol metabolism in overdosed patients. British Journal of Clinical Pharmacology 11, 110-111.
4. Jollow, D.J., Thorgeirsson, S.S., Potter, W.Z., Hashimoto, M. & Mitchell, J.R. (1974). Acetaminophen-induced hepatic necrosis. Pharmacology 12, 251-271.

Lessons Learned

W. H. W. INMAN

In this discussion I shall refer briefly to three incidents which have focussed public attention on drug safety during the last quarter of a century. I shall identify the lessons that have been or, in the most recent example, should have been learned and the action that has resulted from them.

Thalidomide

The thalidomide tragedy taught us our first lesson which was, quite simply, that drugs should be used with care during pregnancy. Fortunately, although the media have caused anguish among mothers who took "Debendox" or "Primodos" during pregnancy and subsequently produced an abnormal baby, there is no evidence that these drugs or any others which have been used frequently in pregnancy have been responsible for congenital abnormality. It is true that some workers have demonstrated statistically significant associations between these drugs and abnormalities, but mere association does not prove causation. After thalidomide, systems for collecting reports of suspected adverse drug reactions (ADRs) were established in several countries and one of the most successful has been the British "Yellow Card" system. This has brought many important problems to light over the years, but it has occasionally failed to give early warning of a previously unrecognised hazard.

Practolol

In 1970, the beta adrenergic blocking agent, practolol, slipped through the net of laboratory animal studies, clinical trials and the "Yellow Card" system. For four years doctors failed to recognise that the syndrome of skin, ocular and visceral signs was drug related. Practolol toxicity turned out to have been fairly common and it taught us our second lesson - that existing systems are not always reliable. Animals are often poor predictors of human toxicity, clinical trials are too small and too short to reveal uncommon or slowly developing reactions, and many ADRs are clinically indistinguishable from spontaneous non-drug events.

Benoxaprofen

In August 1982, the licence for benoxaprofen ("Opren") was withdrawn by the DHSS because there had been a small number of reports of death from jaundice or other adverse effects. The reported incidence of deaths was low, probably in the order of one in 25,000, and jaundice was exclusively encountered among very elderly patients. In spite of their rarity, these ADRs were blown up by the media to the proportions of thalidomide or practolol, even though there was no evidence that benoxaprofen is any more dangerous than the majority of non-steroidal anti-inflammatory agents.

Incredibly, we find that not only were the ADRs predictable because of the drug's slow elimination by elderly patients, but that the need to reduce the dosage had indeed been predicted at least 14 months before its withdrawal from the market. A series of papers were published at a symposium on benoxaprofen during the 15th International Congress of Rheumatology, held in Paris in June 1981. Among these were several papers drawing attention to the slow excretion rate. The half-life of benoxaprofen in elderly patients was more than four days. The manufacturers cannot be accused of concealing these results, since they sponsored the symposium, and several of their employees were co-authors of the papers which gave all the necessary clues. Moreover, in September 1981, 11 months before the withdrawal of the drug and at least six months before the jaundice cases were reported, a pamphlet summarising the results of the symposium and giving warning of the need to reduce doses in elderly patients was distributed to prescribers by the manufacturers. If more attention had been paid to its pharmacodynamics in the elderly, benoxaprofen would probably have a respected place on the market today.

Our third lesson is obvious. Drugs that are intended for elderly patients or, for that matter the very young, must be tested in those groups most likely to use them when they are marketed. The very old and frail and the very young are often deliberately excluded from clinical trials because they are more liable to ADRs.

PRESCRIPTION-EVENT MONITORING (PEM)

PEM was developed in order to supplement the "Yellow Card" system, but it was introduced too late to prevent the benoxaprofen debacle. Apart from the "Yellow Card" system, it is the only scheme for post-marketing surveillance functioning on a national scale. PEM is based on the concept of "event monitoring" proposed by Professor David Finney in the early 1960s. If "events", rather than merely suspected ADRs, are reported in defined populations exposed to various drugs, differences in the pattern of the "events" may reveal problems that would not otherwise emerge if reporting is limited to positive medical opinions that the "events" are drug related. If, for example, more patients treated with drug A suffer limb fractures than those treated for the same diseases with drug B, it is possible that drug A is causing hypotension, dizziness or softening of the bones.

THE DRUG SURVEILLANCE RESEARCH UNIT (DSRU)

I established the DSRU at the University of Southampton in June 1980. With the help of the Prescription Pricing Authority, we tested PEM as a method for generating hypotheses about the risks and benefits of new drugs. Using nearly a million prescriptions for 16 drugs already included in the scheme, we are building up very large cohorts for future study. We can reliably identify the 1st, 2nd, 100th, and 10,000th patient who received a new drug. Each prescription identifies a doctor and a patient for whom the drug has been prescribed. Questionnaires (green forms) are sent to large numbers of general practitioners and they are invited to copy the key words already used to describe patients' complaints in the practice notes. Since no medical opinions are required, they may delegate this to a secretary or practice nurse. We chose benoxaprofen and another non-steroidal anti-inflammatory agent, fenbufen, for a pilot study which was aimed at testing the method rather than the drug. In January 1982, we distributed 16,000 green forms to about 9000 doctors and more than half of them were returned. Rapid feedback of results was achieved by means of a personal letter to all general practitioners exactly one month after the green forms had been distributed. The well-known side-effects of benoxaprofen were clearly identified, as well as some problems which had not been reported before. Patients with long-standing disease had clearly benefited from benoxaprofen and many more had reported that they would prefer to use the drug in spite of quite severe side-effects, rather than abandon the pain relief that they had enjoyed. Four cases of jaundice occurred in about 6000 patients taking benoxaprofen, but four more had developed jaundice several months after they had discontinued the drug. This small "signal" of trouble did not justify a special warning at this stage, and while these cases were being investigated we were overtaken by reports from elsewhere which led to the sudden and, in my view, inappropriate, withdrawal of the drug. Fortunately, we will be able to conduct a very much larger enquiry since we had only included about one in six of the patients we had identified by means of prescriptions in the pilot study. This will reveal whether the cases reported to the CSM were merely the tip of an iceberg or whether the drug could safely be reinstated with the proviso that the dosage should be reduced in elderly patients.

Encouraged by the successful outcome of the pilot study, we anticipate that PEM will be expanded to include most or all new chemical entities introduced into general practice. PEM allows us to estimate the incidence of adverse effects and we believe it will also give much greater perspective of the risks and benefits of drugs.

General Discussion

PAUL TURNER

Rapporteur

Professor DOLLERY elaborated on the procedure by which first doses of a new compound were chosen for administration to human volunteers. It is his practice to identify the minimum intravenous dose that produces a measurable pharmacological effect in an animal species, with no evidence of adverse effects. One-sixteenth of that dose is then given orally to the human subject. Depending on the absence or presence of measurable effects, and their nature, a second volunteer may then be given twice that first dose; that is an eighth of the animal dose, and so on, until a measurable effect occurs. Such a study is intensive, involving detailed pharmacokinetic and pharmacodynamic measurements, and extensive laboratory investigation to establish safety in haematological and clinical biochemical tests.

Dr I. NATOFF supported Professor DOLLERY in emphasising the need for tests in conscious as well as anaesthetised animals. He recalled attempts to develop an animal model to investigate the interaction between monoamine oxidase inhibiting antidepressive drugs and tyramine-containing foodstuffs. This interaction could not be reproduced in anaesthetised animals, because the anaesthetic procedure inhibited gastric emptying and so prevented absorption of tyramine.

Several participants, including Dr Susan HAYWOOD and Professor D. CONNING discussed with the speakers the relationship between pharmacological and toxicological studies in animals, particularly the question of whether there is a true distinction between them. In the final analysis, any interaction between a chemical substance and a living organism can be defined in a limited number of ways, whether the result is the basis of a desirable and potentially therapeutic action or of an undesirable toxic effect. There was general agreement that priority should be given to elucidating these basic mechanisms of chemical/organism interaction, and that isolated tissue and cellular models may well prove of value in this research. However, Professor DOLLERY repeatedly emphasised that a living animal, including man, is much more than its constituent parts, and that no amount of isolated tissue research can ever predict the whole profile of a chemical's influence on the function of the intact animal. This is not to say that we are satisfied with present methods of studying adverse effects in animals, particularly where a lethal end-point is involved. New ways must always be sought, which are more economical in numbers of animals used, more productive in the information obtained, and more humane in the treatment of the animals employed.

While there was general acceptance of the need for studying the effects of chemicals in man at an earlier stage than hitherto, concern was expressed that there was reluctance on the part of the community at large to encourage such studies and of ethics committees to approve them. Comparisons were drawn between the opportunities available for testing novel drugs in human volunteers and the difficulty of setting up such studies for other chemicals to which men may be widely exposed or which pose a particular hazard. For example, at least two participants had volunteered in the past to take very small amounts of paraquat under strictly controlled conditions for pharmacokinetic studies, but had been refused permission by ethics committees. Dr M. DRAPER drew particular attention to the need to investigate the effects of drugs and other chemicals in children, whose responses may be very different from those of adults, yet experimental studies involving children were generally positively discouraged by ethics committees and the law. The Chairman informed the Meeting that revised "Guidelines on Toxicology" would be published by the DHSS in the very near future, in which this problem would be discussed. The need for research in children is recognised by many responsible organisations, including the Medical Research Council and the British Paediatric Association. Dr INMAN felt optimistic that the Drug Surveillance Research Unit would be able to give special attention to minority groups such as the young and the old in its analysis of drug-related adverse effects.

Regulatory Aspects

DENNIS V. W. PARKE

Toxicology is a relatively new and rapidly developing science, but the safety evaluation of drugs and chemicals, which has evolved over the past few decades, is predominantly an empirical procedure with only a superficial regard for the scientific principles of toxicology. For example, both the quantitative and qualitative aspects of chemical toxicity show such diverse species differences that the choice of animal species to be used in safety evaluation studies as models for man is of paramount importance. Yet in most cases the choice of animal is more often determined by traditional (more background data available) or commercial (low cost of supply and maintenance, short lifespan) considerations. Furthermore, the selection of doses should be scientifically determined from a knowledge of the quantitative aspects of detoxication and activation of the chemical and of the comparative toxicokinetics in animals and man, and not by the use of empirical formulae of multiples of human dosage and fractions of the LD50 values in the animals studied. To avoid this non-scientific, and often futile, approach to the safety evaluation of chemicals, each chemical to be studied should be regarded as a novel, and often unique, problem that requires a specifically-designed programme of investigation. Regulatory Guidelines should be guidelines and not obligatory requirements.

Following the voluntary or fortuitous ingestion of a drug, food additive, or other chemical, this generally undergoes metabolism in the body to a variety of different metabolites, which may be less toxic (detoxication) or more toxic (reactive intermediates) than the parent chemical (Fig. 1) The parent chemical and/or its metabolites may interact with endogenous molecules or receptors (e.g. enzymes, glutathione, DNA) to elicit pharmacological or toxic activity.

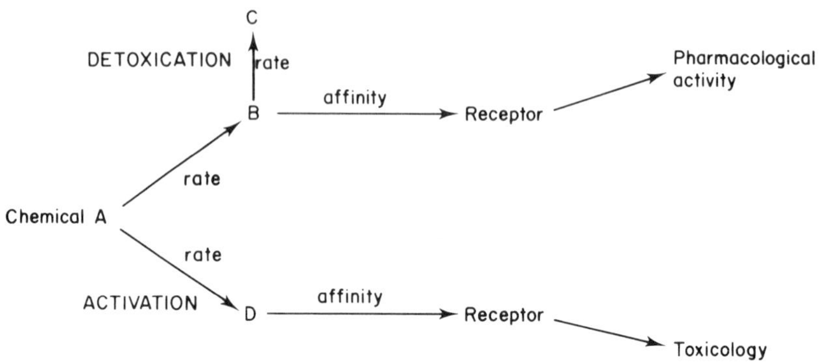

Figure 1 Detoxication and Activation of Chemicals

If, for example, a chemical is metabolised in the rat principally to a metabolite that is not formed in man, there is little point in choosing the rat as the animal model for toxicity testing; if, on the other hand, the dog forms the same major metabolite as man, this would obviously be a more suitable animal model for study. Similarly, the rates of metabolism are also important, perhaps not so much for the selection of animal species for toxicity testing as in the selection of doses and the interpretation of animal toxicity data in terms of its significance to man. Lastly, but not least in importance, are the reactions of the parent chemical and its metabolites with various endogenous receptor molecules which may be involved in the manifestation of toxicity: the quantitative expression of toxicity has been considered to be dependent on the concentration of the reactive chemical at the receptor site, [C], the concentration of the receptors in the tissue, [R], and the affinity of the specific receptor for the chemical concerned, a_R, all of which may vary widely in different species. A quantitative expression for toxicity may thus be expressed as follows:

$$\text{toxicity} \propto [C]\,[R]\,a_R$$

To illustrate the importance of these three fundamental scientific requirements (comparative metabolism, toxicokinetics, and biochemistry - or receptor studies) for safety evaluation studies, I propose to cite a few examples.

The anti-peptic ulcer drug, carbenoxolone, was first evaluated for safety some twenty-five years ago, using a variety of rodent species and rabbits. However, subsequent studies revealed that the drug is metabolised by one pathway (glucuronide conjugation) in man, dogs, ferrets and primates (Fig. 2) and by a distinctly

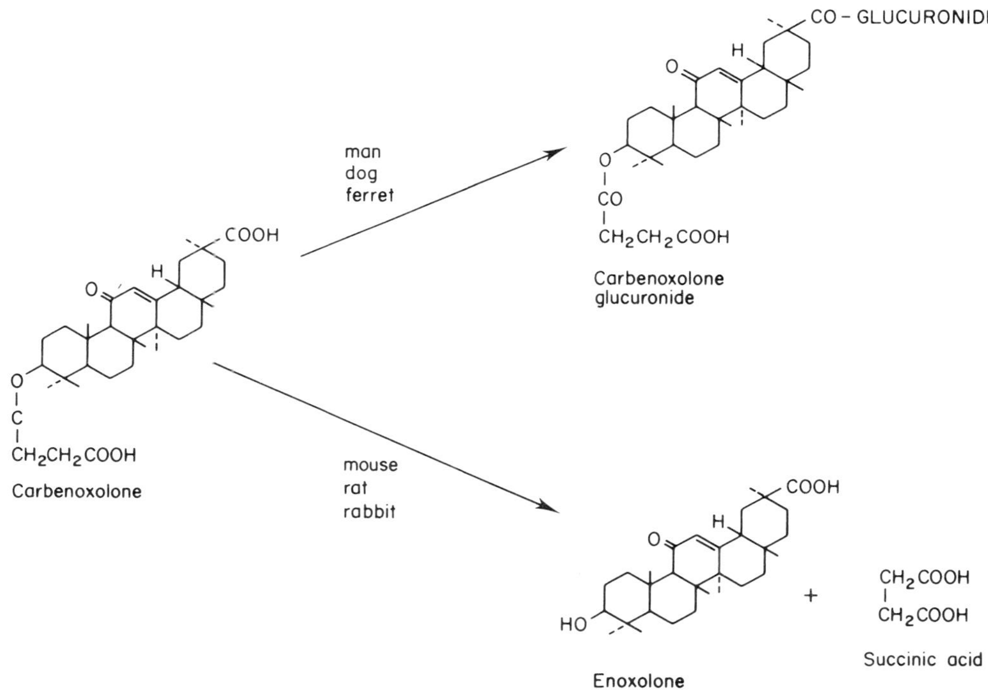

Figure 2 Species Differences in the Metabolism of the Anti-ulcer Drug, Carbenoxolone

different pathway (hydrolysis to enoxolone and succinate, before absorption) in rodents and rabbits, due to the practice of coprophagy in these species (1). As a consequence of these marked species differences, the Food and Drug Administration of the USA considered the rodent studies to be of little value in predicting the safety of the drug in man and required the safety evaluation of the drug to be determined anew in dogs, ferrets and monkeys.

Table I

Species Differences in the Toxicity of Paracetamol

Dose of Paracetamol (mg/kg)	Incidence of Hepatic Necrosis (% of animals)		
	Mice	Hamsters	Rats
150	0	0	0
500	75	100	0
1000	100	100	2

A further example of marked species differences in toxicity resulting from differences in metabolism is that of the well-known drug paracetamol; at a dose-level of 150mg/kg, paracetamol is relatively non-toxic to mice, hamsters and rats, whereas at the higher doses of 500 and 1000mg/kg it results in lethal hepatic necrosis in hamsters and mice, but is still relatively non-toxic to rats (Table I). This is because the liver enzymes of mice and hamsters are readily able to activate paracetamol by N-hydroxylation to the toxic reactive intermediate, whereas the enzymes of rat liver tend to detoxicate the drug; in this case, man behaves more like the mouse and the hamster, and the rat would be a poor model for man in safety evaluation studies of paracetamol. Similarly, the anti-inflammatory drug TA1-284 is readily metabolised by the mouse, but is metabolised extremely slowly by the guinea-pig, and the two species show markedly different patterns of parent drug and metabolites in the plasma concentration/time profile (Fig. 3). This species difference in metabolism has been proposed as the reason for the more prolonged activity of the drug seen in the guinea-pig (2). Yet another recent study has shown that an anti-inflammatory pro-drug that was readily metabolised into an effective anti-inflammatory agent by rat, rabbit, dog and marmoset, was not metabolised into the effective drug by man, primates and the mouse; in this case only the mouse and primates would appear to be suitable models for assessing the pharmacological activity or toxicity of the pro-drug in man (3).

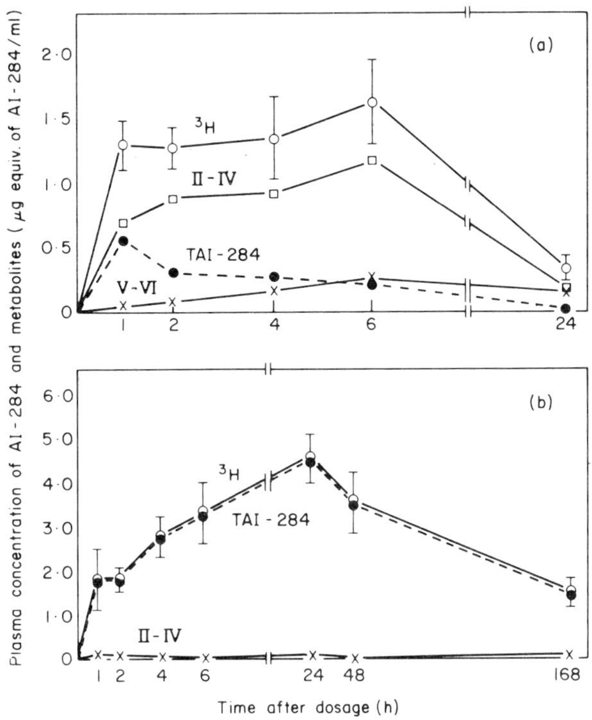

Figure 3 Species differences in the plasma concentrations of the anti-inflammatory drug, ^{3}H-6-chloro-5-cyclohexylindane 1-carboxylic acid (TA1-284) and its metabolites in (a), mouse, and (b), guinea-pig

^{3}H = total radioactivity; TA1-284 is unchanged drug; II-IV = hydroxylated metabolites; V-VI = unidentified polar metabolites.

The importance of the toxicokinetics of a chemical in the selection of animal species and dosage in safety evaluation may be illustrated by the chromone anti-hypersensitivity drug FPL 52757 (4,5). The safety evaluation of this drug was studied in mouse, rat, hamster, rabbit, ferret, squirrel monkey, cynomolgus monkey, stump-tailed macaque, and baboon, and in all these species no overt toxicity was observed at doses many times greater than the intended dose for man. Yet, when administered to patients in clinical trials, hepatoxicity was observed that could be reproduced only in the dog. This has been shown to be due to an anomalous low clearance of the drug in dog and man (Table II), giving rise to higher blood plasma concentrations in dog and man than are seen in other animal species (Fig. 4), so that only the dog would provide a suitable animal model for man in the evaluation of the toxicity of this drug.

Table II

Species Differences in the Plasma Clearance of the Chromone Drug FPL 52757

Species	Dose (mg/kg)	Clearance (ml/kg per hr)
Rat	10	138
Rabbit	10	44
Squirrel Monkey	10	59
Dog	1 - 50	14
Man	1	15

The toxicity of the drug, benoxaprofen, which was recently withdrawn because of the deaths of many patients, was quite unexpected and was not indicated by any of the preclinical toxicity studies in animals. The marked species differences in the route of excretion and in the plasma half-life, with the longest $t\frac{1}{2}$ observed in man (33 hours), should have indicated the need for further kinetic studies in patients and the potential for accumulation and toxicity (6).

The importance of receptor studies (biochemistry) in the safety evaluation of chemicals is, perhaps, best exemplified by the use of enzyme kinetic studies with erythrocyte acetylcholinesterase for the evaluation of the safety in man of various organophosphate anti-cholinesterase pesticides. Receptor studies have also been important in evaluating the significance of carcinoma of the breast seen in beagle dogs used in the carcinogenicity testing of lynestrenol and other oral contraceptive progestational steroids. Determination of the tissue concentration of progestational receptors, of the affinity of these receptors for the synthetic progestational steroids, and of the concentration of the steroids, and their metabolites in the breasts of beagle dogs and humans, indicated that the beagle dog was several orders of magnitude more sensitive to the growth-promoting effects of these chemicals than were humans. The carcinogenicity of these steroids in dogs was therefore considered to be of little or no significance to humans (7). Furthermore, epidemiological studies of humans who had taken oral contraceptives for long periods indicated that there was no significant carcinogenic hazard to women at the dosage used. All that was shown by the very numerous, and often retrospective, animal carcinogenicity studies of the oral contraceptives, with positive results in dogs and equivocal findings in rodents, was that the studies were poorly designed and that the animals chosen for study were unsuitable models for man. In the final event, the carcinogenic potential was studied in humans by epidemiology, and the oral contraceptives were established to be without significant hazard. The animal studies were generally considered to be of little value in establishing safety in humans. Earlier studies of receptors and of the metabolism and toxicokinetics of the oral contraceptive steroids, before undertaking the animal carcinogenicity studies, might have indicated a more appropriate choice of animal species for the carcinogenicity studies, and might have saved the considerable expense and futile use of animals.

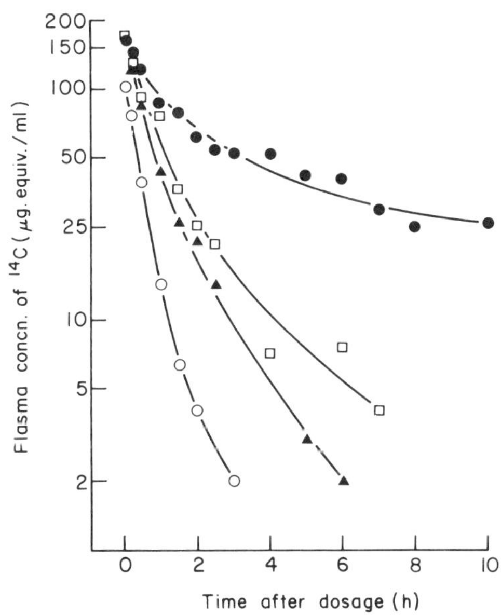

Figure 4 Species Difference in the Plasma Concentrations of ^{14}C Following Intravenous Dosage of the Chromone Drug FPL 52757

Intravenous doses (10mg/kg) were given to the following species: ●——● dog, □——□ rabbit, ▲——▲ squirrel-monkey and ○——○ rat, and the subsequent plasma concentrations are shown above.

The choice of animal species and the selection of doses must therefore be considered from the standpoint of the interaction of the chemical and its active metabolites with susceptible endogenous molecules (receptors) in target organs and tissues. Thus, a knowledge of the metabolism, toxicokinetics and biochemistry (receptor interactions) of the chemical, at varying dosage and in both laboratory animals and humans, becomes essential to the scientific design of safety evaluation studies. By these means, choices of appropriate animal species and doses can be made, which thereby enable animal toxicity data to be evaluated in terms of potential hazard to man. If this procedure were followed, the number of different animal species could be substantially decreased, and the number of different dose-levels decreased, as has recently been allowed by the Committee of Safety of Medicines (CSM) for Clinical Trial Certificates for new drugs.

The determination of acute toxicity by the LD50 test is another example of the empiricism of present safety evaluation procedures. Large numbers of animals are used to quantitatively determine the LD50 values in various species, yet this data is of little value in safety evaluation. Of much greater value, would be a knowledge of the nature of the toxicity, the target organs affected, and the cause of death, all of which could be obtained by clinical and *post-mortem* examinations, using far fewer animals. These principles have been proposed, but were resisted by industry as being too costly.

"The only truly suitable animal species for studying the potential toxicity of chemicals in humans, is man", is a frequently quoted aphorism. With modern analytical technology, it is now possible to detect predictive subclinical changes occurring at very low dosage in man, and to conduct metabolic, toxicokinetic and biochemical studies in human volunteers and patients, which give more-meaningful safety evaluation data and also enable the significance of frank toxicity in animals to be evaluated for potential human risk. Before the present obsession with absolute safety for humans, and the advent of ethical committees, it was common practice - and a relatively safe practice - for not only drugs, but also food additives and pesticides, to be studied in human volunteers, in order to make the animal toxicity studies at higher doses more meaningful. In the safety evaluation of drugs, more extensive studies in patients, especially repeat-dose pharmacokinetic studies, are essential to the safe usage of medicines, but this is seldom satisfactorily undertaken before marketing - or even after marketing. Some aspects of safety evaluation, including immunotoxicity and individual idiosyncrasies - major causes of drug toxicity in man - can be adequately evaluated only by human studies.

A further example of the illogical empiricism of present safety evaluation procedures is the precedence that statistical methodology is given over sound biological reasoning. What is the point of using large groups of animals so as to obtain statistically-meaningful results if the scientific basis of the experiment is unsound because of the inappropriate choice of animal species or dose. The wide variations in toxicity seen in different strains of a single species illustrate the pointlessness of the use of large groups of a single inbred strain of an experimental animal for the safety evaluation of chemicals which are intended for use by such a genetically heterogeneous species as man. Furthermore, without comparative metabolism, toxicokinetic and biochemical data, the biological significance of the animal toxicity data for man, no matter how statistically significant, cannot be evaluated.

Because of all the legislation introduced to ensure the safety of drugs and other chemicals, industry now employs highly competent and experienced toxicologists and other scientific and medical staff. It is to be expected that these scientists would be at least as proficient as academic and government-employed toxicologists in the safety evaluation of their products. Furthermore, it is the industrial company, and its toxicologists and scientists, who are held ultimately responsible in law for the safety of the drugs and chemical products marketed. These industrial scientists and physicians undoubtedly become more familiar with all the diverse properties and problems of their product than can any government-employed toxicologist, with the short time he has at his disposal. Yet the industrial toxicologist's advice on what is necessary to establish the safety of his product, and his interpretation of the significance of the animal toxicity data, is seldom countenanced. The consequence is that guidelines become specific requirements, and each and every aspect of toxicity is routinely studied, so that many unnecessary investigations are undertaken, while other important aspects are not pursued in sufficient depth. The result is that some animals are used unnecessarily. To obviate this undesirable practice, the industrial toxicologist should be allowed more freedom in the design of toxicity studies and in the interpretation of the significance of the results. In this respect, the CSM has again recently changed its procedure for Clinical Trial Certificates and now allows greater participation by industrial toxicologists and physicians and gives them greater responsibility for assessing the safety of their products. This lead by the CSM should be followed by other regulatory bodies concerned with the safety evaluation of non-pharmaceutical chemicals.

The carcinogenic potential of drugs and other chemicals is now considered in very great detail by most regulatory agencies, yet the mutagenic potential, with its far more serious consequences of heritable mutations, is comparatively neglected. The traditional choice of the rat and mouse as species for lifespan carcinogenicity studies is firmly established, no matter how biologically-inappropriate these species may be as animal models for man, for the chemical under test. Comparative metabolism, pharmacokinetic and biochemical data are rarely provided, and even less often considered. When they are considered, as they were in the safety evaluation of the oral contraceptives by the world's numerous regulatory agencies, and in the safety evaluation of pesticides by the Joint Meeting of FAO and WHO on Pesticide Residues (8), the rodent data are frequently seen to be of little value to the prediction of safety of these products in man, and are, therefore, often disregarded. This waste of human effort and expense, and waste of animals lives, should not continue, and the selection of biologically-suitable species with adequate data on metabolism, toxicokinetics and biochemistry to allow interpretation of human risk, should be required before embarking on extensive animal carcinogenicity studies. Even if primates or other species with long lifespans are indicated as appropriate animal models, the use of high doses enables a meaningful assessment of carcinogenic potential to be made in a comparatively short period of exposure (two years). Furthermore, the use of mutagenicity studies, and other short-term tests to cover non-genetic mechanisms of carcinogenicity, are valuable, as the former will predict mutagenicity as well as genotoxic carcinogenicity, and both often offer greater biological significance than is given by rodent lifespan studies. Once again, the CSM has taken the lead in this matter and is allowing a combination of mutagenicity, metabolic, toxicokinetic and histopathological evidence to be substituted, albeit temporarily, for traditional carcinogenicity testing.

Finally, it is imperative in seeking to decrease the number of animal experiments by rationalising the safety evaluation of chemicals on a more scientific basis, to achieve some degree of international harmonisation, as without this, little or nothing can be achieved. When a company initiates safety evaluation studies on a new product, it is seldom considering only the home market, as it would now generally be uneconomic to do so. The major market, and the most exacting when it comes to establishing the safety of the product, is the USA, but regulatory authorities in the EEC and WHO/FAO have also usually to be considered. Fortunately, the requirements of all these different regulatory bodies are fairly similar. However, this means that any major change effected only in the UK would have little effect on the number of animals used in toxicological studies, as the more extensive studies would have to be completed anyway, to satisfy the regulatory authorities of countries overseas. Failure to do this would result in loss of markets, and would ultimately result in the collapse of some of our commercially most successful industries, with consequent loss of employment. Britain has already taken the lead, by virtue of the recent changes initiated by the CSM, to introduce many of the changes I have suggested and the task now is to extend these developments to the world scene.

The safety evaluation of drugs and chemicals is now an

essential aspect of public health, and should in no way be diminished in standards. However, it is possible, by the application of current scientific knowledge and modern technology, to achieve an even greater level of safety at lower cost and with the use of considerably fewer animals. This is already beginning to occur in the UK and we have now to convince other countries, particularly the USA, of the many advantages of applying new scientific methods to this problem.

RECOMMENDATIONS

My recommendations for decreasing the number of animals used in safety evaluation studies of chemicals are therefore:

1. The approach to safety evaluation should be scientific and not empirical or commercial. Each new chemical to be tested should be regarded as a novel problem in toxicology. The choice of animal species as models for man is critical and must be scientifically based on evidence obtained from metabolism, toxicokinetic and biochemical (mechanisms) data. If these principles are followed, one scientifically selected species would be more appropriate than the present two or more empirically selected species and, in many cases, fewer dose-levels might be necessary.

2. More responsibility should be given to industrial toxicologists and physicians to plan and interpret their safety evaluation studies. This should result in animals being used in meaningful studies and not merely to comply with guidelines or standardised requirements.

3. More studies to be undertaken in man, especially metabolism, toxicokinetic and biochemical (mechanisms) studies. With presently available, highly sensitive analytical methods, much truly predictive data can be obtained with low, non-toxic doses. In short, more low-dose studies in man and fewer high-dose studies in experimental animals are needed. This applies not only to drugs, but also to food additives and pesticides which, a few years ago, were more frequently studied in man than they are today.

4. The present requirements for LD50 studies should be replaced with more-detailed acute toxicity studies using fewer animals of each species. The empirical counting of cadavers using large numbers of animals should be replaced by full clinical and <u>post-mortem</u> studies to establish the nature of the toxicity at different doses, the target organ(s) and the cause of death, using fewer animals of each species.

5. Smaller groups of animals should be used, as interspecies and interstrain differences in toxicity are so great that statistical analysis is of small consequence when the biological significance of the animal studies to predicting human toxicity is unknown.

6. The continued choice of large groups of rats and mice for carcinogenicity studies has little or no scientific basis, and the data obtained is frequently misleading and is increasingly being discounted worldwide. These traditional rodent carcinogenicity studies should be replaced by batteries of mutagenicity and other "short-term" tests, and by the use of smaller groups of animal species that have been shown scientifically to be appropriate models for man, for the particular chemical under study.

7. Efforts should be made to obtain harmonisation of the requirements for safety evaluation of chemicals between such organisations as WHO, EEC, OECD and the USA.

REFERENCES

1. Iveson, P., Lindup, W.E., Parke, D.V. & Williams, R.T. (1971). The metabolism of carbenoxolone in the rat. Xenobiotica 1, 79-95.
2. Tanayama, S. (1973). Metabolism of 6-chloro-5-cyclohexylindane-1-carboxylic acid (TAI-284), a new non-steroid anti-inflammatory agent. I. Absorption and distribution and excretion in rats. Xenobiotica 3, 643-656.
3. Marten, T.R., Ruane, R.J., East, P.B. & Malcolm, S.L. (1983). Species variations in the metabolism of the anti-inflammatory cinnamate ester pro-drug, Ro 03-6037. Xenobiotica (in press).
4. Clark, B., Smith, D.A., Eason, C.T. & Parke, D.V. (1982). Metabolism and excretion of a chromone carboxylic acid (FPL 52727) in various animal species. Xenobiotica 12, 147-153.
5. Eason, C.T., Parke, D.V., Clark, B. & Smith, D.A. (1982). The mechanism of hepatotoxicity of a chromone carboxylic acid (FPL 52727) in the dog. Xenobiotica 12, 155-164.
6. Chatfield, D.H. & Green, J.N. (1978). Disposition and metabolism of benoxaprofen in laboratory animals and man. Xenobiotica 8, 133-144.
7. Committee of Safety of Medicines. (1979). Medicines Act Information Letter No. 25, p. 2, London: DHSS
8. Joint Meeting of FAO and WHO on Pesticide Residues (1981). FAO Plant Production and Protection Paper 26, pp. 6-7 and 53-56. Rome: FAO

The Need for Flexibility

ANDREW COCKBURN

Each day we are exposed to a diverse range of chemicals, an exposure which begins to all intents and purposes prior to conception and continues until death. The chemicals include a wide range of food additives, cosmetics, drugs, agrochemicals, household products and industrial chemicals. The level of exposure may be extensive, unavoidable, and is frequently unknown. In these circumstances, it is not surprising that regulatory bodies must exist to control the spread of new chemicals and thereby prevent undue hazard to man and his environment. Governmental agencies worldwide exercise this regulation by legislation, which in part calls for toxicological testing aimed at predicting risk. Such testing, while empirical, has been largely successful and, in the absence of better knowledge, a framework of toxicity tests has evolved which has broad international agreement. National and supranational authorities have not been slow in adopting such testing schemes and most issue their interpretation as guidelines, which in some cases, as in the UK, are guidelines, but which in perhaps the majority of cases are rather inflexible, or even mandatory, requirements.

It is in this context that I believe greater flexibility is the key to the future development, and even survival, of toxicology as a credible science. It is a fascinating paradox that just as too little legislation can jeopardise public safety, so can too much. My plea is that the professional toxicologist should be accorded the flexibility to do only that which is necessary for the most relevant toxicological evaluation of a novel drug or chemical. More tests with more animals do not automatically lead to the development of safer chemicals and yet we are frequently required to repeat studies with minor variations to meet the idiosyncracies of certain regulatory authorities. How safe is safe? The appreciation of risk is a value judgement and can never be absolute.

Each chemical undergoing toxicological evaluation should be subjected to a uniquely tailored programme, developed from a base-set of acute and subacute studies according to the specific properties and intended use of the material. In this respect, the UK has made a notable contribution with its new CTC exemption scheme.

Wherever possible, tests should be performed once and once only with fewer animals, studied for a more appropriate period of time, to a more critical protocol (is the study really necessary?), and with the maximum practicable information being obtained from each animal killed. Alternative tests should not be introduced until they have been fully validated. For drugs, the literature on animal toxicology contains a number of notable false positives and false negatives for predicting effects in man. Thus, early entry into man to establish tolerance and handling is essential, with return to relevant animal species to amplify and extend findings as necessary. Sadly, there are those who say that it is easier to follow regulatory guidelines without a murmur than to challenge redundancy or unnecessary practice. However, safety does not result from inactivity. Any fixed scheme that is employed is likely to become inadequate or excessive as a greater scientific appreciation of the subject is gained. Nevertheless, it is recognised that guidelines do have an important role to play in embracing contemporary wisdom in toxicity testing - the ultimate objective being supranational harmonisation. Above all, however, the safety evaluation of novel chemicals will be improved by understanding the mechanisms of toxicity which must be the fundamental goal in the development of the science. This objective cannot be served by the slavish following of so-called "regulotox" alone. That flexibility and adaptation to change is required cannot be in dispute, particularly with the rapid emergence of the novel and highly potent products of biotechnology and other so-called "biologicals", many of which may be immunogenic and cannot undergo conventional toxicity testing: monoclonal antibodies, for example. Increased scientific exchange between the toxicologist and the regulatory bodies would clearly be a prerequisite in such a system, with the onus very much on the investigator to support his strategy. The advantages of more apposite toxicology would be earlier chemical selection, with shorter development times, which would in turn make more resources available for fundamental research into mechanisms of toxicity and into therapeutic areas which are currently of less commercial interest, but of great medical importance.

Lastly, how would a more mechanistic and flexible approach to toxicity testing impinge on the objectives of FRAME? History has shown that where mechanism becomes known animals frequently become redundant, as in the case of the miner's canary and the frog for pregnancy testing. Our present dilemma was summed up most eloquently by Sir Peter Medawar in 1971 (1):

> "I think that the use of experimental animals on the present scale is a temporary episode in biological and medical

history..... In the meantime, we must grapple with the paradox that nothing but research on animals will provide us with the knowledge that will make it possible for us, one day, to dispense with the use of them altogether".

REFERENCE

1. Medawar, P.B. (1972). "The Hope of Progress", 86 pp. London: Methuen.

Consultation with the Regulatory Authorities

A. N. WORDEN

In the Annual Lecture to BIBRA on 11 October 1982, Emil Poulsen highlighted one deficiency of the present day system as the lack of good quality scientists within regulatory bodies - ascribing this to inadequate levels of remuneration - pessimistically concluding that there was nothing that could be done about it. His description conjured up visions of human analogues of those improperly fed, overweight, bored, confined and sex-starved rats described earlier in this Meeting by Dr Francis Roe. However, in the contributions of Dr J. Griffin and Dr Wintersgill, for which we are most grateful, we have evidence that in this country it is still possible to receive guidance from this quarter. On a worldwide basis, a greater problem is posed by the barriers so often found between regulatory scientists and those representing industry, contract research organisations and other bodies concerned with providing information relevant to the safe introduction of new materials. My understanding is that, even in the UK, there were immediate repercussions from the placing of the Medicines Act of 1968 upon the Statute Book. Gone, it seemed, were the halcyon days when the revered Sir Derrick Dunlop went out and about to give freely and actively of his advice, even on topics other than drugs. In the early 1960s, I used to visit Washington for free-ranging discussions with the late Arnold Lehmen, senior toxicologist in the Food and Drug Administration, in whose room - as many of you will recall - was the notice "You too can be a toxicologist in two easy lessons, each just ten years long". It was then possible to discuss the toxicological assessment of a candidate drug or other compound before, during and after relevant studies and to receive valuable advice upon the protocol or upon what to do concerning unsuspected interim findings. We may be told by some regulatory bodies, by the departments to which they report, or by their legal advisers, that such approaches are fraught with danger and, at the least, could place their medical and other scientific advisers in a vulnerable position and even lay them open to legal procedures if morbidity and mortality were later attributed to a compound or formulation that escaped the net and was marketed. Discussions did continue with the FDA's scientists and ex-clinicians in the post-thalidomide and post-Delaney amendment era, but for a time they were with somewhat low key trios formed to deal with each category of test material. As I once unkindly remarked after a session, it seemed that one member of the trio had just arrived and professed ignorance of the subject, the second was just about to move on and would not commit himself, while the third had not contributed anything anyway. There are, of course, risks attached to an open approach and also to voluntary notification schemes, such as that under which the original Committee on Safety of Drugs in the UK was allowed to operate. As one concerned almost from the outset in the steps that led up to the voluntary notification scheme for pesticides and other agricultural chemicals in the UK, I subscribe to its many advantages, but wonder whether a statutory scheme might have protected manufacturers from the recent import and sale in Southern England of non-UK approved agricultural chemicals. About a decade ago, industry did moot a statutory scheme, but the advice of government representatives on the Joint Medical Panel was to remain voluntary, on the grounds that they would still be free to discuss problems with industry representatives and to advise upon testing procedures and safety evaluation.

Whatever the drawbacks, we should endorse the views expressed at these meetings that full scientific interchange among all concerned is essential to the development of a more rational toxicology and to better protection of the public. Professor Dollery has emphasised the role of pharmacology in what he rightly terms "safety evaluation". Even at the morphological level, the interpretation of findings in animal toxicity studies demands a background knowledge of species, strain and reaction that can come only from practical experience and a high level of competence beyond the purely technical. It is also pertinent that first-hand advice be given by scientists, clinicians and others familiar with conditions of intended use or exposure. Industry may in the past have been deemed guilty of the sale of useless or even inert materials or of permitting the sale of drugs for purposes for which they were not specifically intended, but no manufacturer is likely to allow the most fervent of its scientific staff to browbeat regulatory scientists into recommending the introduction of what is usually designated "another thalidomide". Restrictions of use or exposure are not easy to make, are even more difficult to enforce, and cannot usually be based upon the result of toxicity testing alone. It needs all the experience and wisdom we can muster to make good safety assessments and to devise sensible and economic, preferably tailored, research programmes and to modify them if deemed justifiable. Much of the thinking and consideration should go into the projects before and during their conduct, especially if we are to follow the recommendations of Dr Purchase, among others, concerning interim monitoring. Evaluation of findings should not be left until the final reports are written and submitted for scrutiny to the relevant committees.

The late John Barnes subscribed to the key role of the investigational toxicologist in forming judgements, and felt that he should be enabled to treat a toxicity study as a serious scientific exercise and to take such steps as were necessary to render it so, being equally free to communicate at that stage with his opposite numbers on the regulatory side. The present Meeting is dedicated to the examination of possible so-called alternatives in toxicity testing and to the better and more refined use of such animals as will continue to be necessary. Neither goal will be readily attainable without the collaboration of those on both sides of the regulatory fence and their advisers. Ideally, as an earlier speaker remarked, the same team should devise and tackle both the toxicity testing of a potential new drug and the early human exposure to it. That may be economically impracticable, but I believe that clinicians should assist with the design and interpretation of animal or alternative tests and that the toxicologist or laboratory pharmacologist should discuss Stage I clinical trials.

Not everyone applauds the French Expert System, but _de facto_ the new Clinical Trial Exemption Certificate in the UK reflects a similar approach and is a welcome step towards peer collaboration. Let us in this country take full advantage of the advice and offers of help given by our regulatory colleagues and, worldwide, let us strive for similar facilities and their extension as part of the harmonisation process.

Improving Legislation

R. S. VINE

Since in the present state of our knowledge animals cannot be dispensed with entirely, my task will be first to outline the development of current legislation regulating the use of animals for experimental purposes and second to indicate where I believe improvements could be made to cope with present-day circumstances. In this I have in mind not only the legitimate and justifiable requirements of scientists, but also the feelings and opinions of the general public who may not be knowledgeable in biological matters. Any changes I may suggest are based on my own experience and opinions and may not be taken to reflect the views and opinions of any government department or of any society to which I might belong.

The motivation for legal controls is for the maximum protection of the public. Whatever the system of controls used, it is likely that the power-wielders will be motivated by expediency rather than by ideal or scientific principles. In the matter of the use of animals for primarily human benefits, two opposing groups seek predominance, one seeking the total prohibition of what is described as "vivisection", and the other the free use of animals in pursuit of knowledge. As in so many other fields of human activity, the resultant will lie somewhere between the two opposing forces, with bias towards one side depending on its stridency and on the prevailing political climate. Experiments on animals can be justified only if they are necessary to increase basic knowledge of life functions, to increase knowledge likely to be of use in combating disease and ill-health, and to teach such knowledge to those for whom it is necessary.

Relevant legislation in Britain has been bedevilled by a confusion of ideas to describe two distinct aspects of our treatment of animals. One concerns ill-treatment by such means as beating, overriding, overdriving, terrorising, etc. The other concerns the infliction of pain in bona fide research aimed at studying life processes generally and at seeking knowledge likely to be useful in combating disease and improving health. Legislation against ill-treatment of cattle (which included horses) began with Martin's Act of 1822 and culminated in the

Cruelty to Animals Act of 1854. Because of the existence of this enactment, it would not have been possible for scientists to inflict pain on animals in the pursuit of physiological knowledge, so a special enabling Act was passed in 1876 after a Royal Commission had considered the question the previous year. Most regrettably, this enabling Act was also called the Cruelty to Animals Act, in spite of the existence during the preceding 22 years of a different Act of the same name. The older Act was not repealed for a further 35 years, when it was replaced by the Protection of Animals Act of 1911 (1912 in Scotland). Ill-treatment of animals either by deliberate actions or through neglect and carelessness is one thing: infliction of pain, discomfort, or ill-health in controlled conditions for the ultimate benefit of animals, both human and others, is quite another. The two should not be confused - an opinion expressed by the Advisory Committee on Animal Experiments in its Report to the Secretary of State in 1981 (1). Experiments of the latter nature are controlled and regulated in the UK by the 1876 Act, which is administered by the Home Office with the help of a cadre of professionally qualified medical and veterinary persons who, in the words of the First Royal Commission of 1875, ".... must be persons of such character and position as to command the confidence of the public no less than that of men of science". The Second Royal Commission (1906-1912) reiterated that, "It is essential that the Inspectors should be qualified medical men of such position as to secure the confidence both of their own profession and that of the public". Veterinary surgeons are now eligible for the post of Inspector and, in a policy statement on animal experimentation by the British Veterinary Association in July 1981, it is written ".... that veterinary surgeons are particularly well-suited to supervise the care and welfare of experimental animals". Since the reasons for doing experiments in the words of the 1876 Act are to advance knowledge in physiology, in saving life, in prolonging life, and in alleviating suffering, and since the Act was originally designed - and clearly remains - for the benefit of the human species (with a spin-off invaluable for veterinary science), judgements regarding any likely benefit to human patients should remain firmly in the hands of the medical profession. Veterinary Inspectors are of great value in this specialised field, where the two professions come closest together, but it must be stressed that the Cruelty to Animals Act (and presumably its successor) is not primarily concerned with animal welfare but with the particular circumstance of the animal actually undergoing an experiment. As professionally qualified medical and veterinary consultants, Inspectors under the Act are not police detectives. One of their principal duties is to get to know their registered places and all that work therein. They advise licensees and potential licensees on points of law relating to the 1876 Act. They are there to prevent inadvertent infringements, rather than to give the impression that they are seeking every opportunity to catch people out. Their vigilance in prevention has largely been responsible for the scarcity of offences committed under the Act.

The first drawback of the 1876 Act is its failure to define the words used in the opening sentence of Clause 2: "A person shall not perform on a living animal any experiment calculated to give pain, except subject to the restrictions imposed by this Act." Since invertebrates are excluded from the last paragraph of the Act, "animal" must be interpreted as applying to vertebrates only. Sophisticated techniques in microsurgery, electronic devices and life-support systems now make it difficult to decide when an animal ceases to be alive in the generally accepted sense; failure to define the word "experiment" tempts licensees to err on the side of safety and to report as an experiment any procedure in which there may be doubts about the possibility of pain and distress, however slight; and the word "calculated" has been interpreted administratively as "liable to". The word "pain" has aroused more bitter argument than any other; non-scientists are apt to put too anthropomorphic an interpretation on it, whereas physiologists regard pain as a normal physiological response (and a vital one) to a disagreeable stimulus, which can be inhibited by a counter stimulus with a net result of little or no pain. It behoves legislators when writing a statute either to avoid ambiguous terms altogether or to define them clearly. Similarly, its title should be appropriate.

Pain. Since pain is a purely subjective symptom, it is difficult to diagnose unless the animal exhibits visible or audible signs. It has been interpreted administratively as any departure from the normal well-being of the animal. This is imprecise. Many experiments, such as testing for colour vision or pattern recognition and testing animal intelligence in locating hidden food rewards, may perhaps be regarded as painless, but inevitably there must be varying degrees of stress until the learning process has been established. Where there is any doubt in relating any possible benefits accruing from potentially painful procedures, perhaps the wisest course to follow is that recommended by Wall (2): "The cause of science and scientists, humanity and animals may be protected by the development of local groups who oversee proposed experiments on animals, just as similar groups examine experiments on man."

Experiments. Following a dictionary definition, this has been interpreted administratively as a test, trial, procedure, action or operation to test a hypothesis or to seek an answer to a problem. Procedures falling outside this definition can scarcely be properly regarded as "experiments". Animals are used not only for the production of antisera (a non-painful procedure), but also as reservoirs of viruses, neoplasms and parasites (which may or may not cause ill-health), and for the supply of "spare parts" in the study of transplantation techniques. These could not have been forseen in 1876, so there was no provision for such uses. This ought to be remedied in any new legislation, and the restrictive word "experiment" should be substituted by "procedure".

Ecological observations. Many experiments in the wild have involved the attachment of small transmitters to study prowling and territorial exploration, and to discover the effects on behaviour due to hormonal disturbances caused by castration or implantation of capsules releasing minute quantities of a substance. A sine qua non of the 1876 Act requires that an animal found to be suffering severely must be killed forthwith. Experiments on non-captive animals cannot properly be regarded as coming within the jurisdiction of the 1876 Act, since this requirement cannot be observed and therefore no licence could be issued. It is well-known that small birds and animals were once taken down mines to give warning of foul air. These could be regarded as experimental procedures, but the 1876 Act was never applied in such circumstances, otherwise all coal mines would have been registered under the Act.

Alternative methods. The situation is adequately summed up in the Littlewood Report (3), that alternative methods ".... are actively sought and when found readily adopted; and the discovery of an in vitro test.... which will satisfactorily replace a test on the living animal is always a welcome event".

Foreign legislation. Regulations of other countries may require specific tests with which British manufacturers must comply if they are to export their products. Rationalisation, standardisation and international harmonisation are essential to achieve a substantial reduction in animal usage. Attempts to co-ordinate the views of the European Community are nearing conclusion, and in a recent written answer the Home Office Minister of State said: "It remains the Government's intention to improve and modernise the 1876 Act when final agreement has been reached on the convention (European) and parliamentary time permits" (4).

British legislation. The Laboratory Animals' Protection Bill, sponsored by the Earl of Halsbury, was published on 16 July 1979 (HMSO 50264) and reprinted on 24 April 1980 (HMSO 50997) after amendment by a Select Committee of the House of Lords. This Bill, successfully piloted through the Upper House on two occasions by Lord Halsbury, could well form the basis of a new Act. Research biologists would be well-advised to study these publications carefully. For the smooth administration of any proposed legislation it is desirable to devise a simple, easily understood system of documentation from which whatever information is desired can be easily retrieved. I visualise the licence as a document not unlike a passport, divided into sections showing personal details, full information on procedures proposed and animals to be used, and any additional information which may be required. Applications for licences should be supported by two sponsors, one senior person of managerial status who has personal knowledge of, or can vouch for the applicant, and the other a professor or person of equivalent status with knowledge and experience of the scientific discipline within which the experimental procedures are to be conducted. If the applicant is a student or a technician or an overseas scientist unfamiliar with our legal requirements, there must be designated a suitable senior person to supervise and be responsible for that person. Assuming all seems to be in order, the Inspector may wish to interview the applicant, and the Home Secretary may or may not grant the licence or call for further information. The precise format of the licence is under review.

The Advisory Committee. This was a body set up on the recommendation of the Second Royal Commission and consisted of distinguished senior medical scientists and consultants selected by the Home Secretary from lists submitted by the Royal Society, the Royal Colleges of Surgeons and Physicians and the Royal College of Veterinary Surgeons, sitting under the chairmanship of a High Court Judge. Difficult technical and other problems which had been referred by the Inspectorate for further opinion were placed by the Home Secretary before this Committee for expert advice. During the 60-odd years of its existence, about 150 cases were considered and certain precedents were established. The new Advisory Committee consists of twelve members, of whom only four are medically qualified and two are veterinarians, and no longer sits under a chairman of the status of a High Court Judge.

I conclude by expressing the view that the total abolition of animal usage for "vivisectional" purposes would be analogous to the outlawing of meat-eating, and those advocating such a policy are either naïve or ignorant of the meaning of "vivisection". All operations done by surgeons, dentists and veterinary surgeons are vivisections, and those wanting "vivisection" abolished should not use this word in their money-raising campaigns to stop the use of animals for scientific research. I believe that in this highly emotive field - which concerns several separate ministries, such as those involved in health and social matters, veterinary and agricultural projects, environmental and educational interests - administration should remain under the auspices of the senior and relatively neutral Home Office to forestall any possible inter-ministerial rivalry and precedence claims. Most cultured people, scientists and non-scientists alike, would support some sensitive system of control. I further believe that FRAME deserves the support of all scientists involved in animal experimentation.

REFERENCES

1. Advisory Committee on Animal Experiments. (1981). Report to the Secretary of State on the Framework for Legislation to Replace the Cruelty to Animals Act 1876, pp. 40. London: Home Office.
2. Wall, P.D. (1982). Editorial. Pain. p. 199.
3. Report of the Departmental Committee on Experiments on Animals. Cmnd 2641, HMSO, para. 71.
4. Hansard. 18 October 1982. p. 29.

General Discussion

D. M. CONNING

Rapporteur

In considering the impact of regulatory needs on the use of experimental animals in toxicology or, more precisely for this session, in safety evaluation, three main issues were identified.

First, the role of the toxicologist as a scientist. Toxicology is a multidisciplinary science and, as a consequence, no individual can command a knowledge of all aspects of the topic in detail. Furthermore, as with all branches of science and technology, continual advances are being made, sometimes rapid, sometimes not, so that the position is never static. In these circumstances, it is essential that some method is found whereby the views of the scientists working on a particular material are considered when the possible hazards of that material are assessed. It is simply not possible to establish by precept the information that will be most pertinent. Several speakers illustrated the difficulty of achieving specialist contribution, when a regulatory system is designed to be administered by those untutored in toxicology (and in some countries untutored in science). On the other hand, it is quite clear that many industrial companies, which need regulatory clearance in order to market their products, are anxious to provide the information that the system demands rather than the information that the science requires. The result has been, in many quarters, a burgeoning of demand for superficial empirical data with the consequent growth of use of experimental animals to produce often quite trivial information. Thus, to improve the scientific quality of the data required for regulatory purposes will, at the least, make the use of animals more effective in generating useful information, and may well reduce the overall numbers used.

The second point, which follows from the first, is the need to introduce flexibility into regulatory demands. There is a tendency for so-called "guidelines", though issued with the best intent, to become rules to be obeyed, and from which any variation is to be accepted only as an additional contribution. This tendency is exacerbated by the increasing cost of toxicological studies, which encourage the industrialists to provide only what is required in order to save costs. Such savings tend not to be in terms of numbers of animals. The resolution of this problem probably requires much more scientific expertise within the regulatory system, and one of the objectives of an organisation like FRAME should be to try to bring this about. In the UK, the use of "independent expert committees" has become established and, although these are frequently attacked by the politically motivated, they command a good deal of scientific respect. Such a system is particularly suited to the UK culture where a constructive discussion between industrialists, independent scientists and government officials is possible and valuable. Elsewhere, more confrontational circumstances prevail and it is rarely possible to achieve a meeting of minds. In recent years, there has been a growing tendency to distrust any relationship whereby industrial expertise is used to enable government control to be effected. The "expert committee" is a possible and valuable safeguard which could be more broadly used.

The third issue again follows from the first two. This is that, given the international nature of business, particularly of those industries marketing products such as medicines and agrochemicals which are the main users of experimental animals, there is little chance of reducing the numbers of animals used for regulatory purposes until there is coherence among the regulatory authorities on an international basis. At the present time, there is a tendency for each authority around the globe to acknowledge the "guidelines" produced by the leaders (e.g. FDA or OECD,) but to require certain other tests which they deem important to local circumstances, a legitimate and reasonable demand, but one that increases the numbers of animals used. If it were possible to bring greater international harmony to regulatory control of chemicals, the use of animals for such purposes could be reduced. It is to be regretted that the WHO, which has been so effective in achieving a common basis for the appraisal of the safety of agricultural chemicals, has paid so little attention to the development of the methodology used.

In summary, a large proportion of the animals used in safety evaluation are used to satisfy regulatory demands. In many cases, these demands result from rigid precepts (euphemistic "guidelines") which, while having a central discernible theme, show much embellishment by different countries. With nearly all of the systems in operation, the introduction of new science merely adds to the list of regulatory demands. Few systems show the flexibility that allows for a reduction of the effort required when the scientific rationale would allow it. The conclusion is that an improvement of the scientific expertise available to governments would allow the use of more-advanced information. This would allow the much more effective use of experimental animals which are currently indispensable, and would certainly lead to a reduction in the numbers used in the foreseeable future. The direct recruitment of scientists to government service is not the only method - the use of the expert committee (which can, if necessary, include consumer representation) can also be of great value.

The FRAME Research Programme

MICHAEL BALLS

INTRODUCTION

When they established the FRAME Toxicity Committee, the FRAME Trustees expected that there would be much more emphasis on the introduction of alternatives in toxicity testing and less on the continued use of animals, albeit at a significantly reduced level and with better-designed and more-humane procedures. However, early on in the Committee's discussions and particularly when the working party on tissue culture first met, it became apparent that there had been few systematic attempts to develop and validate cell culture methods for routine toxicity testing and that premature overemphasis on their introduction would be counterproductive. Although I hope that the next meeting to discuss a report of the FRAME Toxicity Committee will be mainly about alternatives, what is the position today? What can we say when asked to assess the potential of alternative methods as total replacements for animal procedures in toxicity testing? To answer that question I shall make an analogy with the development of human flight. If a sceptical spectator watching Icarus about to make his attempt were asked whether man could ever fly, he might have answered, "I don't know, but we may soon find out!". A few minutes later he would probably have said "No!", though a more thoughtful answer would have been, "Not for the foreseeable future!". We who work with alternatives are beyond the Icarus stage - we know that the alternatives have enormous significance, but not precisely what contributions they will make. This is no time for overoptimism or for dismissive pessimism - our answer to the question, "Will alternatives ever totally obviate the need for animal experiments?", must not be

"Yes!" or "No!" but "Maybe, though not for the foreseeable future!".

While the alternatives are being developed and tested, the science of toxicology will evolve, the precise questions asked in toxicity testing will be altered and refined, and the guidelines governing their use will, it is hoped, be rationalised. We do not aim, therefore, to develop direct alternatives to particular animal tests (e.g. the LD50 test), which may themselves be scientifically suspect or of limited real value, but we hope that the various alternatives will themselves be allowed to evolve. FRAME can play a unique part in this, since we have the co-operation of scientists in academic and applied research, the confidence of various industries and administrative bodies, and the active support of politicians and of thinking members of the public. Our contribution will revolve around the continuing discussions of the FRAME Toxicity Committee, the forum provided for objective reporting on the alternatives by our journal, ATLA (Alternatives to Laboratory Animals), and the FRAME Research Programme and International Trials Scheme.

IN VITRO TECHNIQUES

A range of in vitro techniques have been developed, including: cultures of bacteria, algae, fungi and protozoa; subcellular fractions (mitochondrial, microsomal); short-term cellular systems (cell suspensions, tissue biopsies, tissue slices, whole organ perfusion); and tissue culture (the maintenance of cells, tissues, or the whole or parts of organs in vitro in a nutrient medium for 24 hours or longer), including differentiated and functioning primary cell cultures and organ cultures, and the serial subculture of short-lived diploid cell strains and permanent, usually aneuploid, cell lines.

The advantages of in vitro systems in comparison with in vivo methods include their greater sensitivity, more controllable experimental conditions, greater accessibility to meaningful quantitation, relatively low cost, greater speed, relative simplicity, relative absence of complicating factors, and the greater possibility of studying metabolism of toxicants separately from their effects on response systems.

The limitations of in vitro techniques are well-recognised and include: the absence of the complications which result in vivo from the presence of the nervous, endocrine, immune and blood systems, and the absence of the normal systemic mechanisms of absorption, distribution, and excretion.

Although a number of in vitro techniques are currently used in toxicology (see Bridges (1) for review), the only collaborative interlaboratory attempts to test their validity and usefulness appear to have been those involving in vitro and short-term tests for mutagenicity and carcinogenicity (2) and for biologically-active mineral dusts (3).

QUESTIONS AND STRATEGIES

The strategy to be adopted in developing tissue culture methods for use in toxicity testing depends on whether or not the range of events observed in vivo result from a relatively small number of initiating events, the effects of which are modulated or elaborated by the tissue-type specific properties of the affected tissues. If the number of initiating events is small, it should be possible to identify them and to devise methods for their detection in vitro. Then a range of chemicals of known and different degrees of toxicity could be tested in vitro and the results compared with those obtained in vivo.

It would also be useful to have models of the various target organ systems of the body, incorporating as many as possible of the factors which could influence toxicity. This would make possible the recognition and prediction of organ-specific effects. The possibility that this could be achieved depends on the system under consideration. For example, adequate skin organ culture techniques can be envisaged, and great progress has already been made with the isolated rabbit eye. However, it is unlikely that complete in vitro models could ever be envisaged for the brain or the pregnant uterus.

Serially-cultured cell lines or strains of primary cultures of certain cell types could be used as a primary screen or first-order test system, which would enable large numbers of chemicals to be rapidly and inexpensively screened for general toxicity; standardised methods would be needed, to provide reproducible and reliable results, irrespective of the particular laboratory where they were used. The Ames Test is an analogous example, being a first-order test for genotoxicity. When a sufficiently-large data-base had been established, the development of chemicals of low priority would be discontinued if they were found to be cytotoxic in such a test. High priority chemicals giving positive results and all chemicals intended for human application or ingestion would be subjected to higher-level tests.

Second-order tests would take into account the effects of target organ specificity, interactions between metabolism and response systems, and the influence of species, strain, age and sex, and would involve a range of end-points. In the foreseeable future, such tests could be used either before animal experimentation, so that more-effective tests in animals could be carried out, or to help clarify the basis of adverse effects which were found to arise at a later stage.

The two approaches described above would be used alongside each other and together with other methods in a tier system, including, for the time being, scientifically-justified animal tests.

THE FRAME RESEARCH PROGRAMME

The basis of the FRAME Research Programme is the conviction that these developments will not take place and no confidence in *in vitro* toxicity tests will be generated unless they can be convincingly shown to be reproducible in different laboratories. Such reproducibility can only follow the establishment of standard and straightforward routine procedures for cell culture, exposure to the potential toxicant, and the systematic description and quantification of cell injury.

The Programme initially involves four centres: the Robens Institute of Environmental Health & Safety, University of Surrey; the Department of Biochemistry, St. George's Hospital Medical School, University of London; the departments of Physiology & Pharmacology and Human Morphology, University of Nottingham Medical School; and the Department of Mutagenicity and Cell Biology, Huntingdon Research Centre.

The first part of the Programme involves co-ordinated testing at all four centres of the same chemicals, using cells of the same strain, maintained under standardised conditions, and with the same end-points being used as indicators of cytotoxic effects. The work is designed to identify those toxic effects which could readily and reliably be detected, those which could be detected using modified procedures (e.g. with added metabolising systems), and those types of toxicant or toxic effect for which such tests would be inadequate.

We are currently conducting an *initial trial* with known toxicants, such as cycloheximide, 2,4-dinitrophenol, BCNU, cyclophosphamide, carbon tetrachloride, PCMB, and vincristine, and with cell growth and general morphological effects as the end-points. Once reproducibility between laboratories has been established, a *blind trial* will be undertaken, using chemicals with known and different degrees and mechanisms of toxicity.

The progress of the work will be critically assessed by an *Advisory Committee* composed of independent toxicologists and representatives of the industrial companies giving sustaining support, namely, Avon Products Incorporated, Bristol-Myers Company Limited, Fisons-Boots Company Limited, Hoechst UK Limited, Huntingdon Research Centre, Johnson & Johnson Limited, Rimmel International, May & Baker Limited, and Pfizer Limited.

Each of the four centres will have an *individual approach*, since it is anticipated that certain toxicants will not be detectable using general cell lines or strains. This aspect of the work will include studies on hepatocytes, kidney proximal tubule cells, renal papilla cells, skin and tongue epithelial cells, and bone marrow. Attempts will also be made to realise the potential of mixed-cell systems as tests for metabolism-mediated cytotoxicity (4) and to increase the range of end-points which are available for assessing the toxic effect.

INTERNATIONAL CO-OPERATION

Contacts are being sought and established with workers in other laboratories with complementary techniques or programmes, who will be allowed to use the set of trial chemicals in return for interchange of results. This international blind-trial scheme should speed the identification, validation and, ultimately, acceptance of new procedures. FRAME also invites suggestions for chemicals for inclusion in the scheme. These should include: name and address of submitter, name of chemical, name of a non-toxic analogue (where possible), an outline of known toxicity, an indication of any special handling procedures and precautions, and source of pure chemical or of a standard formulation.

SUMMARY

New products must be tested, and live animal procedures will be necessary until alternative methods have been discovered, validated and accepted. Such developments will be more straightforward if cytotoxicity is based on a limited number of intial events, the effects of which are modified in different cell types, resulting in the expression of different symptoms. *In vitro* methods can be envisaged both for general screening and for studies on specific mechanisms and target organ toxicity. A FRAME Research Programme has been established as a practical contribution to the scientific and objective development of *in vitro* cytotoxicology and toxicity testing.

REFERENCES

1. Bridges, J.W. (1980). An evaluation of the present status and potential application of *in vitro* toxicity tests. In "Towards Better Safety of Drugs and Pharmaceutical Products" (ed. D.D. Breimer), pp. 283-298, Amsterdam: Elsevier/North-Holland.
2. De Serres, F. & Ashby, J. (eds.) (1981). Evaluation of short-term tests for carcinogens. Progress in Mutation Research, vol. I. Amsterdam: Elsevier/North-Holland.
3. Brown, R.C., Chamberlain, M., Davies, R., Morgan, D.M.L., Pooley, F.D. & Richards, R.J. (1980). A comparison of 4 *in vitro* systems applied to 21 dusts. In "The *In Vitro* Effects *of* Mineral Dusts" (ed. R.C. Brown, I.P. Gormley, M. Chamberlain & R. Davies), pp. 47-52, London: Academic Press.
4. Fry, J.R. & Bridges, J.W. (1977). A novel mixed hepatocyte-fibroblast culture system and its use as a test for metabolism-mediated cytotoxicity. Biochemical Pharmacology 26, 969-973.

The Johns Hopkins Center

A. M. GOLDBERG

WHY A CENTRE?

All commercial products have the potential for producing toxicological insults. The scientific and industrial communities have a special interest and a responsibility to assess the nature of toxic effects and to evaluate the safety of products.

Although many approaches to safety evaluation have been developed, most methods use animal models and extrapolate from animal to man. Such methods are often cumbersome and expensive. Approaches using in vitro methods would be preferred, and with the many recent advances in biomedical research there are opportunities, as never before, to explore such possibilities. Moreover, during the past several years there has been increasing pressure to decrease or to prevent the use of animals in toxicity testing and safety evaluation. Thus, it is in everyone's best interest to develop appropriate alternative methods to diminish, as rapidly as is feasible, the need for animals in testing. The primary mission of this Center is to develop the fundamental knowledge base that will provide alternative methods to whole animal testing.

GOAL AND PURPOSES

The goal of the Center is to develop appropriate basic scientific knowledge for innovative methods to evaluate fully the safety of commercial and/or therapeutic products. The specific purposes of the Center are:

1. to encourage fundamental research needed for the development of in vitro test procedures or other non-whole-animal test procedures to examine the toxicity of chemicals and chemical compositions;

2. to develop and validate methodology that will provide alternative approaches to whole animal studies for the evaluation of safety;

3. to encourage and promote the acceptance of applicable methods of non-whole-animal safety testing;

4. to provide the best available practical methodological approaches for safety evaluation.

RESEARCH APPROACH

The research approach focuses on developing fundamental knowledge to provide alternative methods for animal tests, and examing the cellular and biochemical mechanisms responsible for tissue damage; and then will develop appropriate in vitro correlative tests as substitutes for whole animal studies.

The research programmes are both intramural and extramural programmes of grants and projects that are reviewed scientifically and awarded on the basis of quality and appropriateness to the mission of the Center.

SYMPOSIA

In order to shape the research approach and identify the research programme, symposia will examine the currently available alternatives to whole animal testing. Each symposium will have several objectives:

a. understanding the state of the art of appropriate research areas;
b. targeting specific research areas for development;
c. stimulating research in alternative approaches to whole animal testing;
d. identifying ways to reduce or replace animals in testing.

The proceedings of the symposia will be published as a monograph which will serve to disseminate knowledge on mechanisms of toxicity and methods of safety evaluation, and to stimulate further research.

The symposium mechanism was chosen as an initial and an ongoing activity, because it will identify the important areas of research need and thereby establish the focus of the research programme of the Center. The second and subsequent symposia will in addition provide a mechanism to evaluate the progress of the Center's programmes.

THE ADVISORY BOARD

A distinguished Advisory Board of voting and non-voting members has been established. The voting members of the Advisory Board are charged with setting and approving the policies of the programme including the selection of research projects to be funded. Non-voting representatives from the animal rights movement and the US government have agreed to serve. In addition, sponsors serve on the Advisory Board as liaison representatives.

THE INTRAMURAL PROGRAMME

The Center Director co-ordinates and manages a programme of focussed research areas in which expertise exists at the Johns Hopkins University. The Center integrates ongoing activities and provides additional funds to target, expand and create new programmes. Applications are reviewed by the solicited grant review process. It is anticipated that through the identification of existing expertise and programmes within the Johns Hopkins University, effective utilisation of the funds for new research will be achieved.

THE EXTRAMURAL PROGRAMME

Once the intramural programme was established, the areas not covered therein were identified and targeted for funds in the extramural programme. Specific scientists with proven accomplishments and expertise were then requested to submit proposals for review and at the same time applications were solicited by advertising in professional journals. The research programmes are chosen on the basis of quality and appropriateness to the mission of the Center.

REVIEW OF SMALL GRANT PROPOSALS

Written reviews of grant proposals are solicited by the Center Director from qualified scientists without conflict of interest. Outside reviewers are requested to provide detailed evaluations, critiques, and suggestions for improvement of each grant. The Advisory Board evaluates the proposals and the solicited reviews and makes recommendations for funding.

GRANTS MANAGEMENT

The monitoring and quality control of the funded applications is through the grants management and evaluation process. Renewal and review mechanisms evaluate quality and stimulate conceptual and productive development. As part of this process, the regularly scheduled symposia allow grantees to present progress reports to members of the Advisory Board and the sponsors of the Center. Further, written reports of programme progress are required of all grantees at six-monthly intervals, and progress reports are submitted by the Center Director to its sponsors.

SUMMARY

The guiding principles of the Center and its programmes will be scientific excellence and credibility.

The approach presented seeks to develop a highly visible and creative International Center to examine alternatives to whole animal testing. This research programme is developed through a process of familiarisation with the needs of its members; identification of areas of research need; development of intramural and extramural research programmes; and dissemination of its research findings.

The Johns Hopkins Center was established by a grant from the Cosmetic, Toiletry and Fragrance Association, Inc. Additional funding for organ specific toxicity was provided by the Bristol-Myers Corporation. The Center is an international resource dealing with the development of *in vitro* product safety evaluation methodology. The full address of the Center is: The Johns Hopkins Center for Alternatives to Animal Testing, Department of Environmental Health Sciences, School of Hygiene and Public Health, 615 North Wolfe Street, Baltimore, Maryland 21205, USA.

Round Table Discussion

K. J. ÖBRINK

Chairman

Chairman: I suggest that we should not discuss the topics one by one as they have appeared during the past three days but instead try to make an overall summary. The title of this symposium is "Animals and Alternatives in Safety Evaluation". It is therefore appropriate that before starting the discussion we try to define what we mean by "alternatives". An alternative method must be a choice between at least two different methods. If method A can be considered an alternative to method B, then method B is an alternative to method A. It should be realised that study of a problem of a cellular event, e.g. a receptor mechanism, may be possible only by using in vitro systems. We would not be able to get the same answer by using an intact animal, so that is not an alternative method. Therefore, cell culture is not, in itself, an alternative method, but an alternative method may very well involve cell culture. As a matter of fact, when we are looking for new biological knowledge, we may need to use in vitro systems, but then these methods, if they are the only possible ones, cannot be called alternative methods. In my view, alternative methods never provide us with new basic knowledge. We can use them to test for carcinogenicity because we know what we are looking for; we can use them for vaccine production, because we know what product we want. However, if we want to study the cellular mechanisms of action of a carcinogenic substance, i.e. to find the intracellular biochemical events induced by the substance, then the studies of enzymes, membranes and receptors are basic knowledge obtained by what should be called complementary methods, not alternatives.

This Meeting has been arranged because of two driving forces, namely, scientific problems and ethical problems. If it were not for the ethical problems, I don't think that FRAME would ever have arranged a discussion of this kind. It is therefore inevitable that ethics must come into the discussion, even if it has not been a main topic during the last three days. Let us, however, remember the definition of the three R's, i.e. Replacing, Reducing and Refining. The discussions in this symposium have clearly shown that a total replacement is not possible in very many cases. However, reduction of the numbers of animals employed, and especially refinement of the experiments carried out, are actions that can be taken immediately. Let me remind you of the last FRAME meeting on "The Use of Alternatives in Drug Research", where in the Introduction by Drs Rowan & Stratmann it was estimated that the number of animals in 273 published papers could have been reduced by up to 40% if the experiments had been properly planned. Maybe it would also be possible to refine the experiments to the extent that animals could be used without any suffering or distress at all. Would that be a desirable development?

Dr M. BALLS: I think that all animal welfare organisations, among which you can include FRAME, want to completely get rid of animal houses in connection with laboratory work. That is the ultimate goal of all animal welfare work in this context. That means that we hope for a time when we could use a battery of non-animal methods to find all the information we need before a product can safely be used by man.

Dr Susan HAYWOOD: I came to this conference of FRAME's because I am interested in animal welfare. As an experimental pathologist and as a veterinary surgeon I am aware of the needs of animals. I am experienced in assessing animal distress and I am also interested in mechanisms of toxicity. I know that it is possible to study mechanisms of toxicity in whole animals, and that by observing a very careful protocol with regard to dosage, sampling, route of administration and termination of the experiment, it is possible to do this without there being any overt discomfort to the animal. I look at my animals every day during an experiment and I know it is possible to discern signs of ill-health and discomfort.

Chairman: Very little has been said about the quality of the animals used in toxicity testing, but wouldn't it be better if one used defined animals from inbred strains? May I call upon Professor Bridges to elaborate on that, because it must be a matter of concern in his work on pharmacokinetics.

Professor J.W. BRIDGES: If we are talking about quantitation in pharmacokinetics, which I think is the area you are asking me about, then it is certainly a great advantage to have animals which are as reproducible as possible, and that usually means inbred strains. But if we are talking in the more general context of pharmacokinetics in toxicology, then it is much more important to use the animals that the toxicologists are using now.

Dr I.F.H. PURCHASE: The problem of the selection of strain is one which is frequently discussed by toxicologists. There are lots of different strains of animals which can be used for carcinogenicity tests. Because animals are inbred, they are not necessarily better models than others. Some inbred strains have a very high incidence for a particular cancer or are particularly susceptible to a carcinogen. In such cases the relevance to man has not been established. The second point is that a genetic definition does not necessarily require inbreeding per se, and as you know, the National Toxicology Program in the United States uses f_1 generation animals, which I personally would prefer if one was to try to select defined animals. It has been shown in nutritional experiments that f_1 and, particularly, f_2 generation animals enormously reduced the standard errors of estimate of body weight, food consumption, etc.

Professor D.V.W. PARKE: I agree with Professor Bridges. The genetics of an animal are very important when you are studying basic mechanisms, for example in carcinogenicity, but to demand defined strains of animals when all you are doing is seeking a general model for man is, I think, quite irrelevant.

Dr I. NATOFF: The point which crosses my mind is that all testing done in laboratory animals involves strains which were developed for laboratory purposes, so we are dealing with relatively pure strains. But we are trying to predict the effects of the compounds we study in man or in animal populations in general, which are very heterogeneous. Ideally, of course, we should use heterogeneous animals for testing our compounds, so that we can give some sort of prediction of the variability we are going to see in the human population in general. This is, however, totally impracticable, because we would get too much variability and be unable to make any meaningful conclusions. So we are left with the need to use pure strains of animals to get meaningful results, but these results can only be relevant to those particular animals. So there is an inherent risk in extrapolating our observations to a heterogeneous population.

Chairman: I have just received a question from Dr Jennie Gwynn to Professor Parke, who stated that one should choose a model which is as close as possible to man before one starts doing tests on a new compound. Dr Gwynn's question is, "How can you do that before you have ever tested the compound in man?"

Professor PARKE: If you gave me a couple of hours I could certainly answer that. This is a question we always get when kinetics and metabolism are discussed. The answer is that you have to progress from animals to man, back to animals and then back to man again. You start by doing, say, 7- or 14-day toxicity tests in one species, probably the rat, and then you do your kinetics on a very low dose in humans. Then you go back for longer studies in several species. It is a very elaborate procedure that every toxicologist here knows and practices, so I am amazed that this question has come up again.

Dr PURCHASE: I'd like to add to Professor Parke's comments. If you work with industrial chemicals and agrochemicals, the opportunity to go into man is rarely available. Therefore, the point he makes is rather an academic one for us.

Dr P. HODGES: There is a requirement in the UK for two species toxicology before going to clinical trial. From what Professor Parke has said, it would appear that one is ethically justified in going into volunteers with less toxicology studies than one would need before using patients. There seems to be an inconsistency in this different treatment of patients and volunteers.

Professor PARKE: You are quite right. It was the Minister of Health who decided that his responsibility was to the patient and not to the general public. Thus, the law applies to patients and does not apply to human volunteers. However, anyone carrying out an experiment in humans realises he has to take the responsibility for it, and I do not know of any example where this responsibility has been inappropriately exercised.

Chairman: There are many things that can cause variability in toxicity tests, such as environmental conditions and nutrition. Dr Warren has asked if and how you can allow for circadian rhythms in your animals. Do you have standards for light and darkness? Are the environmental conditions in animal rooms standardised?

Dr R. HEYWOOD: We are standardising the conditions of our animal rooms as best we can, in terms of temperature control, humidity, and light cycles. However, there are lots of factors in animal rooms which cannot be controlled. This gives me an opportunity to mention the importance of animal technicians. They are the vital people in toxicological work, since they are handling the animals day by day and treating them in a humane manner. We must pay considerable attention to the animal technicians, who represent a variable that we otherwise cannot control.

Those of us who are doing toxicology to international standards are now working to GLP regulations. We report the conditions within the animal rooms twice daily with respect to temperature, humidity and the controllable variables. The number of animals per cage is clearly stated in any protocol before the start of any study. We are also defining the diet as best we can. We are having our diets analysed in detail, not just once, but throughout the course of the study; we also analyse the water. Thus, we know as much about the variables as we possibly can, and some of us include these data when we publish our toxicological studies.

Chairman: You heard the arguments by Dr Roe about the nutrition of rats. Besides protein content, etc., we all know that the fibre content is very important for the absorption of many things after an oral administration. The more fibres the less the absorption. How is that controlled?

Professor D.M. CONNING: It is extremely difficult to decide what is meant by fibre. It goes without saying that there is a considerable bulk of fibre in all animal diets, because they are largely based on cereal proteins. There is, however, an added aspect to this question which is extremely important. That is the content of bacteria in the gut. We know that the toxicological response of many experimental animals varies considerably according to the state of the bacterial flora in the gut. It is known that the state and quantity of these bacteria are related to such things as fibre, but there are also other factors. It is certainly true that there is a considerable amount of work to be done to define and refine our understanding of the impact of diets.

Dr J.S.L. FOWLER: Dr Heywood suggested that an indication of toxicity was reduced body-weight gain and, I assume, also diet consumed. Dr Roe proposed that the diet influenced the tumour incidence. It has also been suggested here that one could perhaps combine toxicity testing and searching for tumours, but how can you choose doses which will not affect the body weight and therefore the tumour incidence and yet still evaluate toxicity? I do not see how these tests can be combined and I do not know how you would save a significant number of animals by trying to combine them. To do so would simply frustrate the objects of both types of study.

Dr A. COCKBURN: I do believe we have a duty to try and refine studies and get as much as we can from each. I have seen it suggested that one could in fact incorporate fertility, teratology, and prenatal and postnatal studies into carcinogenicity studies. I wonder what the views of the Round Table would be on that suggestion?

Dr PURCHASE: The conduct of most of the toxicity studies is complicated enough when we only have one end-point in them. I consider that trying to combine too many things leads to extreme difficulties.

Professor C.L. BERRY: I would entirely agree with Dr Purchase that if you attempt too much in one study you end up without answering anything satisfactorily; but I think that any toxicity test should be critically looked at before going on to the next one, because it may have given you information that you should take into account in subsequent designs.

Dr HODGES: I have a question relating to the use of human material for toxicological studies. This sort of material could provide some very attractive alternative methods. However, I wonder if anybody would care to speculate on the ethical, practical, moral and, indeed, scientific implications of trying to turn this sort of hospital research technique into methods that industry could use on a day-to-day basis. One can imagine patients not minding a clinician in a hospital medical school taking a little bit of liver tissue, for instance, during the course of an operation, but I think the reaction to being asked for some material for an industrial company just down the road might be entirely different.

Professor BERRY: I am a large provider of material in one sense, in that the kind of operation that I do as a pathologist results in considerable amounts of material being available without much comment from the patients. In fact, these circumstances are quite properly governed by law and in obtaining tissue from autopsy proper permission must be obtained. Indeed, there are difficulties, for instance, in obtaining human pituitary glands from cadavers for extraction of growth hormone. In my own experience, for example, in asking for material for establishing fibroblast cultures, when the matter is discussed with a patient, in the majority of cases there will be no problems. There is usually an enthusiastic response. I am sure most would not object to a company using the material, but I think the practical point is that it must always be done as a matter of informed consent, as in a clinical trial.

Dr BALLS: I would like to make the point that if tissue is taken from a patient, one would tend not to have enough information about it. For example, questions relating to alcohol consumption, use of drugs and what diseases the patient may have had.

Professor BERRY: I think you will never find human beings as adequate as laboratory animals, simply because we are a rather capricious species. You raised the problem of alcohol: it is practically impossible to get anybody to tell you how much alcohol they actually drink!

Chairman: Dr Warren has given me another question. We are often talking about using "lower" animals, such as invertebrates, which are not included in the British Cruelty to Animals Act (1876). However, many of them have nervous systems, so what about the ethics of using these lower animals?

Dr BALLS: Some of the invertebrates, including the higher molluscs, have very advanced nervous systems, and if we are going to take on the complex issue of pain in lower vertebrates, I think we have to very seriously consider these animals, too. I noticed that the Home Office Advisory Committee felt that there was a need to consider certain invertebrates if the legislation is revised. We should not look on developing stages of vertebrates as being casually expendable material. We should also give more thought to the ethics of their use.

Dr A. WARREN: If you want a totally acceptable alternative, it has got to be something that has not got an organised nervous system. I don't think anybody can say whether or not a cell line or tissue culture could feel anything. As philosophers say - nobody can feel anybody else's pain.

Dr BALLS: I think having a nervous system should not be the critical point. Earthworms have nervous systems. If you cut them in half, one half will generate new parts and will be able to live and reproduce. However, I am not advocating that earthworms should be widely used. I do not think that present-day cell cultures can feel pain, although it may be that one day we shall have cultures which could. Then we shall have another kind of problem. By that time I hope that we shall have such good alternatives that we shall not need animals.

Chairman: It is not the existence of a nervous system that is important. We are already at the point where cell cultures can conduct nerve impulses. The question is whether they feel and how they react, i.e. whether they can have symptoms. What we are dealing with is whether or not the lower animal has well-developed associative brain functions.

Now let me turn to another topic. I have received many questions about the LD50 test. I would like to call on Dr Johnson to expand on his question.

Dr A.W. JOHNSON: My question relates to the use of the Limit test. I think that if we accept that the full classical LD50 test is not necessary, then you do a screening test on a few animals to obtain an approximate idea of toxicity, and you have some idea of what amount of material could be harmful. However, if you use a limit test, unless you happen to produce effects at the dose that you choose, you may not have any idea about what amount of the substance would be harmful, but merely that a certain amount would not be harmful. If you take a small child of 12.5kg body weight and give it 2ml/kg, that would be 25ml; 5ml/kg represents something in the region of 65ml and if we went to a high limit of 10ml/kg that would represent 125ml. Many of the products which we have in our homes, whether they be cleaning products, toiletries, products in the garage, chemicals for the garden, and so on, are sold in amounts very much greater than 50 or 100ml. So my question would be - do we need to know, in the case of such consumer products, whether a retail pack contains an amount which could be potentially lethal for a small child, and, if we do, how do we go about testing in the case where testing is necessary? What sort of test should we use? Do we use a screening test or a limit test? If a limit test, then what dose should we select as our limit?

Dr V.K.H. BROWN: The question raised is a very provocative one. As in all experimentation, you must define the question that you want answered before you do the test. I think one should be very cautious about making quantum jumps. One has to take into account the fact that your tests are going to be transferred from, let us say, the laboratory rat to humans; but there can be enormous differences in sensitivity between children and adults, sensitivities which are not solely dependent on body weight, but other factors as well. You have to look at the purpose of your experiment. Pitch your upper limit with those things in mind. However, sometimes this upper limit is fixed at ludicrously high levels by legislation, and I know one western European country where, for example, the sort of oil you put in your cars has to be tested up to 50ml/kg. Otherwise a hazard warning label has to be on it. I think this is absolutely ludicrous, but how one sets about getting this changed, I don't know.

Dr HODGES: We heard a certain amount this morning about the necessity for harmonisation of guidelines. I wonder if I could ask someone who has been talking about regulations how we should avoid the convoy syndrome in which everything is rounded down to the lowest common denominator rather than up to the highest standard of science.

Professor CONNING: There is no simple solution to this problem, because it means bringing about the kind of toxicological enlightenment that we share in this room to the regulatory authorities around the globe. It is just not possible at this time to equate the purposes of the regulatory system with the purposes of the science of toxicology. The question we have heard asked is, "How do I improve my toxicology and satisfy the regulations at the same time?", when the real question should be, "How do I ensure that the chemical that I am working with and that I want to sell is not going to hurt anybody or kill anybody?". My view is that all of us have an obligation to educate and train toxicologists so that they will ask sensible questions even if they are employed by regulatory authorities. In many respects the regulatory system has become a kind of job creation system for those who say "No" and only extremely rarely say "Yes". The only way forward is to recognise that toxicology is a science and as such deserves the respect given to other sciences.

Chairman: May I in this context ask whether we should fight to get rid of the LD50 test?

Professor CONNING: I would not like to put the question like that. I am ducking the issue in a sense, but it seems to me that the LD50 test when it was first devised and for the first 30 years of its existence fulfilled an extremely valuable service, which was to enable pharmacologists to compare the relative efficiences or relative hazards of newly developed drugs. The great problem with the LD50 is that it has been taken over by the safety evaluation people as a means of comparing toxicities of chemicals which are going to get into the market or into the environment. But this has given rise to certain absurdities. For example, take a substance which is not going to kill, but can cause severe scarring of the oesophagus so that you will be crippled for life. Measurement of the LD50 is not going to give you any idea of what hazard is involved in exposure to that material. As was said a few minutes ago, you have really got to design your experiment with a view to what it is you want to find out.

Dr PURCHASE: I think that the problem needs further definition because the question you are actually asking is: "Should we be doing acute toxicity tests where the only end-point is the counting of the number of dead animals (the traditional LD50)?" I don't think that any laboratory in this country is now doing LD50 tests of that sort. Other pathological and clinical observations are made, so in that sense we have already abandoned the LD50 test.

Dr HODGES: I wonder whether anybody in governmental regulatory authorities has ever gone back retrospectively and looked at submissions including LD50 tests and asked the question, "Would it have made any difference to our decision if that LD50 test had not been there?".

Professor BERRY: I think it would be unfair to ask anybody who is here from the various authorities to try and answer the question. From the data submitted it would very often be impossible to tell. They are not formulated in a way similar to that for a paper written for a scientific journal. I am sure it could be done from the basic data and perhaps this could be a matter for co-operation between the industry and the authorities - to give us some factual basis for the assertions which many people make about LD50 tests.

Chairman: We still have some other questions, for instance, on the Draize test. Dr Natoff, will you please explain your point.

Dr NATOFF: The ocular toxicity working party felt that prostaglandin potentiation of histamine release might aggravate irritation when a foreign chemical was applied to the eye of a rabbit, so it would be more humane to apply an antihistamine to block the effect of the histamine. But that would block the effect of the compound itself, and this seems curious to me, because the test you are going to make is to see what effect the compound has on the eye surface. I am not going to deal with the morals or the acceptability of the Draize test, but the application of an antihistamine is going to block a secondary effect, which is perhaps triggered off by the primary application of the chemical. Now, if we are going to apply antihistamines to every compound we test, then we may get a number of false negatives. Consequently, when you present that compound to the population at large, which again I emphasise we are trying to protect, then are we going to tell them before we hand them these compounds that they must apply an antihistamine to themselves? Of course not! But that is what the recommendation seems to imply.

Mr D.W. SWANSTON: I agree with the speaker to some extent. We have no experimental results on this; we just thought that it would be one of the things that would be worth investigation.

Dr Olga UVAROV: Throughout this symposium it has been quite clear that FRAME, in addition to wishing to reduce the number of animal experiments or the use of animals, is also recognising the need to protect laboratory animals by other means. I think we can protect our animals by recognising the emergence of a new science, Laboratory Animal Science. It is a science in its own right. A great deal has been learnt about laboratory animals, their anatomy, nutrition, physiology, genetics, and diseases. I was surprised to hear that there were overfed animals, flabby animals, sex-starved animals, and so on. I don't think it is necessary to have such animals. Using animal technicians, who should be trained, is another means of protecting these animals. The need is to recognise the importance of purpose-bred animals, animals defined genetically and microbiologically. All these conditions exist in this country and there are a number of guidelines issued by different organisations. Dr Rowsell of Canada has in fact added another R to the three R's, "The Right animal for the Right experiment". The importance of ethical committees, the ethical guidelines of all our professions and organisations must be stressed; they are all there and I think it should be realised that the breeding and care of laboratory animals are of a very high standard in the pharmaceutical industry in this country and, I am sure, in others. When you, Chairman, wanted to pressurise some of our colleagues into wishing to know the fibre content of rat diets, I can assure you that lots of people from this country have submitted this type of information, and sizes of cages and so on, to the Council of Europe Convention on Laboratory Animals in Strasbourg.

Chairman: Thank you. I appreciate your summary very much. All these things make it possible to refine and reduce animal experiments. Let me add also Carol Newton's "3S" principle, which stands for: "Good Science", "Good Sense" and "Good Sensibility".

Dr D.M. FOULKES: I would like to comment on what Dr Purchase said about the doubtful value of the mouse as a predictor of human carcinogenicity. Assuming that the questionable relevance of the mouse is not a consequence of the "background noise" referred to by Dr Roe, is there some way, through FRAME or otherwise, that evidence can be presented to regulators to dissuade them from demanding studies which annually consume thousands of mice?

Dr PURCHASE: Unfortunately, it is by no means a universal view that the mouse is an inadequate species for studying carcinogenicity of chemicals. The mouse is still an integral part of the National Toxicology Program, so there is still a body of opinion which does not agree with our view. I am not sure how you start advancing this view except by collecting the data.

Chairman: It is time to close this discussion and I would like to summarise a few issues. The demand from Society that the potential hazards and toxicities of new drugs and chemicals be evaluated seems to have resulted in two aims in toxicology, one to fulfil regulatory demands, giving figures on hazard and toxicity so as to satisfy the regulators acting on behalf of Society, the other to develop toxicology as a biological science. Unfortunately, these two lines seem to involve conflicts. I have got a feeling that if toxicity testing does not give up the trend toward the blind obeying of bureaucratic rules, it is going to be discredited in the near future. I have a feeling that all the participants in this discussion are dissatisfied with the present state of things. It has frequently been pointed out that there should be more thought behind the tests. The scientists must convince the regulators that a more scientific approach to toxicity testing is vital. That is the feeling that I, as a non-toxicologist, get from these three days of presentations on the present state of toxicology and toxicity testing.

May I also advocate the need for the greater refinement of all animal experiments and for increasing the quality of all laboratory work with animals in order to reduce the number of animal experiments which are necessary. This is something that can be done today and I make a plea to all of you present to actively consider this responsibility that we all have to our laboratory animals.

Finally, may I thank all the participants in this discussion, especially the members of the Panel, and may I express our thanks to FRAME for arranging this symposium, which has been of immense value.

Summing-up

LEON GOLBERG

Dr Balls, Ladies and Gentlemen: I should like to thank FRAME for the opportunity to attend this Meeting, although I should perhaps not echo the words of André Gide, who began a speech as follows: "All I have to say has been said already; but, since no one was listening, it should be said again." On this occasion, however, I have been struck by the patience, persistence and care that the audience has devoted to these very interesting discussions. So all I can do at this point is give you some personal reflections on what I have heard, just skimming the surface of the tips of the icebergs.

I have found this meeting to be a remarkably valuable and effective stocktaking of the present situation in toxicology, including many points which those of us who are toxicologists should take to heart and apply in our work, as has been mentioned by Professor Öbrink. I also look forward to the published proceedings, which I think will be of great value.

The question is: what comes next? I think that, in the case of FRAME, there is a long haul ahead, and I get the impression that everyone realises this. There are really two ways forward. One can emphasise new and innovative approaches, but one is handicapped when trying to apply these directly on the basis of the tightly-structured classical categories of tests that we have been considering. I think it is inevitable that a programme like this should be arranged in such a manner; but the fact is that if we aim more at the discovery of types of biological knowledge and insights into the properties of chemicals and other materials, such as actions on membranes or DNA or other defined end-points of this sort, in the long run I feel that this approach has the greater promise. In other words, we can accept cakes as an alternative to bread, but perhaps what is needed is a revolution - in thinking and in strategy - or, as Dr Clark put it, "to use our brains." In fact, if one reviews the present scene, and one has only to pick up each week's issue of Nature to realise it, the revolution is upon us. The molecular biologists and the biotechnologists and everyone else in that field are pressing on hard at a pace which is really breathtaking. The application of this new scientific knowledge is bound to have a tremendous impact on our field. If one looks at monoclonal antibodies and what they are capable of doing in the way of detecting and measuring DNA adducts and other products of importance to the toxicologists, one realises that here is the start of something very, very great.

Many speakers have pointed to the huge and increasing cost of animal work, and that also is a factor that will provide impetus for change. The issue of mechanisms of toxic action has been emphasised again and again. I think the Report of the Royal Society Study Group, entitled "Long-term Toxic Effects" published in July, 1978, put this issue extremely well:

> "Toxicology is not adequately supported as a scientific discipline; it is swamped by routine tests of limited value and governed by regulations rather than by rational thought...... This activity (toxicity testing) tends, however, to be diverted into a sterile routine of exposure of many animals, without attention to mechanisms. Only if mechanisms are understood is it possible to extrapolate toxicological measurements across species and from the large doses used in experimental animals to the exposures experienced by man, commonly a thousand-fold smaller".

The question is, how can FRAME help progress in the direction of mechanistic approaches and the use of a scientific basis for many of the methods of assessment of safety? It has been emphasised, for instance, that studies of metabolism, pharmacokinetics, and receptors are of key importance in the validation of animal studies, and also in the development of new tests. Equally important in such validation is the selection of materials to be tested. Dr Longstaff used the term "awkward carcinogens", and I think that is a very expressive statement of our dilemma in reconciling the results of short-term and carcinogenicity tests. There is also the question of backing all this up with epidemiology. I was somewhat disappointed that the emphasis was excessively in the direction of drug toxicity and development, and perhaps not sufficiently on other areas of chemical study, industrial chemicals and so forth, where there is also considerable use of animals. We have to have a broad perspective to keep this whole field in mind. I am sure that those in the audience who are not toxicologists have begun to realise what a vast amount of ground we have to cover and integrate in trying to achieve risk assessments in this field. We are exploring the potential of chemicals, as well as their potency; and, as Dr Williams mentioned, this potency - the measure of adverse response of a biological system - is not an inherent property of the chemical, but depends so much on the test system and the conditions of the test. The enthusiasts of the Ames test have discovered this to their cost. We have to be very much clearer with regard to the anticipated level of exposure when dealing in areas other than drug applications.

The whole question of susceptibility of groups and individuals, and genetically determined factors like a1-antitrypsin deficiency, are becoming more and more important in whatever field these chemicals tend to be used. Professor McLean said that we are dealing with a wide variety of people, and that toxicology has to be correspondingly crude. I agree that hitherto it has had to be so, but to an increasing degree we can discern in the human population, sub-groups of more specific susceptibilities, and we can do something to protect those groups. Finally, there is the question of mixtures and interactions between their components, an issue which has not been dealt with. Here is one of the most serious problems in toxicology, the fact that exposures rarely occur to one material at a time. The necessary methods have not been developed sufficiently. We know of instances of synergisms and antagonisms, and while we have to keep these matters in mind, we often cannot do much about them.

We have heard a great deal of discussion about acute toxicity and I don't wish to repeat it. I would merely echo Professor Turner's advice, when he said, "Don't look at the regulatory requirements - by the time the alternatives are available, they will have changed - and don't look for packages of tests corresponding to the packages which are in use today". Here is a profound statement, because the kinds of techniques - starting with analytical chemistry and going all the way to molecular biology and genetics - the kinds of techniques which are becoming available are going to change everything in the long run. Of course there is the inbuilt inertia of governmental regulatory bodies to be considered, as has been mentioned; but it is up to the scientist to provide the leadership in this matter. The authorities will change when we can demonstrate that we have convincingly improved and validated techniques.

Always remembering that the final assessment concerns safety to man, the use of human tissue banks assumes great importance. The problem is that very often the tissues, especially from autopsies, are not particularly effective metabolically; all kinds of problems arise, and these were touched upon. I found the discussion of pharmacokinetics extremely useful and interesting. Professor Parke's comments on what is needed for translation of animal data to man, deal with absolute fundamentals. It is to be regretted that, in so many instances, the study of metabolism and pharmacokinetics is still an afterthought, relegated to a minor role by many current regulatory bodies. Nevertheless, one has to say that to someone who believes in metabolism and pharmacokinetics, as I do, there are many instances where we are caused great grief by events that occur. To take just a few examples; the question of coumarin, a compound that is still widely used, is typical. This compound differs materially in its metabolism between rodents on the one hand, and man and primates on the other. This issue has recently been reviewed by the Joint FAO/WHO Expert Committee on Food Additives who, after dealing with and accepting all these metabolic differences, reached the final conclusion and recommendation that another lifetime study in rats was required. One wonders just when the "new" thinking will have an impact. A similar example has recently occurred in connection with the National Toxicology Program in the United States. This touches upon the issue of carcinogenicity testing. I detected a rather touching faith, expressed by some speakers, in the reliability and fundamental value of carcinogenicity testing as it is practiced today. Sad to say, in the case of benzyl acetate, which is a material whose metabolism is well known, and can in no way lead anyone to imagine that this could be a carcinogen, the National Toxicology Program nevertheless concluded that it was a carcinogen, and no one on the Committee questioned the end-result. In actual fact, a host of similar results have emanated from the administration of these materials dissolved in corn oil in very high concentrations, and delivered by gavage into the stomachs of rats. There seems to be some association between particular batches of corn oil and the development of pancreatic acinar cell adenomas. The confused situation that exists at the moment is being looked into, but it illustrates the complexities that are apt to arise. Another material in the same general area is ethylene, which under normal circumstances is not metabolised in man nor in animals. However, if one administers Aroclor 1254 to rats at a dose of 500mg/kg (which is a staggering amount), one can produce liver damage with subsequent exposure to high concentrations of ethylene. If one lowers the dose of Aroclor to 250mg/kg (which is still a staggering dose), nothing happens: the liver appears to be perfectly normal. And yet, on that basis, Ehrenberg and others have said, "Aha, here is a manifestation of the fact that ethylene is converted to ethylene oxide in the body, and hence is really a carcinogen". Well, these brief comments on metabolism and pharmacokinetics will have to suffice. I was very glad to see that this aspect is stressed so much in Great Britain. Alas, there is still a lack of enlightenment in this area among some American circles!

As regards subchronic and long-term toxicity, the phrase used by Professor Davies was that we were "obsessed with structure and neglected function". There is much justification for that pithy comment. He emphasised that the study of toxicity should approach clinical medicine more closely. Certainly, observation of the animals, coupled with an increasing repertoire of tests of function (especially now that there are analytical machines that utilise far smaller volumes of body fluids), is a step forward that could readily be made.

When we turn to carcinogenicity, I can sympathise with the crie de coeur that we heard from Dr Roe. The situation in carcinogenicity testing today is perhaps the greatest incentive to change. Exactly how such a change will come about, and how long it will take, is difficult to predict. We need to devote a great deal of effort to this goal, and I hope that FRAME will bear this in mind. There was insufficient emphasis on the short-comings of the present procedure. For example, the use of the "Maximum Tolerated Dose" is a monstrosity that unfortunately we have learned to accept, having become inured to it. The fact of the matter is, as we know very well, that in many instances the enormous dose greatly distorts the metabolism and pharmaco-kinetics of the test material, saturates normal metabolic pathways, and generally wreaks havoc. So we are dealing with artefacts; but the underlying philosophy seems to be that one ignores all those minutiae if the results are positive, so that the material under test can be labelled a carcinogen. Even though definitions of the maximum tolerated dose do exist (it must not cause more than a 10% reduction in body-weight gain), nevertheless, many tests are carried out with reductions of body-weight gain of 30% or 40%, or more. As long as enough animals survive, and the result is positive, then nobody worries. Saccharin has taught us a lesson in this respect, and there have been many others, but yet we don't seem to be able to get this point of view, concerning saturation of metabolic and excretory pathways, across to the people that matter. Dr Roe's suggestion, that we should take just a small first step in trying to achieve healthy old animals, is worth considering by FRAME and others. He talked about the endocrinological imbalances that are apt to result in the course of these tests. Also, the question of hepatocellular carcinomas in male mice has been mentioned - a most serious matter that has led to many compounds being classified as animal carcinogens when it is inconceivable that they could be carcinogenic. One example is that of cinnamyl anthranilate. Both cinnamyl alcohol and anthranilic acid have been tested and found to be non-carcinogenic. We know that cinnamyl anthranilate is hydrolysed very readily when it reaches the gastrointestinal tract; nevertheless, the ester was found to be carcinogenic and industry promptly disposed of it without any further ado. Scientifically, however, this result raises a very interesting question that should be pursued.

I thought that the session devoted to mathematical modelling was excellent. I have rarely heard such a clear and concise presentation of the question of quantitative structure-activity relationships as that presented by Dr Tute and his colleagues. They felt somewhat despondent about the utility of this approach from the standpoint of toxicology. This outlook was largely occasioned by some unfortunate experiences with commercial undertakings that have claimed the ability to predict toxicities, including LD50s, on the basis of structure. I think this is just a false start, and we should not feel disheartened. This is a field of very great promise and will ultimately - it may only be a few years down the road - permit us to forecast with considerable accuracy the likely properties of a member of a congeneric series, thus saving much testing and utilisation of animals. This area is very definitely worth pursuing further. Coming to the statistical contributions, I liked the phrase "statistics is the midwife of science". We had two opposing views, the statisticians themselves saying that we need collaboration, not isolation; we need close involvement of statisticians at every stage of the design of protocols and the interpretation of results, in order to maximise the information from the experiments. There was a rather different suggestion, to downgrade statistics; but I think that, particularly with the power of today's computerised packages, there is no question that the statistician should be brought in at the earliest possible stage to help us design the experiments as effectively as possible, and with the lowest effective number of animals.

With regard to reproductive toxicity, the emphasis was placed on reproductive failure as an aspect that was as important, if not more important, than dysmorphogenesis. One gained the impression that we need to guard against the generals fighting the battles of the last war when they are preparing for the next one, referring to the case of thalidomide. There are, however, wider aspects of this problem that were not touched upon, such as exposure of women in the workplace, and, of course, of men too. A more recent issue that has arisen is the large volume of literature emanating from eastern bloc countries asserting - often with minute occupational exposures to formaldehyde, ethylene oxide or carbon disulphide (to name only a few industrial chemicals) - that women are apt to suffer menstrual irregularities, dysmenorrhea, amenorrhea or "heavy menstruation", spontaneous abortions and other gynaecological disorders. There is a possibility that in all this may be the germ of some observations that we should be searching for.

I thought the session on neurotoxicity was extremely good. The concept has been advanced in the United States of what has been called "cumulative neurotoxicity", an idea that really corresponds to the view held for carcinogens, namely, that our environment is full of neurotoxins and that each molecule of neurotoxin adds to the action of each other molecule of neurotoxin, so that we ought to guard against this cumulative influence. I think that one can only weigh the validity of this idea by having a very clear understanding of the metabolism and mechanism of action of each of these neurotoxins. As was pointed out by Dr Dewar, there is a wide variety of such mechanisms. One can possibly only envisage a cumulative action if two or more such compounds are acting along the same pathway by the same mechanism. Epidemiology has an important role to play in the detection of these combined effects.

We had useful presentations on inhalation toxicity, unfortunately very brief, but pointing out that there are promising in vitro preparations with which to do preliminary screening and save a considerable amount of animal work. The same applies to dermal toxicity. I was disappointed in the way that the role of human volunteer testing was downplayed somewhat. Tremendous value has been derived from the use of human volunteers for studying potential contact sensitisers and photosensitisers. Over 1600 compounds in the fragrance series have been tested by a standard technique, the Kligman maximisation test, in human volunteers, over the past 10 years. Accordingly, we have this data-base on a wide range of compounds, and to a very large extent the results correspond with clinical experience. There are a few exceptions, for instance, in the case of musk ambrette that yielded negative results on volunteers; the few observed cases of photosensitisation may arise from its application to skin subjected to the abrasion that is involved in repeated shaving. Phenomena have been discovered in the course of this human work that appear to have no counterpart in experimental animals such as the guinea-pig; the principal new finding has been called "quenching". This process involves a quite potent skin sensitiser, like citral, which may be present in an essential oil at a level of 85%, and yet the essential oil itself does not bring about sensitisation. Addition of various other terpenes to the citral "quenches" its sensitising capability, and the same holds true for cinnamaldehyde, phenylacetaldehyde, and a number of other sensitising compounds. Here we have a very interesting phenomenon whose mechanism is unknown.

I should like to touch very quickly on the short-term tests for genotoxicity. A very important aspect today is that of promoters and non-genotoxic modulators of carcinogenesis, areas which offer a great opportunity and challenge to develop short-term screening methods. The C3H/10T½ cell line is very promising in this direction, but a great deal more remains to be done, particularly with the methods emerging from the new advances in biotechnology. I was fascinated by Dr Parry's system of testing for aneuploidy. I hope that it will be effective in classifying those carcinogens which are not genotoxic into some sort of order.

Talking about human studies, I had a sense of déja vu because, as you may be aware, studies in human subjects - including prison volunteers - have been carried on for many years. It is unfortunate, in my opinion, that an excessive enthusiasm has led to most of these arrangements being banned. Long-term prisoners welcomed an opportunity to participate in studies of this sort, and they were carried out in accordance with the highest standards and concern for the protection from harm of the people involved. Some very valuable information was obtained. Studies are still being carried out with volunteers such as medical students. I think that we should seek as much information as possible in man. To a great degree that was emphasised here too, but the tendency is to think of such work only in terms of drugs. For instance, with organophosphate pesticides there is no reliable way of foretelling what dose or what level of exposure is going to affect the serum and the red cell acetylcholinesterase activities. With proper precautions, these can be readily determined in human subjects, thus affording valuable information for human protection.

Finally, we went over the regulatory aspects and dilemmas at great length, and that is something for which I am not particularly expert at suggesting solutions. But I do feel that the programme that FRAME has in mind, and the implementation of many of the suggestions that we have heard here over the last three days, promise great advances, provided that we are patient enough to give these matters a chance to evolve. It is unlikely that they will undergo radical changes in the very near future.

Thank you very much for your attention.

REPORT OF THE FRAME TOXICITY COMMITTEE

CONTENTS

I. INTRODUCTION

1. FRAME

1. FRAME was founded in 1969 to seek a significant reduction in the need for live animal experimentation by promoting an objective and scientific reappraisal of the aims and methodologies of biomedical science and the development, validation and adoption of alternative techniques. FRAME is not an anti-vivisection society and considers that the immediate and total banning of all live animal experimentation is an unrealistic and unachievable goal, since continued progress in medical and veterinary research, diagnosis and treatment is necessary if the remaining diseases which lessen the length and quality of human and animal life are to be overcome. FRAME also recognises that new chemicals, including drugs, cosmetics and toiletries, household chemicals, and agrochemicals, must be tested, so that possible hazard to those involved in their manufacture or use, or who may be accidentally exposed to them, can be recognised and suitable precautions taken.

2. FRAME is an independent charitable trust and has no formal links with any other organisation. In the belief that progress toward the material reduction and possible eventual elimination of the need for animal experimentation will be achieved only through collaboration between those who desire such progress and those with the training, experience and imagination to make it possible, FRAME seeks to avoid confrontation and to work positively with scientists in academic institutions, in industry, and in government departments, including the regulatory authorities.

3. Following a successful conference, held at the Royal Society of London in 1978, on "The Use of Alternatives in Drug Research" (ed. A.N. Rowan & C.J. Stratmann; Macmillan, London, 1980), the FRAME Trustees decided to set up an expert Toxicity Committee, since there seemed to be a widespread feeling among toxicologists and others concerned with safety evaluation that a review of routine toxicity testing would be timely, and that some of the procedures involved were of dubious scientific merit and involved unnecessary and wasteful use of animals. It was decided that the Committee should also review the potential role and application of alternative testing procedures.

2. The FRAME Toxicity Committee

4. The FRAME Toxicity Committee held its first meeting on 12 October 1979, with the following terms of reference:

a. to conduct a thorough review of current toxicity testing procedures, to assess their reliability and suitability, and to make recommendations for their modification;
b. to assess the prospects of developing *in vitro*, target organ and theoretical model systems which would lead to a reduction in studies on live animals;
c. to act as an advisory group to a FRAME Research Fund for the support of projects aimed at the development and validation of alternative methods for use in toxicity testing.

5. The Committee met twenty-seven times between October 1979 and November 1982, and there were also numerous other meetings of its working parties to consider specific aspects of toxicity testing. The conclusions and recommendations contained in this Report represent the consensus views of the members of the Committee as individuals, and are not necessarily representative of the views of the organisations with which they are primarily affiliated or of the FRAME Trustees.

6. The background to the conclusions and recommendations included in this Report was presented at a Meeting held at the Royal Society of London on 1-3 November, 1982, when a number of other toxicologists provided independent comment in the light of their own experience. The Proceedings of the Meeting will be published by Academic Press Inc. (London) Limited in 1983.

7. Although recognising that complex issues of ethics and morality are involved in considering the use of animals by man for any purpose, the Committee deliberately refrained from the following:

a. discussions based on animal rights or the sanctity of animal life;
b. making value judgements concerning the need for new products, such as cosmetics, since its members took the view that whenever any new chemical is introduced into the environment of man, domestic animals and wildlife, appropriate steps must be taken to identify and reduce any hazard involved.

3. Committee Membership

Dr Michael Balls, Senior Lecturer, Department of Human Morphology, University of Nottingham, Queen's Medical Centre, Nottingham (Chairman)

Professor C.L. Berry, Professor of Morbid Anatomy & Director of the Pathological Institute, London Hospital Medical College, London

Professor J.W. Bridges, Professor of Toxicology & Director of the Robens Institute of Industrial and Environmental Health and Safety, University of Surrey, Guildford, Surrey

Dr V.K.H. Brown, Head of Experimental Toxicology Division, Shell Toxicology Laboratory (Tunstall), Sittingbourne Research Centre, Sittingbourne, Kent

Professor D.M. Conning, Director, British Industrial Biological Research Association, Woodmansterne Road, Carshalton, Surrey

Dr T.A. Connors, Director, Medical Research Council Toxicology Unit, Woodmansterne Road, Carshalton, Surrey

Dr J.W. Daniel, Director of Metabolic Studies, Life Science Research, Stock, Essex

Mr B.J. Dean, Head of Chemical Mutagenesis Section, Shell Toxicology Laboratory (Tunstall), Sittingbourne Research Centre, Sittingbourne, Kent

Dr A.J. Dewar, Technologist in Group Planning, Shell International Petroleum Company, London

Dr Rosemary Hawkins, Senior Manager, British Industrial Biological Research Association, Woodmansterne Road, Carshalton, Surrey

Dr Ralph Heywood, Veterinary Director & Principal Toxicologist, Huntingdon Research Centre, Huntingdon, Cambridgeshire

Dr Peter Hodges, Product Registration Officer, Pfizer Central Research, Sandwich, Kent

Dr Peter Knox, Senior Lecturer, Department of Biochemistry, St. George's Hospital Medical School, London

Professor Ronald Marks, Professor of Dermatology, Welsh National School of Medicine, Heath Park, Cardiff

Professor D.V.W. Parke, Professor of Biochemistry, University of Surrey, Guildford, Surrey

Dr I.F.H. Purchase, Director, Central Toxicology Laboratory, ICI, Alderley Park, Macclesfield, Cheshire

Ms Rosemary Riddell, Scientific Officer, FRAME, 5b The Poultry, Bank Place, Nottingham (Administrative Secretary)

Dr N.W. Shephard, Director, Medical Science Research, 19 London End, Beaconsfield, Buckinghamshire

Mr D.W. Swanston, Principal Scientific Officer (Toxicology), Medical Division, Chemical Defence Establishment, Porton Down, Salisbury, Wiltshire

Dr M.S. Tute, Senior Research Associate, Pfizer Central Research, Sandwich, Kent

Colonel R.S. Vine, Shola, Fielden Road, Crowborough, East Sussex (formerly Chief Inspector, Home Office)

Mr Colin Walker, Lecturer, Department of Physiology & Biochemistry, University of Reading, Whiteknights, Reading, Berkshire

Dr S.R. Walker, Director, Centre for Medicines Research, Woodmansterne Road, Carshalton, Surrey

Professor A.N. Worden, Co-ordinator of Environmental Studies, Wolfson College, Cambridge and Professor of Toxicology, University of Bath (Scientific Secretary)

4. Acknowledgements

We are grateful to the following for their assistance:

Dr John Baldwin, Beecham Group Limited, Medicinal Research Centre, Coldharbour Road, The Pinnacles, Harlow, Essex

Dr L.F. Chasseaud, Huntingdon Research Centre, Huntingdon, Cambridgeshire

Dr G.M. Cohen, School of Pharmacy, Brunswick Square, London

Dr A.D. Dayan, Wellcome Research Laboratories, Beckenham, Kent

Dr Alan Ebbutt, CIBA-GEIGY (representing PSI), Horsham, West Sussex

Dr A.M. Sincock, Quest, Woodbury, Harlow Road, Roydon, Essex

Mrs Carole Taylor, FRAME, 5b The Poultry, Bank Place, Nottingham

5. Background

8. There is a paradox implicit in the growing public demand for safer drugs and other products <u>and</u> for the phasing out of live animal methods used in toxicity testing.

9. There is specific public disquiet at the use of certain tests, such as the LD50 and Draize Eye Irritancy tests, and there is evidence that legislators in many countries are under great pressure to modify the legislation that requires such tests to be carried out.

10. There is also a growing realisation that some of the current toxicity testing procedures are far from satisfactory. There is widespread feeling among toxicologists that the empirical approach needs to be replaced by a more scientific one.

11. The present scale of animal toxicity testing is widely regarded as undesirable in terms of the technical resources consumed, the financial cost involved, and the time required, particularly for long-term and carcinogenicity studies.

12. Companies introducing new products to the market are faced with laws, requirements and regulations which vary from country to country. This multiplicity of requirements results in unnecessary duplication of animal studies.

13. We have considered those alternative methods which could lead to a reduction in the need for live animal experimentation, or could act in a complementary manner, thus adding to the value or specificity of conventional toxicological procedures.

II. GENERAL CONCLUSIONS AND RECOMMENDATIONS

Although animal models are of limited value in predicting toxic hazards for man, there is as yet little evidence that it will be possible in the foreseeable future to dispense entirely with live animal testing. The immediate prospect for a significant reduction in the scale of live animal experimentation stems from a reappraisal of current animal procedures, better experimental design and analysis, better use of available data on the toxicity of previously investigated compounds, and a refinement of the questions being asked in toxicological investigations. Current methods in toxicity testing have evolved over several decades. Each chemical or series to be studied should be regarded as a novel, often unique, problem requiring a specifically-designed programme of investigation. Total abolition of the need for animal experimentation is a longer term goal, since, with few exceptions, alternative approaches and methodologies are not yet developed to the point where they could conceivably be considered as adequate total replacements. More effort should be put into the development and validation of alternative techniques.

The general conclusions and main recommendations of the Committee are as follows:

14. Until valid alternative methods have been developed and approved, maximum scientific use should be made of every animal that has to be used in any form of toxicity testing.

15. In many animal studies an insistence on numerical indices (e.g the LD50 value) results in rigid protocols and the use of excessively large numbers of animals. More-detailed, qualitative acute toxicity studies should be carried out on smaller numbers of animals, where appropriate, in more than one species.

16. In the case of most pharmaceuticals and many other chemicals, formal LD50 tests should not be required, but should be replaced by more-meaningful acute toxicity studies involving the use of fewer animals.

17. Metabolic and pharmacokinetic investigations should become an integral part of toxicological testing procedures. This would reduce the number of inappropriate toxicological studies, and facilitate more reliable extrapolations of animal findings to the likely human situation. In the case of new drugs, the most pressing need is to obtain very early information in man so that

relevant animal toxicity studies for identifying possible toxic risk can be designed. Reliable human data on the kinetics of existing industrial chemicals need to be obtained so that suitable safety standards for their use can be developed.

18. Banks of human and animal tissues should be established to serve as references for drug metabolism and toxicological research.

19. Meticulous, systematic comparisons should be made between the in vivo and the in vitro biotransformation of xenobiotics. The relevance of early biochemical changes in vivo should be evaluated, so that the relationship between in vitro biotransformation, tissue binding and toxicity can be established.

20. The species employed in long-term toxicity tests should be selected on the basis of appropriate in vitro procedures and carefully conducted short-term tests.

21. Except when carcinogenicity is being investigated, or where there is good scientific evidence to suggest to the contrary, the routine long-term toxicity test should not exceed 6 months in duration.

22. Animals in long-term toxicity tests should be maintained on defined dietary regimes, since diet may profoundly affect responses.

23. The design of carcinogenicity tests should depend upon information derived from earlier in vitro studies and other relevant information. An animal study in a single appropriate species (usually the rat), combined with short-term tests, would normally be adequate for the assessment of carcinogenicity. Species other than rodents should be used only when there are valid scientific reasons for their selection.

24. Studies should be carried out to establish just how appropriate are the presently employed parameters (both physicochemical and structural) for the development of reliable quantitative structure-activity relationships (QSARs). Attempts should also be made to clarify the steric and conformational aspects of interactions between compounds and biological macromolecules, and thereafter to develop suitable parameters for these particular effects.

25. Statistical advice should be sought at the planning stage as well as during the analysis of results, in order to derive maximum information from the eventual study.

26. The numbers of animals used in neurotoxicity testing should be minimised, by obtaining information relating to neurotoxicity from standard short-term and long-term tests. To achieve this, experimental protocols should be sufficiently flexible to allow specialised neurotoxicity detection techniques to be employed.

27. More effort should be put into the development of *in vitro* biochemical tests for certain well-defined types of neurotoxic phenomena. Basic research should be encouraged on the culture of nervous tissues so that rational judgements can be made concerning their potential, both in preliminary screening and in the investigation of specific mechanisms of toxicity.

28. Preliminary data from standard short-term tests should always be used in selecting doses for reproductive toxicity testing, which should be initiated shortly after preliminary subacute studies.

29. The development of alternative methods for identifying mechanisms of teratogenesis should be encouraged, since increased knowledge of these mechanisms will improve our understanding of how results obtained from animal experiments and from alternative techniques can be extrapolated to man and can be of predictive value in identifying potential teratogens.

30. For substances of low or medium toxicity, quantitative assessment of skin irritation should be carried out in man, prefaced only by limited screening tests in animals. Pending the development of standardised techniques, stronger irritants should be evaluated with the aid of whole skin taken from cadavers or operation specimens, and with the use of human skin culture techniques.

31. Appropriate instrumentation should be employed to measure skin reactions accurately and in a reproducible manner. Standard test conditions *in vivo* in man should be worked out.

32. A reduction in the scale of live animal ocular irritancy testing and the avoidance of severe reactions in the eye should be sought by: the greater use of available physicochemical data; a requirement that skin irritancy tests precede eye testing; the

use where appropriate of isolated eyes as irritancy models; a ten-fold reduction in the standard dose applied, and the use of a more descriptive, rather than a purely numerical classification of irritant potential.

33. Research should be encouraged on biochemical tests for binding or denaturation of proteins and inactivation of enzyme systems concerned in tissue homeostasis, on validation of techniques employing isolated eyes, on primary cell and organ cultures of eye-derived tissues, and on general cell culture lines and strains.

34. Where appropriate, and particularly where compound structure suggests intrinsic mutagenic activity or the generation of genotoxic metabolites, <u>in vitro</u> genotoxicity studies should be initiated early in compound development, e.g. in parallel with acute toxicity studies. Results may influence the design and priority of subsequent animal studies and the selection of criteria (e.g. chromosome analysis) to be observed in long-term experiments. Specific <u>in vivo</u> tests for mutagenicity should only be used where it is deemed necessary to confirm or clarify <u>in vitro</u> findings. Appropriate observations should be incorporated into acute, long-term or reproductive toxicity studies.

35. There should be greater emphasis on attempts to develop mammalian cell assays to supersede the existing bacterial tests for genotoxicity, including the development of <u>in vivo/in vitro</u> (e.g primary culture) techniques to investigate the critical cellular, genetic and molecular events associated with neoplastic transformation, the development of sensitive, inexpensive short-term procedures for detecting chemically-induced heritable (germ cell) mutations, e.g. based on DNA adduct formation, etc., the introduction of <u>in vivo</u> chromosome assays of greater sensitivity and relevance than the existing bone marrow cell procedures, and the wider use and refinement of techniques for detecting non-genotoxic carcinogens and promoters.

36. The monitoring of experience in man should be considerably extended in relation to new environmental chemicals. Epidemiological studies should be encouraged as an indirect way of reducing the requirement for animal experiments.

37. Unnecessary duplication of animal experimentation should be avoided by the wider dissemination of data. A time limit should

be set on the maintenance of confidentiality of results obtained. The results of all toxicological investigations should be published or otherwise made available, e.g. in a central register of toxic effects.

38. Although toxicity testing must be conducted according to codes of practice that are acceptable to the regulatory authorities, efforts should be made to harmonise the requirements of different countries. However, such harmonisation should not be allowed to result in the perpetration of methods that are scientifically inadequate or unnecessary or that substitute numerical indices for proper toxicological investigations.

39. Regulatory authorities should always have medical, veterinary and other scientists with appropriate experience available for the evaluation of studies and for discussions with those undertaking them.

40. During toxicity tests, all animals must be maintained with high standards of care and management, and they must be subject to skilled surveillance.

41. We broadly support the conclusions of the Advisory Committee on Animal Experiments with regard to legislation to replace the Cruelty to Animals Act of 1876 (Home Office, London, 1981) and the British Veterinary Association Policy on Animal Experimentation (July, 1981).

42. The development of in vitro and other alternative techniques should be actively encouraged by governments, industries and research institutions; such techniques should be independently evaluated in inter-laboratory trials, including the "blind" testing of coded compounds of known toxicity. The FRAME Toxicity Committee is willing to act as a clearing house for all relevant information, and from 1983 a revised series of FRAME's journal ATLA (Alternatives to Laboratory Animals) will help serve this role by providing a forum for all those who wish to take part in meaningful research and discussion on the complex issues involved.

43. We recognise the immense scale of the problems we have attempted to consider and are fully aware that progress toward the eventual replacement of live animal procedures in toxicity testing, as in other areas of biomedical research, will be achieved only by degrees. However, we believe that our recom-

mendations could lead to a more constructive and more considerate use of those animals which will necessarily be required while the search for suitable alternatives is in progress, are commensurate with a logical approach that will improve the quality of toxicity testing and the resultant benefit to man, domestic animals and wildlife, and should avoid unnecessary wastage and repetition of animal studies.

III. SUMMARIES OF WORKING PARTY REPORTS

6. Acute Toxicity

Summary

44. Acute toxicity testing is essentially concerned with short-term exposure of the test species to the product under investigation and the resulting response.

45. For reasons that are more related to expediency than to science, there has been an overemphasis on numerical indices in acute toxicity testing, often at the expense of more-detailed qualitative studies involving smaller numbers of animals.

46. A reduction in the numbers of animals used in acute toxicity testing could often be achieved by the application of improved experimental design.

47. In some instances, other methods utilising only small numbers of animals (e.g. limit tests) could replace the LD50 test.

48. Current *in vitro* methodology offers useful ancillary information, but not, as yet, a total alternative to *in vivo* procedures.

Recommendations

49. A thorough investigation of the consequences of not acquiring or possessing knowledge of the acute toxicity of products in laboratory animals should be undertaken.

50. Where acute toxicity data in animals are required, the relevance of statistical precision should be carefully assessed, and procedures involving the smallest numbers of animals commensurate with achieving the required information should be used.

51. In the case of most pharmaceuticals and many other chemicals (though not necessarily pesticides and other compounds that are designed to be toxic to specified targets), formal LD50 tests should not be required, but should be replaced by more-meaningful acute toxicity studies with emphasis on interpretation of the nature of the effects observed.

52. The search for alternatives to the *in vivo* procedures used in acute toxicity testing should be encouraged, but must progress in a systematic and orderly fashion so that any potential alternatives can be objectively validated.

7. Application of Pharmacokinetics

Summary

53. Toxic responses may vary both between species and between individuals of the same species. The principal cause of this variation can often be differences in the pharmacokinetic phase. Proper characterisation of the pharmacokinetic phase is therefore essential for the prediction of likely toxic effects in one organism from the known toxic response in another.

54. Direct sampling of the target cell type or tissue component is the relevant approach for determining the concentration of a xenobiotic and its metabolites at the site of action, although it is generally not possible for practical and ethical reasons to take such samples. The best alternative is to sample the blood which perfuses these tissues. Blood levels of unbound xenobiotic are usually more directly related to the magnitude of the toxic effect than is the dose administered.

55. Although the routes of transformation can usually be predicted from the structure of a xenobiotic, it is rarely possible to predict the relative rates of formation of particular metabolites or the rate of formation of an individual metabolite in different species. Thus, it is usually important to obtain some information on the pharmacokinetics of each xenobiotic in the species concerned, especially on the extent and rate of absorption and biotransformation.

56. *In vitro* preparations can be used:

a. to identify the metabolites of a xenobiotic which may be formed, including reactive metabolites;
b. to obtain information on species differences in biotransformation or tissue binding which may explain differences in toxicity;
c. to identify likely human variability in the biotransformation or tissue binding of the xenobiotic which may result in human differences in toxicity.

57. It is not possible to entirely replace *in vivo* pharmacokinetic studies with *in vitro* ones, because at present it is not possible to mimic all *in vivo* rate-controlling processes *in vitro*. Judicious use of *in vitro* studies could reduce the number of *in vivo* pharmacokinetic studies which are required. However, *in vivo* pharmacokinetic studies can also be used in the design of more-relevant models for toxicity testing.

Recommendations

58. More studies on the absorption, distribution, biotransformation and excretion of drugs and other xenobiotics in man should be carried out. These must utilise suitable sampling and analytical methods, and be reported with relevant details on the exact dose, subject characteristics, etc. In the case of new drugs and other products, the most pressing need is to obtain very early information in man in order to select the most relevant animal toxicity studies for identifying possible toxic risk to man. For existing industrial chemicals, the need is to obtain reliable human data on their pharmacokinetics in order to set relevant safety standards for their use. Appropriate studies should also be carried out on beneficial organisms, especially in the case of pesticides and compounds used for veterinary purposes.

59. Pharmacokinetic investigations must become an integral part of toxicological testing procedures. This would reduce the number of inappropriate toxicological studies which are conducted and facilitate more reliable extrapolation of animal findings to the likely human situation.

60. Methodology for preparing and storing *in vitro* preparations of human and animal tissues and of conditions for using such preparations for investigations of biotransformation, etc., should be standardised. This would enable ready comparison of data between laboratories to be made and would greatly facilitate the establishment of a data-bank, but would require interlaboratory collaborative studies. FRAME should undertake the co-ordination of such studies and should serve as an information source on *in vitro* methodology.

61. Banks of properly characterised preparations of human and animal tissues should be established in several centres in the UK, to serve as reference points for drug metabolism and toxicological research.

62. Meticulous, systematic comparisons should be made between the *in vivo* and the *in vitro* biotransformation of xenobiotics. Initially, these should concentrate particularly on the relationship between the apparent *in vivo* and *in vitro* (hepatic) K_m and V_{max} values for the elimination of xenobiotics by metabolism.

63. Studies aimed at understanding the relationship between the physicochemical properties of xenobiotics and their absorption, distribution, biotransformation and excretion should be carried out.

64. Ready access to pharmacokinetic and other unpublished data relevant to toxicological investigations of xenobiotics should be permitted. Perhaps a time limit should be set on the maintenance of confidentiality of results obtained from safety studies.

65. The relevance of early biochemical changes resulting from *in vitro* exposure to a xenobiotic to the toxic events observed *in vivo* should be evaluated, so that the relationship between biotransformation, tissue binding and toxicity can be established.

8. Long-term Toxicity

Summary

66. A long-term toxicity test is essentially comparative in that the spontaneous and induced pathological manifestations are compared in control and test animals simultaneously: it is essential to determine whether an observation or finding is attributable to the test compound and, if so, whether its incidence is dose-related.

67. It is the investigational and observational aspects of long-term toxicity testing that are of significance, including those related to absorption, distribution, site and mode of action. Sensitive criteria of toxicity have been shown to be simple characteristics, such as clinical observation, growth and organ weight analysis, liver and kidney function tests, and histological examination of selected tissues.

68. Manifestations of toxicity are of significance in the context of dose and duration of dosing; correlation with such effects in other species, including man, is not good, and the

demonstration of toxic effects at very high dose-levels may bear little relationship to safety in use.

69. Estimates of safety should be based largely on "no-effect" levels.

70. It is not necessary from the standpoint of safety evaluation to study the long-term effects of massive dose-levels; if more-appropriate dosage levels were studied, the incidence of dramatic and unacceptable manifestations of toxicity, which are often of doubtful relevance to man, would be reduced.

71. In the case of pharmaceutical compounds, studies of some four weeks' duration in two species, usually the dog and the rat, with adequate preliminary metabolic data in man, usually form a sufficient basis for setting up the long-term study.

Recommendations

72. Animals in long-term toxicity tests should be maintained with high standards of care and management and on defined dietary regimes, since diet may profoundly affect responses.

73. The species employed should be selected on the basis of appropriate *in vitro* procedures and carefully conducted short-term tests, including metabolic and pharmacokinetic investigations.

74. Except when carcinogenicity is being investigated, or when there is good scientific evidence to suggest to the contrary, the routine long-term toxicity test need not exceed 6 months in duration.

75. Particular emphasis should be placed on "no-effect" levels, since they are of greater predictive value than manifestations of toxicity induced at high dose-levels.

76. Compounds should be investigated on their merit; it should be possible to make general safety assessments in one species only. Such toxicological assessments would then be supplemented with further experiments in other species when it was necessary to answer specific questions about the toxicological activity of a particular compound.

77. Toxicological data should be published or otherwise made

available, and a critical evaluation of the predictive value of current methods of long-term toxicity testing should be undertaken.

78. *In vitro* techniques have a significant potential role for screening candidate compounds and identifying their modes of action. However, further basic research is necessary before the precise usefulness of *in vitro* methods and other alternatives can be realistically assessed.

9. Carcinogenicity

Summary

79. Cancer is a major cause of death in man. In developed countries 1 in 5 people die of cancer. Diagnosis and treatment, although improving, cannot be considered a satisfactory means of controlling the disease. The identification of those factors which contribute to the incidence of cancer would allow prevention to become a realistic goal.

80. Carcinogenic chemicals, both organic and inorganic, natural and synthetic, are known to be one of the many environmental causes of cancer. Their identification is an important task in the process of controlling the incidence of cancer.

81. Since 1913, when the carcinogenic effects of coal tar after application to rabbit skin were discovered, animal experiments have been the primary means of identifying carcinogenicity of both existing and new chemicals. This reliance on animal models is based on the similarity of the carcinogenic process in mammalian species. The fact that the majority (about 90%) of known human carcinogens are also carcinogenic to animals emphasises the usefulness of animal studies in identifying carcinogens.

82. Animal carcinogenicity studies suffer from several drawbacks. They are expensive and time-consuming and use relatively large numbers of animals (usually several hundred). There is only an 80% co-incidence of carcinogenicity between rats and mice, and many chemicals known to be carcinogenic in animals have not been confirmed as human carcinogens. Nevertheless, animal studies currently provide the most reliable method for the detection of carcinogenic potential.

83. Alternative *in vitro* methods have been developed in recent

years; for example, microbial mutation assays and mammalian cell culture techniques. The results show a correspondence with animal carcinogenicity studies of between 50% and 90%, depending on the type of chemical. They suffer from the disadvantages inherent in *in vitro* tests for toxicity evaluation, particularly their unrepresentative metabolic systems and the absence of complex immunological and physiological processes present in the whole animal. Their use is most beneficial for:

a. testing of chemicals used on a small scale;
b. selecting new chemicals for development, thereby giving a higher probability that animal carcinogenicity studies will be negative;
c. providing a better selection of existing natural and synthetic chemicals for submission to animal studies;
d. providing information on mechanisms of action.

These *in vitro* assays are not substitutes for carcinogenicity studies, as they provide data of a different nature; however, they do improve the power of conventional animal studies.

84. High quality in the protocol, conduct, reporting and interpretation of a study is critical to the justification of animal carcinogenicity studies.

Recommendations

85. Although there is at present no adequate alternative to long-term animal studies for the assessment of the carcinogenicity of chemicals, an animal study in a single appropriate species (usually the rat), combined with short-term tests, would normally be adequate for the assessment of carcinogenicity.

86. Species other than rodents should be used for carcinogenicity studies only if there are valid scientific reasons for their selection.

87. Since the complexity of animal carcinogenicity studies makes them extremely difficult to conduct adequately and to interpret accurately, attention should be given to:

a. Protocols. Sufficient animals should be used to meet the objectives of the experiment; both too few and too many are wasteful and unnecessary. Careful consideration should be given to selection of doses, so that unnecessarily large doses which disrupt the normal metabolism and physiology are avoided. Procedures should be designed to avoid confounding factors which might frustrate the purpose of the experiment; in particular, environmental conditions, diet, disease control and avoidance of contamination by other chemicals on test, require careful attention. The recording of data should be meticulous, so that the maximum information is obtained from a particular study.

b. Reporting. An assessment of carcinogenicity and potency requires data on number of animals, survival, gross pathology and histopathology, in such a way that a life table can be constructed. Many studies are inadequately reported and are therefore invalid as a means of predicting carcinogenic risk.

c. Strategy. Different strategies may be required, depending on the purpose of the testing procedure. The rat is the species of choice for carcinogenicity testing and, when supported by the results of short-term tests, provides adequate data for the assessment of carcinogenicity. The other commonly-used species is the mouse but, increasingly, difficulties in interpreting mouse studies mitigate against their routine use. Other species should only be used when there are specific scientific reasons for preferring them to rats.

88. The search for better short-term or *in vitro* tests suitable for the rapid screening of chemicals for carcinogenicity should be encouraged.

10. Mathematical Modelling

Summary

89. Over the last twenty years, the explosive growth in computer technology and resources has stimulated the development of sophisticated mathematical models of structure-activity relationships. Although these models have at present limited applicability for explaining or predicting biological response - on the basis either of physicochemical property or of some index calculated directly from structure - they are capable of further refinement as a greater understanding of the complex interactions which occur between molecules is obtained.

90. Currently, there are two principal types of model. In the

first, changes in physical properties relating to lipid solubility, electronic features, and shape, are correlated with biological response for a series of compounds - the training set. A numerical relationship between property and response is derived and can be used to diagnose the mechanism of response and to predict the likely response of any compound similar to those in the training set. This type of model has been useful for predicting response, including toxic response, to hypnotics, to sedatives, and to certain defined chemical types under controlled conditions. A second type of model does not rely on physical property, but uses indices calculated directly from structure, such as patterns of atom connections, or position and energy of electrons. By the latter technique, excellent progress has been made in understanding some aspects of the mechanism of chemical carcinogenesis.

91. To be viable, all models must make simplifying assumptions. In the complex interactions between a compound and a living organism the usual assumptions are: that conformational changes in a compound or biological receptor can be ignored, that metabolism does not interfere, or that all compounds have the same response-determining step. Approximations are almost always made in the numbers chosen to represent physicochemical or structural effects, especially in those numbers representing changes in size or shape of molecules. Although the simplifying assumptions and approximations of mathematical modelling may appear to be overwhelming, it is emphasised that limitations of this sort are not inherent solely in a mathematical model, but are present also in any other model, e.g. tissue culture, used to predict a human response. The limitations of every alternative must be carefully assessed.

92. The end result of mathematical modelling is an equation known as a QSAR (quantitative structure-activity relationship). As a QSAR can be of both diagnostic and predictive value, there are two ways in which it may be used to limit animal experiments. First, the QSAR can suggest that it is no longer profitable to modify or extend a series of compounds in a particular way. As a result, no more compounds are made and resources - including animals - are not wasted. Secondly, a QSAR can allow the prediction that an available, but untested, compound will elicit a particular response in an animal. Provided there are no regulatory body requirements for <u>animal</u> data, animals need not be used. In this category, the response predicted may be either a beneficial one, a crude indication of overall toxicity (LD50),

or some more specific toxic effect (convulsant, mutagenic, etc.).

93. Much attention has been given to the possibility of deriving a predictive model for acute toxicity, as expressed by the LD50. The prediction of toxic response is a great challenge to modelling, and is probably its most difficult objective. This difficulty arises because lethal toxicity can be the result of many mechanisms, simultaneously involving several target organs and enzyme systems, whereas successful modelling requires that the mechanism by which the response occurs should involve one rate-determining step common to all compounds. Despite this difficulty, models for predicting acute toxicity have been proposed, although at present they cannot replace carefully acquired experimental data. At best they can be used only to set priorities for further testing or to eliminate from further evaluation certain compounds predicted to be highly toxic.

94. In areas other than that of acute toxicity, mathematical models have proven to be of considerable value in rationalising and in predicting biological data for congeneric series of compounds. This has not led directly to a reduction in the use of animals to derive data but has, in many laboratories, led to more careful experimental design, with less wastage of animal resources.

Recommendations

Based on the above comments and conclusions, a number of recommendations can be made in order to widen the range of applicability of modelling and to increase the reliability of models for predicting biological responses.

95. More work should be done to establish just how appropriate are the presently employed parameters - both physicochemical and structural - for the development of reliable quantitative structure-activity relationships.

96. More work should be done to clarify the steric and conformational aspects of interaction between compounds and biological macromolecules, and thereafter to develop suitable parameters for these particular effects.

97. Information exchange should be encouraged. This should include computer programs for data analysis, and information

stored in data-banks. Such exchanges will prevent unnecessary duplication of experiments, and provide raw data with which to test new modelling techniques and new parameters.

98. Care must be taken to ensure that the information stored in data-bases for general use is both reliable and relevant to the user.

11. Statistical Contributions to Experimental Design

Summary

99. Much wastage of animal material could be reduced by improving the design of screening tests for toxicity and efficacy. Many statistical techniques could be applied more frequently than at present. These include factorial designs to maximise information from limited material, and analysis of covariance to reduce experimental variation.

100. The design of an experiment affects its ability to show "statistical significance", but this is only one aspect of the problem. Any result, quantitative or qualitative, can only be properly interpreted if the design has allowed for unmeasurable influences. Thus, it is important to use randomisation, stratification and, where possible, "blind" operation, to allow for systematic bias in the conduct of the study.

101. It is vital that the major sources of variability are identified. These may include inter-laboratory variation and differences between animal strains. The experiment should be designed to allow for such factors.

102. Wastage of animals in testing occurs in several ways. First, the statistical parameters may be inefficiently estimated - in current LD50 testing, sequential methods or survival time analyses can produce better results with fewer animals. Secondly, experiments may give equivocal results and have to be repeated. For example, unless all sources of bias have been removed, and the context of tumour discovery has been recorded, carcinogenicity studies may produce meaningless data. Thirdly, inappropriate replication can occur. In early preclinical efficacy screening, for example, it is unnecessary to aim for statistical significance and hence use large numbers of animals per group. It is merely necessary to ensure that the overall testing system has a reasonably high chance of discovering an active

compound.

103. Good experimental design requires the close collaboration of the statistician with the researcher. Statistical techniques could be applied earlier than at present, including factorial design to investigate the effects of different treatments or factors simultaneously, and the analysis of covariance.

Recommendations

104. Greater attention should be given to the statistical efficiency of experimental designs. This will often require the active participation of a trained statistician, not only at the analytical stage, but also in defining the concept and in the design of the project. The likely outcome of such an approach would be to increase the volume and reliability of the data, with little or no extra expenditure.

105. Results must be unbiased. Randomisation methods should therefore be considered and "blind" assessments should be used in assigning treatments and assessing outcomes.

106. Unnecessary replications should be avoided.

107. Major sources of variation should be identified and taken into account. The technique of blocking and use of concomitant variables should be more widely used to reduce the size of experimental error and the number of animals required.

108. Factorial designs should be used more frequently, since when more than one factor is being investigated this approach allows the researcher to obtain more information from less material than the single factor approach.

109. Sequential methods or survival curves should be used when LD50 testing is required, in order to reduce the numbers of animals used. Where traditional methods must be used, dose-levels should be carefully chosen and data from similar tests should be pooled, to minimise animal wastage.

110. Tumours arising in carcinogenicity experiments should be classified as "incidental" or "the cause of death". Correct statistical analysis is only possible if this is carried out. The scheme for slide reading should remove any treatment-related bias that may arise.

111. Since good experimental design is as important in mutagenicity testing as in any other area, random sampling, adequate controls and estimation of standard errors are essential.

112. In preclinical efficacy testing, highly precise early screens are unnecessary. A statistician should be involved at the design stage, since this will prevent the wastage of biological material without reducing the value of the results obtained.

12. Neurotoxicity

Summary

113. The functional and structural complexity of the nervous system is reflected in the wide range of toxic actions that can be exerted upon it. This diversity of neurotoxic end-point is accompanied by a multiplicity of potential mechanisms of neurotoxicity. For these reasons it is impossible to conceive of a single all-embracing "neurotoxicity test". Neurotoxicity testing strategies must involve both acute and chronic dosing regimes, several species, and both mature and immature animals.

114. Apart from the inappropriately-named hen "demyelination test" for organophosphate-induced neurotoxicity, no neurotoxicity tests *per se* are specified by regulatory authorities - the tacit assumption being that many types of neurotoxic phenomena will be first detectable in the context of standard acute toxicity testing or during chronic feeding or inhalation studies. It cannot be assumed, however, that all types of neurotoxicity can be detected and characterised on the basis of routine acute and chronic toxicity tests in rodents. There will also be a need for more-specialised tests.

115. Animal tests have their limitations, particularly in the extrapolation of data to man. Some types of neurotoxic phenomena found in man are virtually impossible to detect using experimental animals. However, the option of performing neurotoxicity studies directly on man does not really exist, except in some very specialised cases, such as clinical trials of new therapeutic agents. Nevertheless, epidemiological studies have in the past contributed much to neurotoxicology.

116. Valid *in vitro* toxicological testing methods are based either on a detailed knowledge of the mechanism of the toxic

action or on the possession of a good structural model possessing the essential characteristics of the target organ. In view of the many potential mechanisms for neurotoxicity and the fact that no model system could approach the structural complexity of even a simple animal nervous system, there is no realistic prospect of an in vitro test predictive of all in vivo manifestations of neurotoxicity being developed. However, in vitro methods for detecting specific neurotoxic effects of compounds belonging to classes of chemicals whose mechanism of action are understood, and methods for detecting certain well-defined types of neurotoxic phenomena, can be envisaged and have been, and are being, developed.

117. Biochemical methods based on a knowledge of mechanism have considerable power in that they ultimately allow direct prediction of neurotoxicity to man. They have the potential to be performed entirely in vitro (possibly with post-mortem human tissue), thus eliminating the use of live animals. However, complete in vitro testing has a drawback in that it eliminates such critical factors to in vivo toxicity as absorption, metabolism, excretion, etc., and consequently, to overcome this, such methods are often performed in vivo/in vitro, i.e. using tissue from animals dosed with the toxicant. Such an approach requires the use of fewer animals than conventional in vivo methods. At present, only one such method exists for predicting neurotoxicity of the structural type. This is the neurotoxic esterase assay for organophosphate-induced delayed neurotoxicity which has been exceptionally well-validated and is preferable both on scientific and humane grounds to the conventional in vivo hen "demyelination test".

118. Wherever possible, further alternative methods based on mechanism should be developed. However, the difficulties in so doing must not be underestimated - particularly in the area of structural neurotoxicity. Specific biochemical methods are limited in scope, and the effort required for their development may be justified only for families of related compounds of sufficient economic importance. The development and validation of such methods may itself require animal experimentation, although this could be reduced by use of appropriate tissue culture methods or in vivo biochemical techniques, such as the use of brain slices, isolated neurones and glia, or synaptosomes.

119. Techniques for the culture of materials of nervous origin are only now approaching the state of development where they

could be said to be routine, and maintenance of such cultures demands considerable specialised expertise. Neurotoxicological studies where tissue culture techniques have been applied have been primarily concerned with the mechanisms of pathogenesis of known toxicants. The very factors which make tissue cultures useful for the study of mechanisms, e.g. direct exposure of the toxicant to the target tissue, absence of complicating metabolic transformations, absence of blood-brain barrier, etc., limit their effectiveness as predictors of in vivo toxicity. Consequently, although tissue culture techniques could be potentially very useful as a preliminary screening tool, they will only be a valuable adjunct to in vivo testing and not a total replacement.

120. The future of tissue culture as a tool in neurotoxicity testing lies not in the development of ultracomplex culture systems, but in the use of simple systems for answering specific toxicological questions. These include systems containing specific cellular elements, enabling the relative sensitivities of each cell type to be assessed, and the use of organotypic cultures for the testing of specific types of neuropathological damage.

Recommendations

121. Since no single technique is capable of detecting all potential neurotoxic end-points a multidisciplinary approach is necessary, and a structured, but flexible, "scientific" approach tailored to the nature of the neurotoxic phenomenon under investigation should be followed.

122. The numbers of animals used should be minimised by obtaining more information relating to neurotoxicity from standard acute and long-term tests. To achieve this, experimental protocols should be sufficiently flexible to allow specialised neurotoxicity detection techniques to be employed.

123. The numbers of animals required in more-specialised tests should be reduced to a minimum, by ensuring that all tests are designed and executed to the highest standards, so that the maximum information is obtained from each animal used.

124. Epidemiological studies should be encouraged as an indirect way of reducing the requirement for animal experiments.

125. More effort should be put into the development of in vitro biochemical tests for certain well-defined types of neurotoxic phenomena.

126. Basic research should be encouraged on the culture of nervous tissues, so that rational judgements can be made concerning their potential both in preliminary screening and in the investigation of specific mechanisms of toxicity. Straightforward methods should be sought to allow the inexpensive and reproducible production and maintenance of cultures. Each potential technique should be independently validated in several laboratories.

127. Efforts should be made to evaluate the use of lower vertebrate models for neurotoxicity testing.

13. Reproductive Toxicity

Summary

128. The complex nature of the reproductive process, the multiple processes involved in gametogenesis, fertilisation, implantation and embryonic development, and the three metabolic compartments involved (mother, placenta, fetus) make accurate experimental modelling difficult, particularly when interspecies differences act as further confounding factors. As yet, there is no alternative to the use of whole animals in reproductive toxicity testing.

129. The high fetal wastage which normally occurs in man has not been studied extensively and could provide useful data on environmental effects, particularly if linked with employment records, as in Scandinavia, and could facilitate better test design by identifying potential hazards more precisely. This central mechanism, where abnormal conceptuses are eliminated, is of major importance in reducing the consequences of human reproductive failure, but is also very difficult to model realistically in animals, although some approximations can be made.

130. The value of alternative systems was considered by the group to be maximal in determining specific mechanisms of action of teratogens. This is of evident academic value, and the results of such work may come to have widespread general implications - for example, by providing the basis for prediction of toxicological hazard in pregnancy in relation to a particular

chemical structure. In addition, a defined mechanism may be exclusive to man: if a particular system does not operate in man, a valuable compound may be usable, although appearing to be dangerous from other studies. For these reasons this type of work should be encouraged.

131. With regard to current testing procedures, the design of studies varies considerably between countries, and may also vary within countries, where different agencies are responsible for different types of chemical. Some countries change designs at intervals, which must be expected in a developing field, but all these changes and variations result in a considerable duplication of work and inevitably increase the numbers of animals used.

132. Specific factors in relation to detailed aspects of current testing were considered. For example, choice of species is sometimes based on availability rather than on scientific criteria, and pharmacokinetic similarity to man is sometimes presumed without having been demonstrated (e.g. in the choice of primates).

133. The value of work being performed against the background of data that a laboratory might have about its "own" strains of animals should be noted. Problems of dosage regimes, number of animals, routes of administration and timing of treatments were all considered, and the necessity for adequate examination of material was emphasised. In assessing submissions of data on compounds under test, it is surprising how often studies need to be repeated due to the inadequate examination of fetuses, despite the existence of well-established procedures.

134. It was considered that not all agencies evaluate the data presented with equal competence, since some lack assessors with an adequate background of experience, particularly in the evaluation of variations/malformations. This may lead to unnecessary duplication of experiments.

Recommendations

135. There should be harmonisation of international testing requirements wherever possible.

136. These requirements should be interpreted in such a way as to permit the maximal use of the data provided, i.e. if two

parts of an assessment require similar tests, a single study should suffice.

137. Preliminary data from short-term tests should be used in selecting doses for reproductive toxicity testing, which should be initiated shortly after preliminary subacute studies.

138. An attempt should be made to develop a methodology which will give dose-response relationships for teratogens in a variety of species, since such data are lacking for man.

139. The use of alternative methods to identify mechanisms of teratogenesis should be encouraged, since increased knowledge of these mechanisms will improve our understanding of how effectively results obtained from experiments can be extrapolated to man and can be of predictive value in identifying teratogens.

14. Dermal Toxicity

Summary

140. The two aspects of toxic damage to the skin from external application, irritancy and sensitisation, merit separate consideration: irritation is of more significance to the community.

141. There are a wide range of clinical symptoms in dermal irritation, from "stinging" without visible cause to gross erosions with surrounding erythema and oedema.

142. It is by no means certain whether all the reactions encountered represent degrees of severity or whether they are due to separate mechanisms. If the latter were true, a single test would be unlikely to indicate all types equally efficiently.

143. None of the current test systems are ideal, but, for substances of low and medium toxicity, tests using human skin *in vivo* appear to be the best available method.

144. For substances of high toxicity, special tests need to be developed.

145. Limited screening tests on animals may still be necessary to determine the general order of toxicity before tests on human skin are contemplated, although the need for these should be

obviated with the development of reliable _in vitro_ techniques.

146. Among factors that may influence the results of skin tests on man are: individual variation in susceptibility to cutaneous irritation, ambient conditions, season of year, anatomical site chosen for test, age (but not sex) of subject, concentration of test substance, vehicle employed, and method and frequency of application to the skin. Keeping these factors in mind, conditions for a "standard test" methodology should be agreed.

147. LD50 or ID50 determinations are not appropriate for weak irritants; observations on the type and degree of reaction to a test substance are more useful than numerical indices.

148. Studies of the irritancy of stoma application and of dithranol indicate that appropriate instrumentation is necessary in order to obtain reproducible and accurate measurements of skin reactions.

149. _In vitro_ techniques are potentially of great value for many aspects of skin toxicity testing, but, apart from those that relate to phototoxicity, are still at the development stage.

150. The evaluation of stratum corneum barrier function using cell culture methods presents obvious difficulties. For this purpose, whole skin taken either from cadavers or from operation specimens can be employed.

151. Useful methods that are being developed include a chamber technique for the estimation of respiratory enzyme release from skin to which irritant has been applied.

152. Another technique under development utilises suction blisters and the measurement of enzyme activities in the blister fluid after application of the substances under test to the surface.

Recommendations

153. For substances of low and medium toxicity, it is appropriate to undertake quantitative assessment of skin irritation in man, prefaced only by limited screening tests on animals.

154. Pending the development of standardised alternative techniques, stronger irritants may be evaluated with the aid of

whole skin, taken from either cadavers or operation specimens, and with human skin cultures.

155. Appropriate instrumentation should be employed to measure skin reactions accurately and in a reproducible manner.

156. Procedures and conditions for in vivo tests in man should be standardised.

15. Ocular Irritancy

Summary

157. A review of ocular toxicity testing demonstrates that mechanisms of chemical irritation in the eye and consequent responses to such irritation are not necessarily simple processes, but are more often interactions of several factors, which may be modified if the test substance consists of a mixture or formulation, rather than a single substance.

158. In spite of potentially variable mechanisms, a reliable assessment of potential chemical hazard to the eye is necessary, because of the great psychological and physical significance of visual damage, impairment or loss in man. It is therefore not surprising that to date no in vitro methods have yet emerged that in certainty and scope have been judged to be equal, or able to supersede the in vivo model for final safety clearance or hazard evaluation. Even a close approximation, such as the isolated eye preparation, is not seen as a full substitute for the in vivo situation. Nevertheless, the fail-safe eye tests demanded hitherto have tended to be counterproductive, because the aim of eliciting the most potentially severe response, when allied to the variability inherent in their design, made the results difficult to interpret, and virtually guaranteed the exclusion on safety grounds of materials which, in practice, would present only a minor hazard. Variations among the regulatory authorities and codes of practice in terms of procedures and scoring systems have not helped, nor has the tendency to overemphasise the quantitative aspect of what are essentially qualitative data.

159. Although total replacement of in vivo by in vitro testing for ocular irritancy is not yet possible, reduction in the number of animals used in in vivo testing should be sought on the grounds of humanity, and the refinement of any remaining

live animal testing is also necessary on scientific grounds. Whether the aim of complete replacement of in vivo irritancy testing by in vitro techniques could ever be achieved is, for the moment, a matter of conjecture. Reduction of in vivo eye irritancy testing to a practical irreducible minimum by the use of physicochemical data and scientifically-validated in vitro alternatives remains the most practical objective for the present.

Recommendations

160. A reduction in the scale of live animal ocular irritancy testing and the avoidance of severe reactions in the eye should be sought by:

a. the gathering and application of all available physico-chemical data on the test compound relevant to ocular inflammation, as a first step in predicting eye injury potential and eliminating highly irritant compounds;
b. skin testing, which should precede eye testing, so that the data can be used in guiding the approach to subsequent eye testing, should it prove necessary;
c. the use, where appropriate, of isolated eyes as irritancy models, obtained either from laboratory animals or, preferably, from animals already killed for other purposes, e.g. in abattoirs.

161. In those situations where whole animal testing is still deemed necessary, refinement of testing procedures would lead to both a more humane and scientifically more valid test and reduce the need for repeat tests. Under the present procedure, up to eighteen animals may be required, owing to the possibility of repeat groups. The recommendations listed below should increase the possibility of obtaining a result from no more than six animals, thus providing a further means of reducing animal usage. The following refinements of in vivo testing are suggested:

a. a ten-fold reduction in the standard dose to 0.01ml or 0.01g;
b. direct application to the eye rather than to the conjunctival sac;
c. avoidance of irritant overreactions;
d. the use of a more descriptive, rather than a purely numerical classification of irritant potential;

e. since in the rabbit eye, prostaglandin-potentiated histamine causes marked conjunctival inflammation and local tenderness, the feasibility of using antihistamine during testing to reduce both discomfort to the animal and the spurious overreaction of the conjunctiva should be investigated;

f. the use of local anaesthetics in eye testing is considered of doubtful benefit, since their influence on the eye test is not clear and such use may ultimately be counterproductive, by prolonging irritant effects.

162. The considerable investment now being made in the search for alternatives to in vivo testing, including eye irritancy, is certain to bring further advances in the ability of in vitro tests to assist in safety testing or in the investigation of mechanisms. Research should therefore be encouraged on biochemical tests for binding or denaturation of proteins and/or inactivation of enzyme systems concerned in tissue homeostasis, on the validation of techniques employing isolated eyes, on primary cell and organ cultures of eye-derived tissues, and on general cell culture lines and strains.

16. Short-term Tests For Genotoxicity

Summary

163. The last decade has seen the introduction of a series of short-term in vitro and in vivo tests that have been used with varying degrees of success to detect chemicals that are potentially genotoxic to man. The number and diversity of the tests in current use illustrate the short-comings of many of them, and with continuing research it is inevitable that the present generation of short-term assays will be superseded by new tests with better predictive value.

164. Current practice is to use a battery of assays representing different genetic end-points, e.g. point mutations, chromosome aberrations, and incorporating some form of metabolic activation system. The results of such batteries cannot be accepted as firm evidence of the presence or lack of a human genotoxic hazard, but have a number of valuable applications. They can be used to screen new chemicals at an early stage of development - to eliminate those with possible carcinogenic or mutagenic activity. By testing series of analogues, it is feasible to select non-genotoxic compounds as candidates for further

development. Both these applications can produce increased cost-effectiveness in the development of new drugs, food additives and agricultural chemicals. The results of short-term assays on industrial intermediates can be used to establish safe handling procedures in the design of new chemical processes. A further application lies in the testing of existing chemicals to aid the assessment of priorities for animal bioassays. The intelligent use of short-term genotoxicity assays is now an integral part of general toxicity testing. However, the interpretation of these tests in terms of human hazard is not well established and should be approached with caution. Realistic risk analysis is not possible with the present generation of short-term tests.

165. Of all the areas of toxicology, it is probably in the area of testing for genotoxicity that the application of the philosophy of replacement of animals has been most successful. The development of <u>in vitro</u> test systems for mutagenicity testing has resulted in a marked reduction in the use of animal tests such as the dominant lethal assay, host-mediated assays and, to a lesser extent, of <u>in vivo</u> cytogenetics. A major factor in reaching this situation has been the development and utilisation of metabolic activation systems.

166. Further development of short-term tests for the identification of carcinogenic chemicals will be determined to a greater extent by progress in the elucidation of the mechanisms of neoplasia. The major task is to identify the critical events that occur during the transformation of a normal cell to an overt neoplastic state, with the objective of developing techniques based on the mechanisms of neoplasia rather than on numerical correlation between the results of short-term tests and animal bioassays.

167. The whole area of genotoxicity testing is a rapidly developing scene, and the existing array of test systems will certainly be refined and altered, possibly dramatically. Further developments will undoubtedly improve the predictive value of <u>in vitro</u> tests for carcinogenic and mutagenic hazards to man and will possibly extend to cover other toxicological end-points. Every additional refinement added to the <u>in vitro</u> test system will result in better employment of animal resources. Whether scientifically valid <u>in vitro</u> test systems, which will render the orthodox carcinogenicity bioassay redundant, can ever be developed, must remain a matter for conjecture. At the moment such a situation seems unlikely and, in any event, even <u>in vitro</u>

tests are to a greater or lesser extent dependent on the utilisation of animals, e.g. in the provision of metabolic activation systems and mammalian cell cultures.

Recommendations

Based on the above comments on future developments in short-term genotoxicity tests, a number of recommendations and research objectives have been identified, the main emphasis being on the development of mammalian cell assays to supersede the existing bacterial tests:

168. Development of *in vivo/in vitro* (e.g. primary culture) techniques to investigate the critical cellular, genetic and molecular events associated with neoplastic transformation.

169. Isolation and characterisation of more-appropriate mammalian cell lines, particularly of an epithelial-type, that retain representative intrinsic metabolising activity.

170. Development of sensitive, inexpensive short-term procedures for detecting chemically-induced, heritable (germ cell) mutations, e.g. based on DNA adduct formation, etc.

171. Development of *in vitro* mammalian cell assays for detection of chemically-induced aneuploidy.

172. Introduction of *in vivo* chromosome assays of greater sensitivity and relevance that the existing bone marrow cell procedures.

173. Wider use and refinement of techniques for detecting non-genotoxic carcinogens and promoters.

17. Human Studies

Summary

174. Man is always the ultimate experimental animal. Our survival is dependent upon adaptation and trial-and-error in the selection of food and environment. The consideration of gross adaptation phenomena is a vast subject, but some indication of genetic changes and the likelihood of their happening are well characterised, particularly in relation to environmental radioactivity. Considerable progress has been made in studying such

phenomena in bacterial and cell cultures.

175. The aim of evaluating new chemical entities to be used as medicines or added to the environment must be to identify potential hazards, and to reduce their incidence and duration to within acceptable limits. Before any new substance is studied in man (be it medicinal, agrochemical or pharmaceutical), extensive, relevant preliminary studies are necessary, including meaningful animal investigations.

176. Ideally, the animal species selected for toxicological study in depth should be the one which metabolises the substance in a manner close to, or identical with, man. It does not necessarily follow that the species thus selected has pharmacological reactions similar to man, but closer attention to these aspects of preliminary animal screening would reduce the number of animal experiments.

177. The methodology in man can be divided into stages:

Stage 1. Controlled exposure of normal man to the chemical concerned, starting with minute single doses which are gradually increased, progressing to multiple dosing until the maximum exposure likely or needed has been reached, and the tolerance, toxicity, pharmacology, pharmacokinetics and metabolism have been shown to be acceptable and safe within the context of the ultimate usage of the substance.

Stage 2. For medicines, the controlled exposure of the medicine to ill patients, again to confirm all findings in healthy individuals and also to develop and confirm the efficacy of a therapeutic regime.

Stage 3. Controlled monitoring of experience, since the careful observation of those exposed to new chemical entities is easy in the development of a new medicine, but proves to be more difficult in the case of new environmental chemicals, such as agrochemicals. This stage is important in the recognition of toxic effects unique to man, abnormal distribution of the substance in a few people, and idiosyncratic responses. It may also involve additional specialised testing, e.g. for allergy.

Stage 4. Some degree of post-marketing surveillance is undertaken for all substances. This is becoming more of a necessity in medicines, but less so in other areas, where epidemiological retrospective techniques are more common.

Recommendations

178. Improved studies in animals should be undertaken to provide more-meaningful information regarding safety and likely effects in man.

179. Greater emphasis and effort should be put into developing and validating non-animal methods, specifically in relation to their predictive value in man.

180. The monitoring of experience in man should be considerably extended in relation to new environmental chemicals.

18. Regulatory Aspects

181. The approach to safety evaluation should be scientific and not empirical. Regulatory guidelines should be guidelines and not requirements, thus allowing flexibility rather than encouraging the "check-list" approach.

182. There should be a continuing reappraisal of safety evaluation tests in the light of new scientific knowledge. In the case of pharmaceuticals, the extent and nature of preclinical studies should relate to the desired objectives and to the type and severity of the disease to be treated.

183. An intensive and critical examination of animal drug toxicology should be carried out in comparison with data on human adverse drug reactions, with a view to identifying the predictive value of safety studies, thus allowing the subsequent rejection of any tests found to be of limited value. It is unacceptable that existing tests should continue to be applied uncritically and that new animal tests should be added without adequate validation.

184. A mechanism should be established for comparing the drug regulatory procedures of different countries which involve the scientific assessment of animal data and result in the rejection or acceptance of a drug for study in man or for marketing.

185. Animal toxicology should not be repeated for different regulatory authorities unless valid reasons are given. There

should be a positive move towards the mutual recognition of foreign data, and considerable efforts should be made to achieve international harmonisation of the scientific principles and procedures used in regulatory assessment.

186. Routine animal studies alone cannot adequately predict adverse drug reactions in man. There should be increased emphasis on post-marketing surveillance and on the identification of those animal tests or alternative methods which will result in the early diagnosis of potential hazards.

19. Control of Animal Experimentation

187. Experiments in animals are only justifiable if they are necessary to improve human and animal welfare, if they are carried out by persons with appropriate training and experience, and if the animals concerned are maintained in legally-recognised premises where they are given high standards of care.

188. Experiments on animals in the United Kingdom are currently controlled by the Cruelty to Animals Act (1876), but it is anticipated that new legislation will be considered by Parliament, in the light of the recent Report of the Home Office Advisory Committee on Animal Experimentation (1981) and the recommendations of the Council of Europe.

189. With minor reservations, we are in broad agreement with the conclusions of the Advisory Committee and with the British Veterinary Association Policy on Animal Experimentation (July, 1981).

190. We particularly agree that applicants should be required to show not only that their proposed projects are worthwhile, but also that they are technically competent to do the necessary work.

191. We consider that all licence holders should have recieved training in the care and handling of animals, and we welcome the introduction or proposed introduction of courses run by professional bodies such as the Royal Colleges, universities, research institutions, and contract and industrial organisations.

192. We also consider that the supply of animals should be under stringent control, and that, except in special circumstances and

when prior approval is given, the use of individuals of certain species (including the cat and dog) should be permitted only if they are purpose-bred and supplied from registered premises or other approved sources.

SUBJECT INDEX